RESTORING YOUR DIGESTIVE HEALTH

T0007818

RESTORING YOUR DIGESTIVE HEALTH

A Proven Plan to Conquer
Crohn's, Colitis,
and Digestive Diseases

JORDAN S. RUBIN, N.M.D.,
AND JOSEPH BRASCO, M.D.

CITADEL PRESS
Kensington Publishing Corp.
www.kensingtonbooks.com

CITADEL PRESS BOOKS are published by

Kensington Publishing Corp.
119 West 40th Street
New York, NY 10018

Copyright © 2003 Jordan S. Rubin and Joseph Brasco

All rights reserved. No part of this book may be reproduced in any form or by any means without the prior written consent of the publisher, excepting brief quotes used in reviews.

PUBLISHER'S NOTE
This book presents information based upon the research and personal experiences of the authors. It is not intended to be a substitute for a professional consultation with a physician or other healthcare provider. Neither the publisher nor the authors can be held responsible for any adverse effects or consequences resulting from the use of any of the information in this book. They cannot be held responsible for any errors or omissions in the book. If you have a condition that requires medical advice, the publisher and authors urge you to consult a competent healthcare professional.

All Kensington titles, imprints, and distributed lines are available at special quantity discounts for bulk purchases for sales promotions, premiums, fund-raising, educational, or institutional use.

Special book excerpts or customized printings can also be created to fit specific needs. For details, write or phone the office of the Kensington sales manager: Kensington Publishing Corp., 119 West 40th Street, New York, NY 10018, attn: Sales Department; phone 1-800-221-2647.

CITADEL PRESS and the Citadel logo are Reg. U.S. Pat. & TM Off.

ISBN-13: 978-0-8065-4128-0
ISBN-10: 0-8065-4128-8

First Twin Streams printing: May 2003
First Citadel printing: April 2021

31 30 29 28 27 26 25 24

Printed in the United States of America

Electronic edition:

ISBN-13: 978-0-8065-4147-1 (e-book)
ISBN-10: 0-8065-4147-4 (e-book)

*To those who suffer from digestive disorders
and often feel "alone" in their suffering,
we wrote this book for you.*

Contents

Part Two

GUTS AND GLORY:
THE PRACTICE

Foreword

Restoring Your Digestive Health: How the Guts and Glory Program Can Transform Your Life offers new hope and help to the millions of Americans who are suffering from digestive related disorders and are tired of treatments that do not address the causal factors responsible for their disease. In this easy-to-understand manual, Jordan Rubin and Joseph Brasco give not only a guided tour of the major reasons why our guts revolt against our modern ways of living, but step-by-step directions on how to reverse gastrointestinal complaints.

Helping people become self-reliant in taking care of their health problems runs contrary to both most medical and most "alternative" practices, where patients are trained to become dependent on physician care in ways that discourage them from taking control of their own health destiny. Nowhere is this more evident than in the realm of digestive-related disorders. We must acknowledge the fact that gastrointestinal complaints are treated by symptom suppression in the majority of medical offices. Patients are left ignorant of why they became ill and remain subject to increasingly serious health problems as the years go by.

My twenty-five years as a practitioner, a professor of public health, clinical nutrition and gastroenterology, and my personal experiences with digestive-related disorders have made clear to me the immense impact of gastrointestinal function on the development of a wide array of degenerative conditions. From when I first read the brilliant work of Dr. Weston Price in 1966 (*Nutrition and Physical Degeneration*) to my studies in chronic disease epidemiology at the University of Texas to my more than twenty-five years as a practitioner seeing numerous sick people, the message continues to be clear: We are personally and collectively responsible for the vast array of chronic health problems from which we suffer. If we are to escape from our dilemma as a population that has become increasingly burdened with illness, we must understand the importance of efficient gastrointestinal functioning, the many ramifications of our guts' not functioning well, and what steps are needed to reverse these problems. It is in this light that *Restoring Your Digestive Health: How the Guts and Glory Program Can Transform Your Life* can play such an important role.

In this book, the reader has the opportunity to learn from the experiences and perspectives of former patient Jordan Rubin, who suffered with serious, life threatening digestive-related disorders and who, through his own often terrifying trial-and-error experiences, fought his way back to good health. This perspective is reinforced and added to by the insights of medical gastroenterologist Joseph Brasco, who complements his medical training and experience with a natural, causal-oriented outlook that he uses in clinically assisting his own patients. Both authors exhibit the all-too-rare art of independent experience, logic, science, and clear concern for their fellow human beings.

I assure the reader that while each case of illness is different, the wealth of information contained in this book can serve as a foundation for not only an improved understanding of why we become ill, but also as a road map to follow on the way back to better health.

Paul A. Goldberg, M.P.H., D.C., Director
The Goldberg Clinic, Marietta, Georgia

Preface

Opinions vary as to how many people suffer from gastrointestinal disease. People suffering from colds, flu, arthritis, and most other diseases are not hesitant to talk about their illness with their family and friends. They swap war stories and compare notes. They trade ideas about how to get well. But gastrointestinal disease is a taboo subject. The bowel is considered a foul, slimy, repulsive organ. People who have gastrointestinal disease feel a certain amount of shame and are reluctant to talk about their illness. What's more, the onset of many gastrointestinal diseases is gradual. Many sufferers do not realize they have a disease until the symptoms become apparent. Some gastrointestinal diseases are ill defined. Irritable bowel syndrome (IBS), for example, comprises a host of different symptoms, including constipation, diarrhea, and cramping. The lack of a clear definition of IBS has made it difficult to pinpoint how many people have the syndrome (although 20 percent of the population has it by some estimates).

Still, evidence suggests that gastrointestinal disease is widespread in the United States. In some surveys, 40 percent of the patients who visit internists do so because they have a gastrointestinal complaint. Digestive disorders are second to the common cold as the reason why people visit doctors. According to the U.S. Department of Health and Human Services, one-third to one-half of American adults had a digestive illness in 1994. Antacid tablets are the best-selling over-the-counter medication in the United States. The ulcer medication Zantac, with sales of more than $1 billion annually, is the best-selling drug of all time. It appears that gastrointestinal disease is a scourge in the United States.

In some ways, people with gastrointestinal (GI) diseases have it twice as bad as people with other diseases. Because GI-disease sufferers have impaired digestive systems, they cannot absorb food properly. They cannot absorb certain foods at all. The foods in their diet have to be nutritious enough to feed and heal their bodies, but also friendly enough to be absorbed by their impaired digestive systems. We have designed the Guts and Glory Program to meet these dual requirements. Chapters 3 and 9 of this book explain why certain kinds of foods enhance the health of the digestive tract and when to consume these foods to overcome a digestive illness. The Guts and Glory Program offers groundbreaking information. It reveals secrets handed down to us from our ancestors that can completely rejuvenate the gut, the immune system, and the entire body.

The premise of the Guts and Glory Program is that we are genetically programmed to eat the same wholesome foods as our ancestors. Theirs was a high-nutrient, moderate-calorie diet, whereas our diet is high in calories—especially calories from carbohydrates—and low in nutrients. We believe that an improper diet is the primary cause of intestinal disease, and that a diet rich in healing foods can be the primary cure. If you want a quick fix, you came to the wrong place. The Guts and Glory Program doesn't work overnight. The program's principles are based on nothing less than humankind's history of eating food and being nourished successfully. The more you adopt the principles outlined in this book, the better you will feel. The Guts and Glory Program is based on cause-and-effect nutrition. We have carefully examined what has worked for humankind—both in diet and lifestyle—through most of our history. Our program passes these fundamental principles on to modern humans.

When it comes to illness, we prefer the word "overcome" to the word "cure" because the road to better health is a journey that has to be taken one step at a time. We believe that everybody can improve their digestive heath because the principles of good health are as simple and straightforward as the law of gravity. When you change your diet and your lifestyle—thereby transforming yourself—your health always improves. To what extent it improves depends on how long you were ill and other factors, but in the case of gastrointestinal diseases, patients can become symptom-free and restore the tissue in their bowels to a normal, healthy state. To do so, however, they have to make across-the-board changes in their diet and way of life. They have to do the many little things that add up to good health. The way to reconstruct a building that has fallen down is brick by brick. No single act can restore the whole building in one fell swoop. Similarly, a body that has been ravaged by disease and a poor diet has to be reconstructed one step at a time. There is no single cure-all. This book is intended to teach the reader how to conquer digestive problems once and for all. We are not interested in individual symptoms. We'll leave those for other books.

The Guts and Glory Program is the only program we know that takes into account all of the important components involved in regaining and maintaining your digestive health. Our soil, water, and environment are not as healthy as they were in the past. Our food is not as wholesome. We have abandoned the age-old dietary principles that kept our ancestors healthy and have instead taken up practices that are contrary to building a healthy body. The Guts and Glory Program will give readers the tools they need to break free from many life-altering symptoms. This doesn't mean that one particular food or kind of food will heal you. The Guts and Glory Program will teach you to construct a lifestyle that is conducive to health and healing. This program will put *your* health in *your* hands. It is a map to guide you on the path to recovery.

As Chapter 1 describes in detail, coauthor Jordan Rubin survived and conquered a severe case of "incurable" Crohn's disease. Jordan's weight dropped from a healthy 180 pounds to 104 pounds (Jordan is six feet one inch tall). After his remarkable recovery was detailed in health magazines, Jordan was inundated with questions from people who had gastrointestinal diseases. They wanted to know what he ate, what he did, and how he managed to get well.

We decided to write this book in part to answer those questions. Jordan's recovery was extraordinary. However, it was also a hit-or-miss affair. Jordan undertook to cure himself with limited knowledge. By trial and error, he learned how to do it. This book is a record partly of what Jordan learned during his recovery and partly of what he learned in the ensuing seven years about gastrointestinal disease and how to overcome it. One of this book's goals is to give readers the information that Jordan wished he had had during his illness.

This book is unique in that it looks at gastrointestinal disease from the viewpoint of a doctor as well as of a patient. The doctor's perspective comes from coauthor Joseph Brasco, M.D. Dr. Brasco has been a practicing, board-certified gastroenterologist for ten years. As Chapter 1 explains, Dr. Brasco, like Jordan, gradually came to the belief that a primitive diet is the best way to overcome digestive illness. The doctor's innovative, food-based treatments have helped thousands of patients. Dr. Brasco has skillfully combined diet, supplementation, and the judicious use of medications to provide a very comprehensive treatment program that reflects the insight of several different disciplines. The partnership between a patient and a doctor makes this book unique because the authors examine treating gastrointestinal disease from opposite perspectives.

Included in this book are protocols for getting well that complement conventional medicine. In our opinion, alternative medicine has as many shortcomings as conventional medicine. It promises a natural approach to healing, but it usually doesn't deliver. Many alternative practitioners lack an understanding of biology. Their treatment protocols are rarely scrutinized. Many alternative practitioners promise too much (and if it sounds too good to be true, then it probably is). In conventional medicine, by contrast, physicians understand the biology behind diseases, but give dietary and lifestyle changes only lip service. They do not appreciate diet and lifestyle changes for the therapeutic power they possess. In Dr. Brasco's experience, many of the suggestions his colleagues make are superficial and lack the necessary depth to effect change in a disease state.

Our goal with this book is to give every person on the planet the knowledge to avoid or recover from gastrointestinal disease. You will find critiques of treatments, programs, and supplements in this book to help you choose a protocol that will work for you. We don't have an agenda to push. We want to offer the public information about how to get well.

Overcoming a disease takes the determination of a world-class athlete. It takes vision. It takes sacrifice. It takes drive. But if you go at it fast and furiously from the beginning and your life means enough to you, there is hope. You can overcome disease. This book will show you how.

Part One

GUTS AND GLORY:
THE PREMISE

❖ 1 ❖

A Patient and a Doctor

This book brings a unique viewpoint to the subject of treating gastrointestinal disease. It unites the thoughts and ideas of a patient who healed himself of a gastrointestinal disease and a practitioner who works on a daily basis with patients who suffer from gastrointestinal disorders. To provide a background for this book and to give the perspective of the patient and the doctor, we will present our stories in this chapter. Jordan Rubin will explain how, suffering from a severe case of Crohn's disease, he put himself on the road to wellness and eventually managed to heal himself with what he now calls the Guts and Glory Program. Dr. Joseph Brasco will describe his longstanding interest in gastrointestinal health and how he, too, came to the conclusion that improving your diet is the best way to overcome a bowel disease.

The Patient: Jordan Rubin

Getting over an "incurable" disease is hard work. In fact, I liken it to being an Olympic athlete. The percentage of people who overcome incurable diseases is the same as those who become Olympic champions or Most Valuable Players (MVPs) in their sports. It takes that kind of determination. But take heart, there is hope. You can champion disease.

3

This is the story of my struggle with Crohn's disease. In the midst of my disease, I would never have dreamt of writing these words, but my experience with illness happened for a reason. It gave me the opportunity to make a difference in the lives of people who needlessly suffer at the hands of diseases similar to mine. It gave me insights into what it means to have and overcome an "incurable" illness. Ultimately, it led me to develop practical solutions for those who suffer from chronic illnesses. I spent two miserable years battling the disease—and then I found my answer. If I had been lucky and stumbled upon the answer in the first month, I might never have understood what a powerful gift I was given. And I might never have thought to pass along that gift to others.

During my first eighteen years, I never once had a digestive problem. (Well, once or twice I ate ten tacos at a fast-food restaurant and got a case of indigestion.) I never had diarrhea or constipation. Television commercials about Pepto-Bismol mystified me. It never occurred to me that digestive disorders were so prevalent.

My father was a student at National College of Naturopathic Medicine in Portland, Oregon, where I was born. I was born at home, not in a hospital. Four naturopathic students delivered me. Naturopathic medicine takes an unconventional approach to health. Practitioners are taught to recognize the integrity of the whole person in their diagnoses and treatments. They are supposed to treat patients by noninvasive means and without medications. Until I was hospitalized for Crohn's disease at age nineteen, I had never set foot in a hospital.

If I were asked to characterize my diet before my encounter with Crohn's disease, I would say it was healthy. What I really had was a "health-food store" diet. For my first four and half years, I was a vegetarian. After I started school, my lunch usually consisted of a whole wheat bagel with cream cheese, a turkey sandwich, or something similar. I didn't eat junk food or drink Kool Aid like other kids. My family avoided preservatives at all costs. We didn't keep sugar in the house. We made sure that we ate vegetables, and we ate brown rice instead of white. We used whole grain flours, not unbleached or white flour.

But I didn't eat especially nutritious food. Looking back, I realize that we didn't pay enough attention to several key dietary principals. We didn't select the right kinds of fats or oils. And the level of carbohydrates in our diet was extremely high.

I was very healthy until I developed the horrific digestive symptoms of what would later be diagnosed as Crohn's disease. I took antibiotics maybe a handful of times. I hardly ever took medicines. The only time I paid attention to my diet was when I developed acne. As the saying goes, "It's much better to look good than to feel good." People are much more interested in cosmetic appearances than overall health. When I got acne, I asked the question that many teenagers ask: "What can nutrition do to help clear up my skin?"

As a former Crohn's disease sufferer, I am super-cognizant of my bowel habits. As someone who consults with thousands of people who suffer from bowel problems, I know more about others' bowel habits than most people would care to know. I talk to people with bowel diseases nearly every day. In my youth, however, I never paid any attention to my bowels. And I didn't care to know about anyone else's bowels either. If I went away to camp and didn't like the toilets, I would hold it for five days without thinking about it. I didn't know anything about the gastrointestinal tract and that was all right with me.

Setting the Stage for Crohn's Disease

My problems with bowel disease started after my first year of college. I have reflected on this year many times while trying to figure out what caused my illness. The truth is, determining the cause of a bowel disease is difficult. Why does one person stay healthy and another end up with Crohn's disease? In my case, I believe a busy lifestyle, a hereditary predisposition to intestinal problems, a bad diet, and stress set the stage for the disease.

At age eighteen, I went away to Florida State University. The school had awarded me a partial athletic and partial academic scholarship. I was very active in college. In fact, "active" doesn't begin to describe my life as a student at Florida State. I was very busy—and that's putting it mildly.

I occasionally went to class, of course, and I was also a cheerleader. In 1993, Florida State won the national championship in football. The cheerleading team competed nationally. Being on the cheerleading squad was a big commitment. I joined a fraternity. I was a soloist in a traveling music group. (I had been singing and acting since childhood.) I went to church three or four days a week, where I participated in the music program and leadership activities. I played on an intramural football team. I was studying for the American College of Sports Medicine exam. I wanted to be a fitness professional. I saw how sports nutrition made me a better cheerleader and helped me build strength. Amid all my other activities, I was an avid weightlifter.

How I found time for all this, I'm really not sure, although my eating habits permitted me a few extra minutes each day. I always ate on the run. I didn't take the time to eat properly. People used to say to me, "You don't eat your food—you swallow it whole."

My diet strayed in college. Under my parents care, I didn't eat the greatest diet, but it was certainly better than the diet that followed. In college, my diet took a wrong turn. I didn't cook very much. For the first time in my life, I ate junk food. I definitely didn't eat enough vegetables. The only greens I saw were the moldy rice and beans that my roommates left in the refrigerator too long.

I know what my diet was that year because I wanted to have low body fat and I tracked my diet carefully. Blame it on vanity: I intended to participate in the Mr. Florida State University Contest. To keep my body fat percentage low, I went on a high-carbohydrate, low-protein, almost-no-fat diet. Like most Americans, I mistakenly believed that fat is the enemy of humankind. I literally lived on health food muffins, granola bars, and cookies, all of them fat-free. A typical day's intake consisted of 600 to 700 grams of carbohydrates, about 80 grams of protein, and, some days, less than 10 grams of fat. I didn't drink alcohol. I ate a large amount of processed, albeit natural, grains.

❖

Food for Thought

As you read about my health journey, think about your own. Here are some questions for you to consider. Feel free to jot down your answers on this page or to use a notebook or software program to record your comments.

*When did you first show signs of digestive distress?

_____

*What were your eating habits like up to that point?

_____

*Were you experiencing unusual stress in your life at the time?

_____

*What beliefs led you to develop your eating habits?

_____

*What role did your friends and family play in your eating habits?

_____

*Do you believe you can improve your gastrointestinal health by changing your eating habits?

_____

I believe stress also played a part in my disease. I was under a tremendous amount of stress in college. If I missed one cheerleading practice I was off the squad-and I had cheerleading practice six days a week. We cheered for three sports at a time: football, basketball, and volleyball. I would cheer a couple of games on weekends. On Wednesday, my only day off from cheerleading, I played quarterback for my intramural football team.

My busy schedule would have been more manageable if I had had a car. I didn't drive, however, so I always had to arrange rides from one place to another. I remember throwing a touchdown pass for my football team and then running, at the end of the game, off the field and into a car to get to my music group practice. (If I'm going to recall events, they might as well involve touchdowns!) I was stressed from having to fit everything in. I was always dashing from one place to the next.

Like all college students, I didn't get enough sleep. If I wasn't burning the midnight oil studying for an exam, I was staying up to the wee hours with my friends.

Beginnings of Crohn's Disease

I trace the beginning of my Crohn's disease to the summer after my freshman year of college. I had lined up a job as a day-camp counselor. Accompanying the kids on the afternoon bus ride, I'd feel a little sleepy. Sometimes I fell asleep altogether, and that wasn't typical of me. Usually I felt very energetic. I put on a little weight, which wasn't typical of me either. I started getting canker sores, or aphthous ulcers. Whether or not these problems were early symptoms of my Crohn's disease I'm not sure, but my body had begun to break down.

I started to have digestive disturbances. In a three-day period, I was in the bathroom ten to fifteen times a day. Because nothing like this had ever happened to me before, I thought I would be fine. My father gave me some aloe and acidophilus. He tried several natural remedies to help me.

At the end of the summer, my church held a sleep-away camp. Although I didn't feel well, I decided to go to camp. What a mistake! There I was, roasting in the hot Florida sun, drinking glass after glass of sugary iced tea, and eating bad camp food. (What is it about camp food that it always has to be awful?) I spent my time running to the bathroom. Where I had gained weight before, I lost weight—a lot of it. In seven days, I lost twenty pounds. I was dehydrated. On the sixth day, I needed someone to drive me home from camp. My mouth felt like it was stuffed with cotton.

College was starting in ten days. I was looking forward to getting back to school. I wanted to be healthy in time for college, so I broke down and did something that wasn't typical of me—I went to a family practitioner. For me to go to a doctor was unusual. Before I got Crohn's disease, doctors and I had rarely crossed paths.

The doctor performed a battery of tests: a blood test for human immunodeficiency virus (HIV), a stool culture for parasites, you name it. He put me on a broad-spectrum antibiotic and told me I could go to school. I was still having problems, but I wanted to go back to school, so I did my best to ignore them. I weighed about 145 pounds, down from my normal 175 to 180. I was lean and mean. And I didn't want to face the fact that I was becoming increasingly ill.

I went back to Florida State for my sophomore year. I was scared to death of being ill. I was scared as well to tell my parents how sick I was because I didn't want to leave school. But I knew I was starting to deteriorate—I could feel it in my bones. On top of my gastrointestinal problems, my joints began to throb. I would get out of a car and my hip would pop out of its socket. Once, walking to my guitar class, my hip popped out and I couldn't walk another step. At night I ran fevers of 104 degrees Fahrenheit. I was running to the bathroom more than ten times a day and getting up at night to go to the bathroom as well.

My father had sent me to school with a bag full of probiotics, enzymes, and other health supplements. Not that I knew what I was taking—I wasn't into nutrition at the time. I was, however, keen to get well. I started trying all kinds of diets, including the Specific Carbohydrate Diet. But I didn't have a proper understanding of nutrition. I couldn't stay on a diet. Well, I could stay on a diet, but only until my roommate, who worked at a sorority, brought home leftovers from the kitchen. Then, all of the sudden, I wasn't on a diet anymore. I was hungry all the time. I had a ravenous appetite, but I wanted to eat only those foods that tasted good to me.

Right about this time I was introduced to the problem that almost everyone with an intestinal disease has to face: "Where is the bathroom?" I never knew when I would have to use the bathroom. As a consequence, I was reluctant to leave the house for fear of not being able to find a public toilet. Your life can be run by that. In a restaurant, I would take note when somebody went into the bathroom. I wanted to be sure the bathroom was available to me, and I became anxious when the bathroom was occupied. Sometimes just seeing somebody go in the bathroom made me have to go. It was a mental thing. I remember one episode while driving my car in Tallahassee, the home of Florida State University. I kept getting lost. I have a terrible sense of direction. I was desperate to get home to use the bathroom but I couldn't find the way. Fortunately I made it back home just short of having an accident. I can laugh about it now, but it wasn't funny at the time.

Diagnosed with Crohn's Disease

Finally I called my parents and told them how sick I was. I flew home immediately. My temperature was 104. As soon as I arrived, my father put me in an ice-cold bath—literally. He put ice cubes in the bathwater. While I was submerged in the bath (you don't "soak" in water that cold), I heard my father say something on the other side of the bathroom door. His words made me realize how serious my situation was. "My God," he said, "I don't want my son to die."

I was confused. I didn't know what was happening. I had never been around anybody with a severe illness.

Hours later, I found myself in the hospital emergency room. It was the first time I had ever been in a hospital. My visit lasted two weeks. (As anybody who has stayed in a hospital for a long period of time knows, you spend an inordinate amount of time watching television. My first hospitalization occurred during the week of the Oklahoma City bombing. I watched the news coverage of that for hours and hours. My second hospitalization, about a year later, coincided with the O. J. Simpson Bronco chase. Just my luck! I got nothing but bad news from the television while I was suffering in the hospital!)

During my stay in the hospital, I was hooked up to two IVs. I was flooded with intravenous (IV) antibiotics and antiparasitics. To halt the inflammation, I was given the steroid hydrocortisone. The doctors ran a battery of tests on me: upper GI series and lower GI series. They took a biopsy of my colon. X-rays showed that the upper portion of my small intestine was inflamed. I had what is known as marked duodenitis. I later learned that this disease—an inflammation of the duodenum, the first portion of the small intestine—occurs in less than 1 percent of people with Crohn's disease. I had inflammation throughout my small and large intestines. I was diagnosed with Crohn's colitis. Because I was in such bad shape and couldn't absorb food through my intestines, I was put on total parenteral nutrition (TPN), an IV infusion in which nutrients are delivered directly to the bloodstream. My sedimentation rate, a measurement of the inflammatory activity in my body, was 43. The normal sedimentation rate is 10 to 20.

Crohn's colitis, my doctor told me, is a treatable although "incurable" chronic disease. They said I would be on medication for the rest of my life. But, my doctor reassured me, I would be able to live a relatively normal life with a few surgeries and lifelong medication.

According to the medical literature, 85 percent of Americans have had a digestive problem of some kind. Bowel diseases are on the rise. Crohn's disease, the experts say, will surpass ulcers as the number-one digestive problem in the United States. A good 20 percent of Americans have been diagnosed with irritable bowel syndrome. Since I became involved in the health field, I have met thousands of people with gut problems, but as a teenager being discharged from a Florida hospital, I knew no one with Crohn's disease or any other bowel disease. People don't talk about bowel diseases. I've noticed that people don't hesitate to complain about every ache and pain, but most people consider bowel disease a taboo subject. After my diagnosis, I had to deal with all the emotions of having a gastrointestinal disorder. I didn't want to tell my friends because I thought my disease was too embarrassing.

In spite of my Crohn's disease diagnosis, my chief concern was getting back to school. Would it be two weeks? Three weeks? I still believed in a magic medication that I could take to get well instantly. In spite of the fact that I weighed less than 130 pounds and had been in the hospital for two weeks, I still expected to resume my normal life in a matter of days or weeks.

The doctors switched me from IV medications to oral medications. The switch to oral prednisone was hard. I experienced hallucinations for an entire day. I flipped out. I had an emotional breakdown. And that wasn't like me. Besides prednisone, I was on another anti-inflammatory, Asacol; two antibiotics, Cipro and Flagyl; and a drug called Diflucan for thrush (an oral yeast infection). I took an acid-suppression medicine called Zantac. I was a human drugstore.

Even with the medications, I was in the bathroom ten to twelve times a day. Throughout my disease, I had nocturnal diarrhea. From five o'clock in the evening until the following morning, I was in the bathroom every forty-five minutes to an hour. I couldn't sleep for more than one hour at a time. Sometimes I could last two hours without going to the bathroom, but that was all. My life became one long extended nightmare.

Riding the Hamster Wheel of Alternative Medicine

My hamster-wheel journey through alternative medicine began. After I was discharged from the hospital for the first time, I tried just about every alternative medicine, product, and diet. You name it, I tried it. Along with my dad, I began an obsessive search for a cure for Crohn's disease. My dad convinced me that I could beat the disease with alternative medicines. I was luckier than most people. I had a father who was a health practitioner and who could help me make medical decisions and guide me.

I began massive probiotic therapy. And when I say "massive," I am not exaggerating. I took dozens of probiotic products, in doses as large as two bottles of acidophilus a day, two bottles of bifidus a day, and two bottles of bulgaricus a day. I took thirty capsules a day of a combination probiotic in an oil matrix carrier that cost $2 per capsule. One product at $60 a day—that gives you an idea of how much my family spent on my supplements. I must have tried every health product known to man and beast.

Somewhere along the way, I took injectible vitamins and minerals. I injected myself seven times a day. I used an insulin needle to do it. I would often inject myself in the shoulder or the side of my hip. Often I hit bone. That's how thin I was.

My weight had fallen to less than 120 pounds. The iron level in my blood was 0 for fourteen months straight. By laboratory standards, I had the blood of a dead man. At rest, my heart rate was between 115 and 130 beats per minute. My body was tormented by an army of different afflictions:

- *Candidiasis.* A systemic fungal infection from candida that I had in my mouth as well as in my intestinal tract. Candidiasis often occurs in individuals with weakened immune systems who are taking the drug prednisone.
- *Amoebiasis.* An intestinal illness, also known as amebic dysentery, that is caused by a microscopic parasite called *Entamoeba histolytica.*
- *Cryptosporidiosis.* Another intestinal illness, this one caused by a protozoa infection in the gastrointestinal tract. Again, this illness is made worse by a compromised immune system and the drug prednisone.
- *Extreme intestinal dysbiosis.* An overabundance of unfriendly microorganisms in the intestines.
- *Chronic electrolyte imbalance.* An imbalance of the minerals in the body that are responsible for controlling the different metabolic processes.
- *Elevated C-reactive protein.* A condition that is usually part of an inflammatory reaction.
- *Anemia.* A disease that results when too few red blood cells are present in the bloodstream and insufficient oxygen reaches the muscle tissues and organs. In my case I was probably losing small amounts of blood through my intestinal tract on a daily basis.
- *Chronic fatigue.* A condition common in individuals with severe systemic disease. I had unceasing fatigue, headaches, weakness, aches in my muscles and joints, and an inability to concentrate.
- *Arthritis.* A disease that inflames the joints and causes stiffness and pain. The disease can be autoimmune in origin—that is, it may result from the immune system mistakenly attacking itself.

- *Diabetes.* A disease in which the body cannot properly metabolize carbohydrates. I probably got this one as a consequence of malnutrition and my use of prednisone.
- *Hair loss.* A condition I should not have had yet. I was only nineteen! A normal man doesn't start losing his hair till much later.
- *Leukocytosis.* An abnormal increase in the white blood cells.
- *Malabsorption syndrome.* The inability to properly assimilate the nutrients from food.

For the second time, I went on the Specific Carbohydrate Diet, but this time I observed the strictest form of the diet. I consulted person-to-person with Elaine Gottschall, the woman who popularized and refined the Specific Carbohydrate Diet. We spoke on a daily basis. I was on the diet three different times for three to five months each time. The diet is beneficial for some, but it didn't work for me.

I tried other diets. I was a vegetarian for a while. I went on something called the ultraclear detoxification/elimination diet. When one diet didn't work, I switched to another. I lived mostly on chicken soup, butternut squash, and pureed peas with the skins taken off. I longed for tasty food. The foods I ate were never fulfilling. They had almost no flavor. I now understand what it means to have a chronic illness and see all the flavor and fun sucked out of your life.

My search for an answer to my Crohn's disease sent me farther and farther from my home. I traveled to clinics all over the world. I went to the offices of seventy health practitioners in seven different countries—in Europe, South America, Mexico, and Canada. As my search grew more frantic and desperate, it went farther off the beaten path. At times I grasped at straws. I tried two or three treatments that no rational person would consider. I tried more than 300 different "miracle" products. I was the victim—and I chose that word carefully—of many well-meaning network marketing distributors of nutritional products. A lot of nutritional products are promoted through network marketing and multilevel marketing. These products are often promoted shamelessly. Often people are taught that the product they are distributing will cure anything. They make a number of false claims and present all kinds of unsubstantiated testimonials.

I did different IV treatments. I took something called adrenal cortical extract, or ACE (the Food and Drug Administration warned back in 1978 that this extract is obsolete and ineffective). I did cellular therapy, a procedure involving the injection of cells from the embryo of a sheep. The injections were extremely painful, but I endured them because the gentleman who gave me the therapy claimed to have successfully treated 250 cases of Crohn's disease in the United Kingdom.

My dad, through reading health magazines and calling colleagues, found all kinds of clinics and therapies for me to try. The number of machines that were hooked up to my body could fill a science fiction novel! I tried various forms of electro-dermal screening (EDS). In this therapy, an electric probe is placed on different parts of the body and the electrical charges that the probe registers are recorded by a computer. The doctor told me I was sensitive to the electromagnetic fields in my house. He had a steel cage constructed that I had to put around my room. I had to pull the plugs on my television and clocks—all my electrical devices—at night. Another person I visited said I was sensitive to the movements of a certain satellite that orbited the earth every ten years. He said I was one of the rare, unlucky people that the satellite influenced. I assure you I am not exaggerating about the satellite!

I tried applied kinesiology, a chiropractic technique in which different tests are done on points of your body. I utilized acupuncture and homeopathy. I tried something called liquid glandular supplements (don't worry, I'll spare you the details). I tried glutamine therapy.

Of all the oddball therapies I tried, none was more odd than the doctor from outer space. I can laugh about this episode now, but it illustrates how desperate I had become. In the middle of my illness, I heard about a local herbalist who was getting good results with sick people. He made teas. We invited him to our house and engaged his services. He brought the tea in unlabeled jugs. He had supposedly been a doctor in a foreign country and he didn't speak any English.

His son acted as a translator. From time to time the herbalist came to the house to replenish the jugs.

At the start, I felt I was doing a little better thanks to the tea. Probably it was a case of me getting more liquids, as I had been severely dehydrated. I was curious about the ingredients in the tea, but the doctor was hard to reach. The doctor and his son were kind of flaky. They didn't visit as often as I had expected. One day the doctor came to our house and showed photographs to my mother and sister. We thought they were vacation photographs. It turned out they were pictures of other planets he had visited! Desperate times require desperate measures. We tossed him out. Thinking back, the language he spoke didn't really sound much like French or Spanish. Maybe he was speaking Martian.

Taking medicine was my life. Unless I was visiting a doctor, which I did several times a week, I stayed home. I sat in my chair watching talk shows and cooking shows. (Because of my bland diet, I had a sick obsession with cooking shows.) I read every piece of literature and book about health that I could get my hands on. I believe I read 300 to 350 nutrition books during my illness. I continuously puzzled over what products to use and which products could help me.

I didn't just read health books. I often consulted the doctor who wrote the book in person. If I couldn't get the top person, I wasn't interested. All the doctors and health practitioners I visited said they could cure me in a short period of time. They had never failed to cure their patients, they said. All of them made promises they couldn't keep. I'm not saying their claims were hogwash. I'm sure they believed in their work. But my willingness to believe them and put all my faith in them demonstrates what people who are desperately ill go through.

Because I was so weak, traveling from clinic to clinic, especially by airplane, was an ordeal. I oftentimes got bladder infections and pink eye from traveling by plane. At one point, as I sat in my seat waiting for an airplane to take off, I said to myself, "If this plane went down, it wouldn't be that bad." It was a sick thought, but it showed my state of mind during my darkest days.

Arriving at Rock Bottom

I hit rock bottom on a trip to Germany, where I went to take Carnivora, a drug made from the fresh juices of the Venus's-flytrap. I had to go abroad to take the drug because the U.S. Food and Drug Administration does not permit it to be imported.

My timing for the trip couldn't have been worse. I was weaning myself off my medications. I had gotten off prednisone, but I experienced a complete adrenal shock. I couldn't catch my breath. My mother accompanied me to the German clinic. On the way there, a twenty-eight-hour trip including planes and trains, one nightmare event after another occurred. I missed a train by a few minutes because my mom and I couldn't manage to drag our luggage through the station on time. Because we missed the train, we were stuck in the station for six hours. All the time I was running around looking for rest rooms.

The German doctor made an interesting diagnosis. Although Crohn's isn't a classic autoimmune disease, he concluded that my problem rested with my immune system. Certain parts of my immune system were overactive and certain parts were underactive.

My mother, a schoolteacher, had to return to work, and she left me in Germany. I stayed in the clinic for six weeks. Not only did I get no results, the nurses were inattentive. After my six-hour IV treatment, no one would come to help me back to my room. Alone, sitting in the IV chair, shaking with cold chills, feeling like I was about to have a seizure, I would wait for someone to help me. Then I would creep back to my room to sleep.

I slept a lot while I was in Germany. I was on high doses of opium, which made me sleepier. In Germany, doctors prescribe tincture of opium to slow down peristalsis and keep patients from having to go to the bathroom so much. But the opium depressed me. The doctor, like any egocentric alternative practitioner, decided that I wasn't getting well because I had mental problems.

I had reached rock bottom. I was nineteen years old. I had dropped out of college. I was alone, with no friends. My mother had left me in a German health clinic where nobody spoke English.

My feeble attempts at German got me nowhere. I was in what felt like hell. I was miserable and constantly in pain.

Finally my parents and I decided it was time for me to come home. I wanted to get out of the clinic and I decided to leave on my own. To catch my airplane, I had to leave at five o'clock in the morning, but nobody in the clinic was awake that early. I was too frail and thin to carry my own luggage and I needed someone to help me. I couldn't find the switches to turn on the lights in the hallways. I tripped down some stairs in the dark and finally managed to get my suitcases to the lobby. But when the taxi cab showed up, I couldn't open the clinic door. I was locked in. Finally I found a back entrance, managed to wheel my bags out, and tripped down another set of steps. I fell flat on my face.

Too weak to walk on my own, I had to be wheeled into the airport. At the ticket counter, the agent had to summon someone who spoke English, but he couldn't find any record of my ticket. I had no money. My credit card was declined. I was sick. I had a urinary tract infection in addition to my massive bowel problems. I was on opium. It appeared I wouldn't get home. I said a quick prayer: "Lord, I cannot do a single thing. Please help me get out of this situation. I am completely spent." In a couple of minutes I was told that my ticket had been found. I got on the plane. I took a ten-hour flight to the United States, missed a connecting flight, but finally made it to Miami. Getting home was a thirty-hour ordeal.

I cannot describe how excited I was to be home. I remember lying on the couch watching *The Annette Funicello Story* on television. Actually, I was listening to the movie. I had packs over my eyes for my now double conjunctivitis (pink eye in both eyes). I had to run with my eyes closed to the bathroom either for a bowel movement or for painful, burning urination (due to another urinary tract infection). But in spite of my illness and pain, I was thrilled to be home again with my family.

Hospitalized Again

The hamster wheel of alternative medicine beckoned and I could not resist. I climbed aboard the wheel again as soon as I returned from Germany. During a visit to one clinic, my pulse was taken. It climbed from 180 to 200 to 220. The nurse became nervous and ordered me to the hospital.

My second hospitalization began. I was now completely dehydrated. I couldn't keep water down. My weight had dropped to 100 pounds, the lowest ever. The nurses tried to get an IV into me so I could be rehydrated, but they couldn't get a blood return because my veins were so dry and tapped out. It took the nurses and doctors two and a half hours to get an IV into my body. The nurses cried in the hallway. I heard one say, "That boy will not make it through the night."

I prayed. I had then and still have a relationship with God. All along, throughout my illness, I believed that God would heal me. But at this point things looked pretty grim. I thought perhaps it was time for me to move on. I said a prayer: "Lord, I've had a great life. I've had so many wonderful things. It's a shame that I'm going to leave this earth without having fallen in love or been married. But if the time has come, so be it."

Finally, the nurses were able to get a blood return. That night, hooked to an IV, I gained ten pounds, which showed how dehydrated I was. I lived through the night and decided the next morning that there still was hope for me. Unfortunately, the doctors put me on the same medications I had had the first time I was hospitalized—the antibiotics, antiparasitics, and anti-inflammatory steroids. When the time came for me to leave the hospital and I was switched from IV to oral medications, I had hallucinations all over again. I had the same traumatic withdrawal symptoms.

"I want you to take a picture of me," I told my mom while I was in the hospital.

She refused. She couldn't understand why I wanted a memento of my sorry condition. She asked, "Why in the world do you want me to take a picture of you?"

"Because no one will believe me when I get well. No one will believe that I was this sick. I'm getting out of bed and you're going to take a picture."

Climbing out of bed and standing up was a big struggle. The picture on the right is the photograph my mother took. I weighed 114 pounds (with the 10 pounds I gained from the IV). The skin on my legs looked dead. People often compare my appearance in that photo to that of a concentration camp victim or prisoner of war. Today when I tell people that at my lowest I weighed 104 pounds without showing them my picture, I find that they think of someone shorter and thinner. They can't even imagine someone my size weighing 104.

The doctors upgraded my condition from moderate to severe Crohn's disease. We started considering surgery to remove my inflamed colon. I also briefly climbed aboard the hamster wheel again. I went on something called the elemental diet, eating just powders mixed with liquids for ten

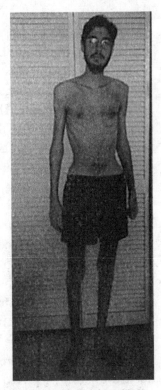

Jordan Rubin, looking like a prisoner of war at 114 pounds.

days. Then I went back to the Specific Carbohydrate Diet. I did that for three months.

But I was exhausted. I was all played out. The quality of my life had deteriorated to such a degree, I didn't consider it a life anymore. Every waking moment I obsessed over my diet or my illness. I had become very jaded. The alternatives weren't working. Along with my family, I decided to go to Mount Sinai in New York and get whatever surgery I needed. I had tried everything.

Getting Well with the Primitive Diet and HSOs

It so happened, however, that I hadn't yet tried the two alternative treatments that would heal me. My father had heard about an eccentric nutritionist in California who might be able to help. My father called this man without my knowing. He didn't want me to get my hopes up so he investigated the man's program himself. The nutritionist told my father why I had become so ill: I was not eating the diet of my ancestors found in the Bible. He said that our bodies are genetically programmed to eat the foods our ancestors ate and that the Bible outlines a plan for us to be healthy. When my father told me about all this, I was curious. It fit into my belief system. I decided to give it a try.

The nutritionist put me on a diet that included raw, fermented goat's milk in the form of kefir, different meats that were organically raised, natural sourdough breads that were yeast-free, whole grains, fruits, and vegetables. I still didn't get well at home. On the idea that leaving behind the place where I had been sick for so long might be good for me, I flew to California. Wheelchair-bound, I went to live with the nutritionist and his family. The nutritionist taught me how to eat.

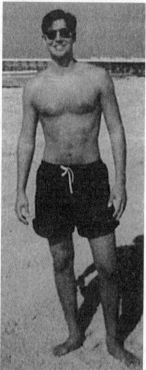

Jordan Rubin, looking healthy and happy at 170 pounds.

Feeling a little healthier, I moved into a motor home on the beach. I thought the ocean air might be good for me. In my motor home, I became something of a bum, an unusual experience for an upper-middle-class kid like me. For a time, I parked my motor home in the parking lot of a health-food store so that I could be nearer to the foods I needed. I started experimenting with other foods that I thought might help me. I drank a lot of vegetable juice. I drank raw-milk kefir and raw-milk cream. I ate raw butter and various free-range and grass-fed meats. Different people stayed in the motor home to take care of me.

Then an amazing thing happened. Although I had told my father not to send any more supplements, he sent me some anyway—black powder in a plastic bag. The black powder, I learned, was described as the missing nutrients from our soil. The literature that came with the powder said it contained nutrients called homeostatic soil organisms (HSOs), which we need to stay healthy. I had already tried more than thirty different probiotics. "Forget it," I thought.

But along with my ancestral diet, I started ingesting the HSOs (which are discussed on page 132). On the thirty-first day, a light started to shine. I had more energy. I went to the bathroom less frequently. During my forty days on the beach, I went from 122 to 151 pounds. I gained 29 pounds in forty days! The photograph of me on page 21 was taken after this period. I was not completely well yet, but I felt revitalized. I felt that good things were happening to my body. On my twenty-first birthday, I weighed 177 pounds. I had gotten sick right after my nineteenth birthday, but now, on my twenty-first, I was back to my normal weight. I was elated. I doubt if anyone in the world was happier than I was. I had rebuilt my intestinal tract and the terrain of my body.

The combination of the ancestral diet and the HSOs had made me well again. Despite my great improvements, I still had a ways to go. In December 1996, I came home to Florida. I was at my normal weight. I was ready to start my life again. I was healthy.

Spreading the Word

I had done what hundreds of thousands of bowel disease suffers desperately want to do—I had recovered my health. And my first idea was to tell the many doctors who had treated me about the primitive diet and HSOs. I sent my before and after pictures to the doctors I had consulted. I thought they would be curious to know what had healed me. I thought the doctors would want to include the primitive diet and HSOs in their treatment programs. Some of the doctors were very excited. Elaine Gottschall, author of *Breaking the Vicious Cycle* (Kirkton Press, 2000), was very happy for me. The doctors all wanted to hear my story, but very few of them wanted to try the primitive diet and HSOs on their patients.

Dr. Morton Walker, a medical jounalist who had sent me to several clinics, suggested that he write an article outlining my story for the *Townsend Letter for Doctors and Patients,* a health publication that focuses on alternative medicines and treatments. The article about my recovery generated two thousand telephone calls from doctors as well as bowel disease sufferers. Overnight, I was forced to find a way to distribute the HSO compound that had helped me get well. I had goals of establishing a clinic where people could come and be treated. I wanted to share the treatments that had helped me. I started Garden of Life, a company that manufactures innovative products designed to help the body heal itself. Our mission is to help people who are ill regain their health, but even more importantly, to help people who are healthy stay there. I pursued and completed certifications in nutrition and sports medicine, and completed a doctorate in naturopathic medicine. I am currently a Ph.D. candidate in nutritional science.

When I was deathly ill, I didn't smile very much. I didn't laugh. And that was completely out of character for me. I'm very outgoing. I was always the class clown. I love to tell jokes. But Crohn's disease sucked the life out of me. I believe the Devil's greatest tool for sucking the life out of people is an illness like the one I had. There can't be anything worse than feeling like you are inside a prison in your own body. I felt if I could help one person who was as sick as I was, it would be worth it.

I went through my ordeal for a reason. I consulted seventy doctors and took five hundred products for a reason. If I had come to the thing that worked first, the people who have the severest bowel diseases might not listen to me. But I can speak as an authority. Doctors said I had the worst case of Crohn's disease they had ever seen. They said I had the worst case of candida they had ever seen. As I have explained, I was a mess.

Today, I've been well for nearly seven years. I have been off medication for eight. People say Crohn's disease is incurable, but from my experience, no disease is incurable. A lot of people are very far gone and may not ever get completely well, but every single disease and every single state of health can be improved through whole-food nutrition and whole-food supplements that bring us back to a diet and a lifestyle that have proven to work for thousands of years.

The Patient Meets the Doctor

We (Jordan Rubin and Dr. Joseph Brasco) met in 1999 at a Designs for Health seminar on clinical nutrition. The seminar was put on by Robert Crayhon, an expert in Paleolithic nutrition. Jordan had come to investigate various nutritional and dietary therapies. Dr. Brasco was there to look into different treatments for gastrointestinal disease. In one lecture, Jordan shared the story of his bout with Crohn's disease. It so happened that Dr. Brasco, sitting in the front row, remembered reading about Jordan's seemingly miraculous recovery in *The Townsend Letter.* "Wow, so this is the guy!" he thought.

After the lecture, we went to lunch, and our partnership was born. It turned out that Dr. Brasco prescribed some of Jordan's health supplements for his patients. What struck Jordan at their first meeting was that, although he was only 23 years old, Dr. Brasco was interested in asking him questions. Jordan found his humility unique in a practitioner.

What impressed Dr. Brasco about Jordan's recovery from Crohn's disease was the importance that food, especially fermented food, had played in the healing process. Over lunch, Dr. Brasco picked Jordan's brain for ideas and theories about how he got well from a gastrointestinal disease by changing his diet. He was intrigued by Jordan's diet of kefir and other fermented foods, and his use of the Specific Carbohydrate Diet and HSOs. In his practice, Dr. Brasco had been playing with the idea of healing patients through diet. He had found that the people who have the willpower to get well by changing their diet inevitably do much better. The problem is convincing the average American that skipping a few meals or simplifying the diet may actually be something healthy.

When the opportunity arose for Jordan to write a book about his story and how to get well from gastrointestinal disease, he realized that he needed an expert to help him with the project and he called on Dr. Brasco. The doctor told the patient that he had been making notes on this very subject and he would gladly help.

The Doctor: Joseph Brasco

Most of the patients who come through my doors do not have inflammatory bowel disease (IBD) or cancer. There is "nothing" wrong with them, yet they come to my office feeling miserable. They have bloating, gas, constipation, loose stools, or hard stools. They come because they need help. They want to feel healthier and enjoy their lives more.

In my practice, I have prescribed the gamut of treatments for these people. And I have discovered that conventional approaches are not terribly effective. To be precise, they work only part of the time. In my practice, I grew frustrated with conventional approaches. For the most part, they are either ineffective or their benefits short-lived.

As a doctor, I felt I had to come up with something that worked more consistently for my gastrointestinal patients. Eventually, I arrived at the primitive diet. My journey isn't epic, but it has a few dramatic twists and turns.

Early Interest in Alternative Medicine

For better or for worse, my mother was one of those people who never trusts authority. She was always a little suspect of doctors—in a healthy way. As a child in New York, I remember very vividly listening to Carleton Fredericks, the grandfather of natural medicine, on radio station WOR. Probably under the influence of Fredericks, my mother had us take a lot of vitamin C. Long before the term "alternative medicine" was coined, my mother had us practicing a variation of it.

In my freshman year of high school, I developed a nasty case of acne. (It's amazing how many alternative physicians were born out of bad skin.) Being a teenager, of course, I was very concerned with my appearance. My mother, to her credit, took me to a dermatologist. He wanted to put me on tetracycline. Tetracycline is an oral antibiotic that is often prescribed for acne. As we now know, antibiotics change the balance of the intestinal microbes. They kill both harmful and helpful bacteria, and leave the territory open to bacteria, viruses, and parasites that are resistant to the antibiotic. My mother knew intuitively that taking tetracycline wasn't necessarily a good thing for me. Instead of letting me take the antibiotic, she advised me to be patient. She said acne isn't so bad and I would grow out of it.

Although I am eternally grateful that she did not agree to put me on chronic antibiotic therapy, I wasn't satisfied with her advice to be patient. I started buying books about ways to treat acne nutritionally with vitamins and whatnot. I cleaned up my diet. I reduced my sugar intake. I stopped drinking soda pop and drank lots of water instead. I ate more fruit. I never developed a china-doll porcelain complexion, but within a month or so, I did notice a marked improvement. The fundamental changes I made back then to my diet have stuck with me for the past twenty-five years.

Off to Medical School

When the time came to start thinking about career choices, I knew I wanted to get involved in medicine and health. And I knew that I wanted to turn people on to natural, alternative approaches. However, I thought the best way to do that was to start by becoming a conventional physician. It's easier to work from the inside out than the outside in.

Medicine as it is practiced in the United States is monolithic. It almost has to be that way. Doctors have to treat many people for many ailments and be 100 percent certain of what they do. Doctors have to be cautious, and trying to introduce new ideas in a conservative environment like that is difficult. It's like trying to turn a battleship around.

The philosopher Thomas Kuhns described advances in science as paradigm shifts. New knowledge is added to the dominant paradigm, but some discoveries don't fit the paradigm. When a critical number of discoveries don't fit, a revolutionary stage develops. The dominant paradigm is overthrown and replaced by a new paradigm. In Kuhns's model, most scientific advances take place during the revolutionary stage, when the paradigm is shifting. In medicine, we are currently in the middle of a paradigm shift. I hope alternative medicine will make inroads during this period.

My primary interest had always been nutrition. But, as I discovered in medical school, "nutrition" as the average person knows it—eating good food for health—is not what "nutrition" means in modern medicine. In medicine, "nutrition" refers to delivering nutrients and vitamins to a person either by intravenous feeding or by nasal tubes or gastric tubes. In medical school, I learned a lot about metabolism and the ways in which nutrients work in the body. But what I learned about nutrition had no bearing on the use of nutrients for a therapeutic effect, which is what I was interested in.

My postgraduate training was in internal medicine and then in gastroenterology. In these fields, I felt I could get closer to my interest in nutritional therapy. During my training, I encountered a book that really changed my outlook: *Life Extension: A Practical Scientific Approach Adding Years to Your Life and Life to Your Years* by Durk Pearson and Sandy Shaw (Warner Books, 1985). The book explains how nutrition can encourage health and longevity. What impressed me was the authors' command of scientific data. They backed up their ideas. Occasionally I challenged my professors with an idea I got from Pearson and Shaw. My professors would reply, "It's an animal study," or "It's not necessarily transcribable to human studies," or "There's no verification." Sometimes a professor declared his or her interest and sometimes a professor conceded, for example, that there probably was a role for increased antioxidants in preventing cancer. Mostly, however, my professors pooh-poohed these ideas.

My professors rendered their decisions about alternative medicine, incidentally, while sipping a diet cola or wolfing down a doughnut! When you wear rose-colored glasses, seeing the world in a different light is very hard. I have noticed that doctors who don't believe in alternative medicine immerse themselves in it when they or one of their children gets an acute illness. All of the sudden they pull research from all over the world and try it on themselves and their families. I know of a researcher whose son developed autism. He delved into the subject and came up with some interesting hypotheses about the interconnection of wheat and autism. The man put his son on a wheat-free diet and noticed dramatic improvements. Of course, his colleagues scoffed at all this in spite of the happy outcome.

My interest in nutrition took me to the University of Illinois at Chicago, where I took a residency to study under someone who was doing beta-carotene studies. Unfortunately, before I could become a senior resident and work with him, he moved on. But by that time I had concluded that gastroenterology was as close as I would get, in conventional medicine, to my interest in nutrition.

Learning the Importance of Diet

During my residency, I worked at an inner-city hospital. It opened my eyes to what is wrong with the American diet. I got an abject lesson in how *not* to eat. My patients were not healthy. They lived on junk food and what I call convenience-store food—potato chips, food in boxes and wrappers, and highly refined carbohydrates with hydrogenated oils. Their diet, to one degree or another, is what most Americans eat. If we are going to improve our health, the food-manufacturing industry needs to be more responsible. I tried to explain basic nutrition to my patients. I asked them to steer clear of fast food and eat more vegetables. I told them that they would feel better if they ate better. In fairness to them, they didn't have many opportunities to shop for nutritious food. Nutritious food seems to be one more "luxury" that escapes the grasp of indigent populations.

My diet wasn't the best either, although my fellow students

thought I was a little odd due to my eating habits. I took vitamins. I skipped the doughnuts. I was a vegetarian (although I ate chicken once in a while). I did a lot of bean-grain combining. I ate whole-grain this and whole-grain that. I followed the high-fiber diet—what I now call the health-food-store diet. I thought I was being healthy. Meanwhile, I was putting in ungodly work hours. I gained weight. I felt bloated and not particularly healthy.

Then I made a remarkable discovery, one that would help me later in my practice: If I stopped eating bananas, oatmeal, and the other high-fiber foods that were supposed to make me healthy, I felt better. A high-fiber diet is supposed to be good for many gastrointestinal disorders, but you feel miserable when you're on it. Like many of my patients, I thought it was my fault. I thought I wasn't combining the right beans or eating the right grains. In fact, I was on the wrong diet. I changed diets. I started eating more chicken and fish. I got more protein from animals. Like a lot of health professionals and people who want a healthy diet, I started out as a vegetarian, but I soon concluded that it just didn't work.

Devising a Treatment Program

By now I was married with one child and another on the way. I decided the time had come to start a private practice and pay back some of my medical school debts. I moved to the suburbs, where I encountered more conventional diseases than the ones I had treated in the inner city. I had quite a few patients with functional bowel diseases, such as chronic constipation, irritable bowel disease, chronic diarrhea, and chronic heartburn.

Treating patients with bowel disease can be a little scary because some of the patients are very sick. Originally, I treated people with the disease by the book. I gave them the traditional drugs— everything from Zantac to prednisone. But then I began noticing that the by-the-book treatment wasn't cutting it. The patients would feel good for a while, but then their problems would recur.

A few years into my practice, I read *Enter the Zone* by Barry Sears (Regan Books, 1995). The book has holes in it, but it made me realize how important reducing carbohydrates in your diet is. As I read more, I got turned on to the work of doctors who favor restricting the amount of carbohydrates in the diet. Most of these books address weight control, not gastrointestinal problems, but I noticed in myself that restricting carbohydrates also reduced bloating and other gastrointestinal symptoms. I noticed that in the Elimination Diet, most of the foods to be eliminated were grain-based. I became an advocate of reducing carbohydrates in the diet.

After I had been in practice for a while, I began to realize that the ten- to fifteen-minute office visit followed by the prescription for medication doesn't work. For medical, legal, and psychological reasons, the patients are given a litany of tests. A patient is given an antispasmodic, for example. It works sometimes, but the patient complains that it doesn't cure all the symptoms. So we do an upper-GI/lower-GI. That's normal. Months pass. The patient still doesn't feel well. Next comes computed tomography imaging, or a CT scan, a high-resolution type of X-ray. At the end of two years, the patient has had literally thousands of dollars' worth of tests for an ailment that we are no closer to curing. I started to realize how futile all the tests I had been ordering and all the pills I had been prescribing really were.

Finally I concluded that you can't treat the gut just with medication. You have to look at the overall lifestyle of the individual. I developed a treatment program of my own. I had enough experience and enough confidence to tell people right from the start that their gastrointestinal disease was a disease of diet. I have a reputation as a doctor who uses natural healing methods. I tell my patients, "We have two ways of looking at this. I'm convinced you have irritable bowel syndrome. I can give you the medication, and it might help a bit, but you're going to be back in my office next month with the same complaints. If you're interested, we can sit down and really try to figure this out, but you have to work with me. I don't want to waste my time or yours if you're not interested in changing your diet."

One hundred percent of my patients would get better by changing their diet. However, only three or four out of ten patients agree to change it. Most people take the path of least resistance—and that includes doctors. Most doctors look at their watches as often as the patients look at theirs. It's a folly of two, to some extent—the doctor and the patient deserve each other. Most patients want to give their doctors a list of complaints and take pills to make their complaints go away. Most doctors prefer to treat a patient by the book and not take a hard look at the patient's diet and lifestyle.

Treating Patients by Changing Their Diet

In standard medicine, you are only as good as your last pill. We don't really cure disease. We treat diabetes with drugs, for example, and if you stop the drugs, the disease returns. By treating diseases with diet, you address the underlying cause of disease. If you put sawdust in the gas tank of your car, the car won't run. Similarly, an improper diet deprives the body of the fuel it needs to be healthy. The medical community believes that the standard American diet is adequate, but a mountain of evidence shows that a primitive diet is what the human body craves.

For me, the last nail in the coffin of the high-carbohydrate diet came when I became familiar with the work of Robert Crayhon, author and chief executive officer of Designs for Health, and Loren Cordain, Ph.D. These men pointed me in the direction of the primitive diet. The fossil record shows a decline in health when humans moved from the hunter-gatherer diet to the agrarian, grain-based diet. During the transition between diets, there is evidence of iron deficiency, bone disease, and different types of infections. Humans became shorter and had less muscle mass after they switched to the agrarian diet. Even the most pristine whole-grain diet is not as healthy as the primitive diet. Humans switched to the agrarian diet because we are creatures of opportunity. A change in the earth's temperature and a decline in the population of large mammals made it necessary to get more protein from grains than meat, but the primitive diet is healthier.

We are naturally inclined to eat a primitive diet that is low in carbohydrates, especially if we come from European ancestry. The different enzymes, which are basically the working mechanisms of your metabolism, are revved up when you are on the diet, so you constantly burn a higher percentage of fat.

Adopting the Primitive Diet

Because I have a reputation as one who advocates natural medicine, I see a lot of patients who are referred by natural doctors. And many of them are no better off than when they first went to see their natural internist. Part of the problem is that the natural doctors are still hooked in to the idea of providing a diagnosis and doing tests. Patients are still caught up in looking at symptoms, running tests, and finding the perfect medicine. Most natural doctors only pay lip service to diet. They prescribe herbs and vitamins as medicines. They are stuck in the same trap as conventional doctors, but they are using different words and different diagnoses.

As I treat more GI patients and do more research, the primitive diet makes more and more sense to me. Many food allergies, for example, come down to eating excessive grains, legumes, and other carbohydrates that are *not* part of the primitive diet. The primitive diet is more physiologic—it helps the human body. As I adopted the diet in my own life, I began to notice benefits in terms of fatigue and weight control. The primitive diet is good for everyone, not just people who have gastrointestinal ailments. When something works for you personally, it becomes much easier to pass it on to your patients.

Most people with any gastrointestinal disorder will improve on the primitive diet. Whether it's as straightforward as irritable bowel syndrome or as severe as Crohn's, they will feel better. The same level of success cannot be guaranteed, but almost everybody notices some improvement after giving the primitive diet an honest try.

❖ 2 ❖

Getting Back to
Your Roots

This chapter lays the groundwork for the rest of the book. It details the workings of the digestive system. It explains how food is broken down and absorbed, and how waste is expelled. Along the way, we explain how various gastrointestinal disorders occur in different parts of the digestive tract. We also look at what causes gastrointestinal disease. There is still much to learn about this subject. Why one person gets a disease and the next person doesn't is still mostly a matter of speculation. However, we examine in this chapter the different factors that promote GI diseases. Finally, we take you to the drugstore, as we look at the two dozen or more drugs that doctors prescribe for different GI disorders. We believe you should know precisely what these drugs do, what their side effects are, and why they are necessary or unnecessary.

Exploring the Digestive System

The gastrointestinal tract, also known as the alimentary canal, is expertly designed to help the body break down food and absorb its nutrients. Not that anyone would want to, but if you stretch the digestive tract from end to end, it would measure 25 to 35 feet long. The digestive tract needs that distance to break down food and to pass the food's nutrients through its walls to the bloodstream. The nutrients are then distributed throughout the body by way of the bloodstream. What is left over after the digestive process is expelled as feces or urine.

To propel food through the digestive system, muscles in the wall of the esophagus, stomach, and intestine rhythmically expand and contract in a wavelike motion called *peristalsis*. You can see what peristalsis is by observing a snake eating a mouse. The principle is the same: As the muscles expand and contract, the food is pushed deeper into the digestive tract and pulverized. Saliva, acids in the stomach, enzymes, gastric juices, bile, and other substances all play important roles in digestion. Everything is designed to break down food and extract what the body needs for nourishment.

Starting at the Nose and Mouth

Most people don't realize it, but digestion doesn't begin in the mouth. It begins with the nose and to some extent the eyes. Before you take the first bite of food, you smell and see it. Especially if the food is appetizing, the salivary glands in your mouth go to work and produce saliva. By the time the food enters your mouth, saliva is ready and waiting to start the digestive process.

Saliva dissolves food. The mucus in saliva adheres to food to make it slippery. It lubricates food so that the food doesn't damage the lining of the esophagus as it passes through. Saliva washes food debris from the mouth and keeps the mouth clean. (During sleep, the flow of saliva diminishes. Because saliva doesn't clean the mouth as thoroughly at night, bacteria build up. This is why most people wake up in the morning with so-called dragon breath.) Like other parts of the digestive system, saliva contains enzymes that break down food. One enzyme in saliva, called salivary *amylase*, breaks down carbohydrates. As this book points out again and again, undigested carbohydrates in the gut are a source of many intestinal ailments. By chewing your food thoroughly, you not only lower your risk of getting an intestinal disease, you avoid the ubiquitous upset stomach, or as the Italians call it, *agita*.

Consider what happens if you *don't* chew your food well. You're in a hurry to get to work. Instead of sitting at the breakfast table to eat, you gulp down your breakfast at the kitchen sink. To wash the food down, you swallow juice or coffee. The food arrives in your stomach in chunks. The acid in the stomach has a more difficult time breaking down chunks of food than it does properly chewed food. Subsequently, the enzymes in the small intestine cannot attack the food adequately, the food isn't properly digested, and the nutrients in the food are not properly absorbed.

The longer you chew your food, the more saliva enters your mouth. And as more saliva enters, more enzymes go to work on the food you are chewing. Chewing increases the surface area of food and makes it easier to digest. What's more, chewing strengthens the immune system. The movement of the jaw stimulates the parotid glands, located behind the ears, which release hormones that tell the thymus gland to produce T-cells. The T-cell, a white blood cell, is crucial for fighting infections.

Into the Esophagus

After you swallow, the food enters your esophagus, a ten-inch-long muscular tube that leads to the stomach. How long the food spends in the esophagus depends on how well it was chewed. Well-chewed food makes the journey in about seven seconds, but dry food that was not properly chewed can take a full minute to move through the esophagus.

At the bottom of the esophagus, where food enters the stomach, is a strong ring of muscles called the esophageal sphincter. At rest, the esophageal sphincter is closed, opening just to let food and liquid pass into the stomach. Sometimes, however, the stomach puts too much pressure on the esophageal sphincter, causing the sphincter muscle to open and letting acid from the stomach invade the esophagus. The result is heartburn. Nearly everyone gets this painful condition from time to time, usually from overeating. Severe, persistent heartburn, a condition called gastroesophageal reflux disease (GERD), can damage the lining of the esophagus. Usually doctors recommend changes in diet and lifestyle as well as pharmaceutical medications to treat GERD.

Through the Stomach

Now we're getting somewhere. The stomach is where digestion begins in earnest. The food that spent a minute in the mouth and a dozen seconds in the esophagus stays in the stomach for two to four hours—two hours for a low-fat meal and longer if the meal included significant amounts of fat. Stress is also a factor in stomach digestion. Acute, temporary stress shortens the amount of time that food remains in the stomach. The stomach seems to register stress more intensely than other organs. After all, you can have butterflies in your stomach, turn your stomach, have an awful feeling in the pit of your stomach, or if you are impervious to stress, have a cast-iron stomach.

The muscle action of the stomach and the stomach's digestive juices churn food into a soupy substance called *chyme*. The primary digestive juice is a substance called hydrochloric acid. It breaks down proteins and kills disease-causing bacteria in food. Hydrochloric acid is extremely caustic. If it were to touch your skin, it would burn you. To put it another way, if your stomach was made out of cast iron like the proverbial cast-iron stomach, hydrochloric acid would eat through the iron in a matter of weeks. Hydrochloric acid doesn't burn the lining of the stomach because the stomach is protected by a thick coating of mucus. The mucus acts as a barrier to keep the stomach from harm. Aspirin and aspirin-related products can weaken this mucosal barrier, allow acid to damage the stomach lining, and cause an ulcer.

Hydrochloric acid is produced by parietal cells in the stomach lining. The older you get, the less the parietal cells are able to function, and the more susceptible you are to hydrochloric acid deficiency, a condition called hypochlorhydria. Physicians used to believe that hypochlorhydria was a natural part of aging, but they believe now that hydrochloric acid deficiency may be a consequence of a chronic infection with the bacterium *Helicobacter pylori* (more about that later). Half of the people over sixty years old have hypo-chlorhydria. Some researchers believe that low levels of hydrochloric acid in the stomach may cause food allergies and enhance the likeli-hood of infections. Normally, the acidic environment of the stom-ach kills harmful bacteria, but a deficiency of hydrochloric acid permits harmful bacteria to pass through the stomach, enter the intestines, pollute them, and cause dysbiosis.

If the mucus coating that protects the stomach from hydrochlo-ric acid fails to do its job, the acid may erode the surface of the stomach and produce a peptic ulcer. Ulcers can also be caused by *Helicobacter pylori*, which can burrow into the lining of the stomach and cause inflammation. By improving your dietary habits and in-cluding probiotics in your diet, you can help prevent *Helicobacter pylori* and other bacteria from damaging your stomach.

As everyone who has eaten Thanksgiving dinner knows, the stomach is capable of stretching to accommodate a second or third piece of pumpkin pie. Likewise, the stomach is capable of contract-ing when you fast or go for long periods without eating. A full stomach can hold about a gallon of food. On the lining of the stom-ach are millions of tiny wrinkles called *rugae* that permit the stom-ach to expand and contract. If you were to smooth out all the wrinkles in your stomach and lay your stomach flat (we don't rec-ommend doing it), your stomach would be the size of a tennis court.

Except from alcohol, caffeine, water, and some kinds of salt, the nutrients in food in the stomach are not absorbed. Candy is dandy but liquor is quicker, as the saying goes, because alcohol *is* absorbed through the lining of the stomach. Most nutrients, however, are absorbed in the small intestine.

In the Small Intestine

Chyme, the churned-up food from the stomach, is gradually re-leased through the pyloric sphincter into the small intestine, where most of the absorbing of nutrients is done. The chyme that isn't absorbed by the small intestine is passed into the large intestine as waste. The small intestine doesn't deserve its diminutive name. In fact, the small intestine is longer than the large intestine. It is 17 to 24 feet long compared to the large intestine's 5 to 7 feet.

Along the walls of the small intestine are thousands of tiny, finger-like protrusions called villi. The villi project from the mucus-membrane walls of the small intestine to absorb nutrients. The villi have been compared to the plants in an aquarium. As they wave back and forth, they acquire nutrients from passing food. Atop each villi are millions of microvilli. Under a microscope, the villi and microvilli look something like the bristles of a brush. Together, the villi and microvilli:

- Activate the digestive enzymes that break down carbohydrates, proteins, and fats so these nutrients are small enough to pass through the walls of the intestine.
- Absorb the nutrients from food and pass those nutrients through the intestinal lining to the bloodstream and lymphatic system. The nutrients then travel through the bloodstream and the lymphatic system to the different parts of the body.
- Act like a strainer to prevent bacteria, large undigested molecules, and foreign substances that aren't nutritious from being absorbed.

The small intestine is divided into three sections: the duodenum, which is about 10 inches long; the jejunum, which is about 8 feet long; and the ileum, which is about 12 feet long. The majority of nutrients are absorbed in the jejunum, the second part of the small intestine. The ileum, and the large intestine as well, is populated by intestinal flora, the bacterial microorganisms that aid in health (Chapter 5 discusses these microorganisms in detail).

The duodenum, the first part of the small intestine, has the same acidic environment as the stomach. The duodenum receives secretions from the pancreas and liver. These organs also play a role in digestion. The pancreas produces bicarbonates, a substance that neutralizes the acid from the stomach and prevents it from burning the walls of the small intestine. The pancreas also produces powerful enzymes that break down proteins, carbohydrates, and fats so they can be digested. The liver manufactures bile, a thick greenish substance that emulsifies fat to help with its digestion. It takes the body longer to break down fats than any other food. Bile is stored in the gallbladder until it is needed. When you eat a big, hearty meal loaded with fat, your liver prepares for the assault by producing bile and storing it in the gallbladder.

When the lining of the small intestine is damaged, it produces excessive mucus as a defense mechanism. But the extra layers of mucus make it harder for the small intestine to absorb nutrients. Nutrients must pass through the mucus as well as the lining of the intestine before they can be absorbed. Digestive enzymes on the intestinal wall, which normally break down foods so they can be absorbed, are blocked by mucus from doing their job.

When nutrients are not absorbed in the small intestine, they can create all kinds of trouble. One hypothesis of the cause of gastrointestinal disorders focuses on carbohydrate malabsorption. Bacteria in the normally sparsely populated small intestine feed on the undigested carbohydrates. This leads to an overgrowth of bacterial organisms in the small intestine. What's more, bacteria (and yeast for that matter) can alter the carbohydrates in such a way that they cause injury to the small intestine. The injured intestine then produces more mucus. More mucus means that carbohydrates become even harder to absorb and are more likely to remain in the intestine. The cycle—of mucus production leading to carbohydrate malabsorption leading to mucosal injury leading to more mucus—continues. The net result of all this chaos is a host of digestive complaints, including bloating, cramping, diarrhea, and the subsequent development of dysbiosis in the large intestine. We believe that this cycle is the primary cause of most gastrointestinal maladies. (For a further discussion of the problem with undigested carbohydrates, see page 40.)

Out the Large Intestine

What the body cannot make use of in the small intestine is passed into the large intestine, also known as the colon. Chiefly, digestive by-products such as bile, fiber, water, and bacteria are all that are

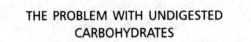

THE PROBLEM WITH UNDIGESTED CARBOHYDRATES

Science has yet to determine the cause of intestinal disorders, but many blame unabsorbed carbohydrates in the small intestine. Carbohydrates are not absorbed for different reasons:

◆ In a person with diarrhea, food travels too quickly through the intestinal tract to be absorbed. Enzymes do not have sufficient time to break down the large molecules with which starch, fat, and protein are made, so their absorption is incomplete and they don't deliver nutrients to the body.

◆ If the pancreas is functioning improperly, the small intestine doesn't get the enzymes it requires to digest food. The pancreas produces enzymes that break down carbohydrates so they can pass through the walls of the small intestine to the bloodstream.

In a person with a severe intestinal disease, carbohydrates can't be absorbed because the structure of the intestinal surface has been dramatically changed. To be specific, the villi and microvilli have been damaged such that they cannot absorb nutrients or, at the very least, cannot absorb them well. Normally, the microvilli assist in digestion by storing enzymes and passing nutrients to the bloodstream. But in people who suffer from severe intestinal diseases, the microvilli are damaged. The tiny hairs are blunted and injured. They can't hold enzymes in place properly, and consequently, the enzymes can't do the job of breaking down food. The result is malabsorption. Nutrients cannot enter the bloodstream and feed the body. In fact, the large molecules of undigested carbohydrates enter the colon and feed the ''unfriendly'' microorganisms.

Microvilli can be damaged due to a number of reasons:

◆ A deficiency of folic acid or vitamin B_1.
◆ Food allergies or sensitivities.
◆ Celiac sprue (gluten enteropathy).

- Excess mucus on the intestinal walls. The body creates mucus as a defense mechanism to lubricate the intestine, but excess mucus comes between enzymes and the carbohydrates they are supposed to break down.
- Infection (primarily from bacteria and viruses).
- Damage from the toxins emitted by bacteria, parasites, and yeast. These toxic substances can also damage the villi.

Lactase is the most fragile of the microvilli enzymes. It is the first to be impaired when the villi on the lining of the small intestine are damaged and the last to return to normal when intestinal health is restored. The lactase enzyme breaks down lactose, the two-molecule disaccharide sugar found in milk. People who are lactose intolerant can't digest milk because they can't produce the lactase enzyme. In severe diseases of the intestinal tract such as a gastroenteritis, the body's ability to produce the lactase enzyme is temporarily lost. However, many adults' production of lactase does not return to its previous level after the infection is cleared. That is why many people find they have "suddenly" developed lactose intolerance after an acute gastrointestinal disorder.

When undigested sugars from carbohydrates remain in the small intestine, the body sends water into the intestine—water that will eventually exit through the colon. Because the water carries nutrients, those nutrients are lost to the body. Vitamins and minerals that would normally be absorbed to increase body energy are lost in the stool.

left. The large intestine absorbs much of the water so that waste material can solidify and form stools. On average, the large intestine absorbs two and a half gallons of water per day. Stools are evacuated from the body through the anus, the last stop in the digestive tract.

Although water is removed from the stools, they retain some water. A healthy stool is made of water, undigested fiber, and living and dead bacteria. A stool that stays too long in the large intestine can dry out and be difficult to evacuate. It can cause constipation. By contrast, a stool that contains too much water can pass too quickly through the large intestine and cause diarrhea.

The best way to prevent constipation is to drink plenty of water and include fibrous and enzyme-rich foods—vegetables, fruits, and raw fermented foods—in your diet. Doctors recommend drinking six to eight glasses of water a day. The body cannot digest fiber, the cellulose and other fibers found in plant food that also goes by the name *roughage*. Fiber passes through the stomach and small intestine to the large intestine. By including fiber in your diet, you increase the volume of waste matter in your large intestine and put more pressure on the muscles of the rectum to loosen and release waste. Another way to prevent constipation is to exercise regularly. Exercise massages the intestines and encourages peristalsis, the rhythmic expanding and contracting of the digestive tract that pushes waste matter to its final, inevitable conclusion. By raising your knees in a proper squatting position during elimination, you can properly align the colon for smooth and easy elimination (Chapter 4 explains this in more detail).

In a healthy digestive tract, twelve to twenty-four hours pass between the moment food is swallowed and the moment waste is released at the other end. The amount of time that food stays in the digestive tract before waste is expelled is called *bowel transit time*. Food that leaves in less than twelve hours cannot be adequately absorbed. The body cannot extract the nutrients it needs in so short a time. Food that stays longer than twenty-four hours may pollute the large intestine. When waste material remains too long in the GI tract, putrid substances that the body normally expels may be absorbed through the intestinal lining to the bloodstream. One theory says that the absorption of damaged estrogen molecules in this manner accounts for the development of breast tumors in some women.

Of the trillions of cells in the human body, 90 percent are found in the large intestine in the form of bacterial microbes called intestinal flora. Altogether, you carry three to five pounds of intestinal flora in your gut. In healthy people, most of the microbes are so-called friendly bacteria that encourage good health and prevent illness. Chapter 5 explains the intestinal flora of the large intestine in some detail.

What Causes Gastrointestinal Disease?

It is hard to assign a single cause to a gastrointestinal disease. Saying for certain why one person got a GI disease and the next person was spared is hard. Often many different factors—diet, the environment, stress, the use of medications, and heredity, to name a few—come into play.

We believe that a poor diet plays a role in the cause of most GI disorders. If you try to fuel a car with sawdust, the car will soon break down and quit running. In the same manner, the standard American diet (sometimes known by its acronym, SAD) is not conducive to intestinal health. As the next chapter explains in some detail, the processed foods Americans eat are low in nutrients and high in calories and sugar. They provide short-term energy but not the deep-seated nutrition the body needs for repair, muscle building, and digestion. Processed food strains the gut. The gut must work harder to extract nutrients from what is essentially skeletalized food. This undigested, processed food remains in the intestines, where it can ferment and cause serious bowel disorders.

However, processed foods are not the only culprits. Here is a list of other causes of GI disease:

- *High intake of carbohydrates.* Many carbohydrates are not digested, but undigested carbohydrates do not pass harmlessly through the small intestine. They stay in the gut, where they can potentially feed "bad" bacteria. As a result, fermenting bacteria and yeasts damage the intestinal wall and digestion is impaired.
- *High intake of sugar.* Refined white sugar, like carbohydrates, can feed the "bad" microorganisms in the intestines. One such organism, a yeast called *Candida albicans,* is a big fan of sugar. Eating too much white sugar can cause candida and thrush. Sugar can also feed bacteria that irritate the lining of the GI tract.
- *Hydrogenated oils.* Margarine and vegetable shortening are examples of hydrogenated oils. These oils are found in potato chips, crackers, and most commercially prepared baked goods, where they preserve food and make it last longer on the shelf.

In the hydrogenation process, liquid (polyunsaturated) oils are saturated with hydrogen atoms to make them solid at room temperature. Hydrogenation has the effect of turning polyunsaturated fats into toxic, unnatural fats called trans fatty acids. These fats raise cholesterol levels, can exacerbate and worsen sugar control in type II diabetes, and raise the risk of getting cardiovascular disease.

◆ *Artificial sweeteners.* Sweeteners that include sorbitol, mannitol, or xylitol can aggravate irritable bowel syndrome and cause diarrhea in sensitive individuals. Diet foods, chewing gum, vitamins, and medicines such as cough syrup and antacids contain sorbitol. These items are often overlooked as potentiators of gastrointestinal distress.

◆ *Alcohol.* The excessive drinking of alcoholic beverages damages the intestinal tract and strains the liver. The liver is responsible for producing bile, the substance that breaks down fat in the digestive process.

◆ *Nicotine and caffeine.* These substances injure the stomach and esophagus. They relax the sphincter muscle that controls the passage of food from the esophagus to the stomach. Consequently, hydrochloric acid from the stomach can splash into the esophagus to cause heartburn and gastroesophageal reflux disease.

◆ *Antibiotics.* Antibiotics can have a devastating effect on the gut. They wipe out bacteria, friendly and unfriendly. Harmful bacteria, yeast, and fungi that were kept in check by friendly bacteria suddenly have a free reign and can proliferate in the intestines. What's more, some strains of bacteria are resistant to antibiotics. These powerful strains remain in the gut to cause all kinds of trouble.

◆ *Vaccinations.* Some scientists have suggested that there is a link between MMR (measles, mumps, and rubella) vaccinations and inflammatory bowel disease. This subject is controversial but it is worth monitoring for future developments.

◆ *Corticosteroids.* These medications—chiefly prednisone—are prescribed for arthritis, asthma, Crohn's disease, ulcerative colitis, and other conditions. They effectively reduce painful inflammation, but they do so at a price because corticosteroids also depress the immune system and provide sustenance for microorganisms such as *Candida albicans* that can damage the intestinal lining.

- *Oral contraceptives.* Over time, birth control pills alter the environment of the intestines. They make it more alkaline than acidic. The alkaline environment encourages the growth of pathogens and yeasts that are harmful to the intestines. If you use oral contraceptives, be sure to take probiotics to encourage the growth of healthy bacteria in your gut. (Chapter 5 explains probiotics.)

- *Heredity.* Bowel diseases do not have a solid genetic link, but bowel problems seem to run in families. Many people who suffer from Crohn's disease or ulcerative colitis have a parent or a sibling with the same disease. Although a susceptibility to bowel disease may be passed down from parents, the genetic component doesn't guarantee that someone will get a GI disease. By following the principals outlined in the Guts and Glory Program, you can prevent or cure the disease no matter what your genetic makeup.

- *Chlorine.* The skin is a great vehicle for absorption. In fact, many pharmaceuticals are being designed in the form of patches to exploit the skin's ability to absorb chemicals. Chlorine kills bacteria, both friendly and unfriendly. People exposed to chlorinated water in showers and baths, and especially chlorinated drinking water, put the natural beneficial bacteria on and the natural pH (acid/alkaline balance) of their skin and GI tracts at risk. Coauthor Jordan Rubin has known several competitive swimmers who suffered from serious digestive disorders. He believes that the large amount of time they spend in chlorinated water was a major cause of their diseases.

- *Stress.* As anyone who has had butterflies in the stomach knows, the GI tract is more sensitive to stress than other parts of the body. Nerve impulses and hormone signals regulate digestion and the movement of food throughout the GI tract. Stress alters nerve impulses and hormone signals. It has been associated with heartburn, constipation, ulcers, and irritable bowel syndrome.

Conventional Drug Treatments for GI Disorders

These pages survey the conventional drugs for treating gastrointestinal disorders. We warn you, however, that in many cases we paint our descriptions of these drugs in broad strokes. Each GI doctor has his or her own approach. Each patient is different. Especially where a combination of drugs is prescribed, the treatment is individual to the patient.

We do not want to be overly critical of these drugs. In some books and articles, the writers present a worst-case scenario, but we prefer not to do that. We have met with many patients whose GI diseases were controlled by taking modest doses of these medications and by changing their diets. The 5-aminosalicylic acid (5-ASA) products and low doses of prednisone, for example, don't necessarily have horrific side effects. If taking these and other drugs works for a patient, we endorse it. People do very well on some of these drugs. They can go about their lives with no obvious complications.

However, if you can control a bowel disease with modest amounts of medicine, why not try to control it with no medicine at all? Nobody knows what the long-term, low-grade side effects of these drugs are. Most of them suppress the immune system in one way or another. All of them alter the biochemistry of the body. While these drugs undoubtedly work, we don't know how they alter the chemistry of the body in terms of its optimal health. Some studies suggest, for example, that proton pump inhibitors can cause an overgrowth of bacteria in the small intestine. What negative long-term consequences does an overgrowth of bacteria have? No one can say as yet, but the law of unintended consequences may well provide an answer someday.

A lot of people take medications without thinking about it, but others take them with great trepidation because they understand that drugs merely keep their symptoms in check. Drugs don't address the underlying health problems. We would like to encourage people to strive for a level of health above and beyond what is needed to have fit, functional bowels. That usually means weaning yourself from drugs and treating your GI disease by changing your diet. In our experience, the best patient—the one who is most likely to attain good health—is the one who says, "I want to beat this disease without drugs." Although drugs are often necessary in the early going, we wholly endorse this attitude. The kernel of this book is that human beings are biologically and spiritually intended to live a certain way and we should embrace that way. We feel there is a right way to live and that, all things considered, drugs like the ones described on these pages are not always necessary.

Antacids

Antacid tablets are the best-selling over-the-counter medication in the United States. The purpose of antacids is to neutralize the hydrochloric acid in the stomach. This caustic substance kills the bacteria in food and helps break down proteins. However, if hydrochloric acid backs up into the esophagus, it can cause heartburn, also known as gastroesophageal reflux disease. Drugs such as birth control pills and nitroglycerine can precipitate heartburn. Heartburn can also be exacerbated by stress, wearing clothes that are too tight, lying down too soon after eating, consuming alcohol or caffeinated beverages, and eating certain kinds of spicy food.

Calcium, magnesium, and probably aluminum are the active ingredients in most antacids. Taking an occasional antacid tablet does no harm, but habitually using antacids can have negative consequences:

◆ Antacids reduce the natural defense against bacteria. Hydrochloric acid kills bacteria in the stomach, but taking antacids decreases the amount of hydrochloric acid and allows some bacteria to survive. In one study done with a simulated digestive tract, a poisonous bacterium found in oysters called *Vibrio vulnificus* that normally is killed by hydrochloric acid was able to survive in the presence of antacids.

- Decreasing the acidity in the stomach keeps the protein-digesting enzymes from doing their work. Pepsin, one of the most important of these enzymes, requires a low pH environment, but antacids increase pH.
- The aluminum in antacids is difficult to absorb. It remains in the intestines, where it can cause dryness and constipation. Aluminum has been implicated in Alzheimer's disease and may contribute to osteoporosis.

Ironically, the symptoms of heartburn—a burning sensation and the feeling of being full—can be caused by insufficient hydrochloric acid in the stomach. This relative hydrochloric-acid insufficiency can lead to inadequate digestion, which subsequently may be at the root of reflux for many individuals. Obviously, taking antacids for a lack of hydrochloric acid is self-defeating. You need hydrochloric acid to digest protein and to kill bacteria and parasites. Instead of taking antacids, try swallowing two tablespoons of lemon juice or apple cider vinegar right after a meal. If this relieves or prevents your discomfort, you likely have a deficiency in hydrochloric-acid secretion.

Be careful about taking medications along with antacid tablets. Most medications are designed to break down and be absorbed in a certain part of the digestive tract. Taking antacids decreases the acidity of the stomach and keeps it from breaking down food, including medications, as readily. If you take a medication along with antacid tablets, the medication may break down later than intended and be rendered ineffective.

The best remedy for heartburn is to eat simple foods that don't upset the stomach, chew your food carefully, and eat less at each sitting. Antacids are a classic example of a drug that masks the symptoms of a disease instead of treating its causes. Drinking chamomile tea, incidentally, is an excellent way to calm the stomach without resorting to antacid tablets.

Anticholinergics

In gastrointestinal patients, anticholinergics, also known as antispasmodics, are used to treat abdominal cramps, nausea, acute diarrhea, and other symptoms associated with irritable bowel syndrome. The drugs block certain nerve impulses and thereby prevent muscles in the abdomen from contracting. They are used to quiet overactive and convulsive digestive systems and are very popular in the treatment of IBS.

From the gastrointestinal perspective, the problem with these drugs is that they stop gastric progress. Food may remain too long in the intestines, where it can ferment and cause bloating or gas. The side effects of anticholinergics include drowsiness and fatigue. Anticholinergics are another example of a medicine that should not be taken too soon before or after taking antacid tablets. Antacids have the effect of neutralizing the drug.

Antidiarrheal Drugs

It is important to remember that diarrhea is a symptom, not a disease. Diarrhea can have any number of causes, such as taking medications, lactose intolerance, stress, diet, or drinking water contaminated with bacteria. If you find yourself taking an antidiarrheal medicine for more than two days, consult your doctor. Your diarrhea is probably a symptom of a disease that needs treating on its own.

Antidiarrheal drugs come in these broad categories:

- *Loperamide (Imodium A-D).* This drug acts on the muscles of the intestinal tract to slow down the passage of stools through the intestines. Because the stools stay in the intestines longer, their water content has more time to be reabsorbed. This gives the stools more content and makes them bulkier.
- *Attapulgite (Kaopectate).* This clay-like mineral absorbs the bacteria, toxins, or germs that cause diarrhea. However, important nutrients and enzymes are also absorbed. "Good" bacteria

needed for proper digestion may be absorbed as well. Whether attapulgite really absorbs bacteria is a subject of debate.

- *Bismuth subsalicylate (Pepto-Bismal).* This mineral decreases the fluid secretion in the intestine and kills some bacteria that may cause diarrhea. Bismuth sometimes causes stools to be darker than normal, but this isn't something to be concerned about.
- *Diphenoxylate (Lomotil).* Like loperamide, this drug slows down the intestinal-tract muscles so that stools remain longer in the intestines and their water can be absorbed. The drug has a mild narcotic effect and can be addictive. For this reason, it is combined with a drug called atropine in Lomotil and in some other antidiarrheal medications.

Whatever manner you choose to treat diarrhea, be sure to drink plenty of clean water. Diarrhea is very dehydrating. It robs the body of water. Avoid fruit juices, soda pop, and coffee, however, because these liquids aggravate diarrhea.

Antifungal Drugs

The antifungal drugs Nystatin, Diflucan, Nizoral, and Sporanox are used to treat yeast and fungal infections such as candida and thrush. Although these drugs are necessary and have saved the lives of some individuals, "alternatively minded" healthcare providers have dispensed these drugs with reckless abandon. While we acknowledge the negative effects of chronic candidiasis, we do not believe that every nonspecific malady is caused by a yeast. Furthermore, a better way to treat fungal infections is to reinoculate the gut with fermented foods such as yogurt and kefir. By doing so, you promote the beneficial bacteria and produce an environment in the gut that is unfavorable to fungal infections.

Bismuth

Bismuth subsalicylate, a mineral that is the major component of Pepto-Bismol, the popular over-the-counter drug, is used to treat heartburn, upset stomach, abdominal cramps, indigestion, and diarrhea. It protects the stomach lining from hydrochloric acid and kills *Helicobacter pylori*. Bismuth compounds have been used to treat gastrointestinal diseases for centuries.

Bismuth is fine for what it is—a short-term remedy for digestive discomfort and diarrhea. But if you find yourself taking bismuth for more than a week at a time, you likely have a digestive disorder that requires more care and treatment than an over-the-counter drug can provide. Bismuth sometimes causes stools to be darker than normal. The drug may also cause a temporary and harmless darkening of the tongue.

5-Aminosalicylic Acid Drugs

The 5-ASA family of drugs are so named because they have compounds containing 5-aminosalicyclic acid. These drugs are used topically and orally to reduce inflammation in the colon and rectum. Doctors prescribe the drugs for people who have ulcerative colitis and Crohn's disease. The 5-ASA drugs are easily absorbed by the stomach and the upper part of the small intestine. Because they must be delivered lower down, to the ileum and colon, the drugs are chemically modified in different ways to make sure they pass unharmed through the stomach and upper small intestine to the colon. The 5-ASA drugs are similar to aspirin in their chemical makeup. For this reason, people who are allergic to aspirin should not take these drugs.

Popular drugs in the 5-ASA family include Asacol, Azulfidine (sulfasalazine), Colazal, Dipentum, Pentasa, and Rowasa. These drugs are relatively safe. The side effects include nausea, headaches, and heartburn. Some of the drugs (specifically Azulfidine) lower the sperm count in men. Many people gain control of their bowel disease by taking a 5-ASA drug. However, patients should be weaned from these drugs as soon as they become habituated to the Guts and Glory Program. No one knows what the long-term effects of these drugs are.

H_2 Receptor Antagonists

H_2 receptors on the lining of the stomach regulate the secretion of hydrochloric acid. H_2 receptor antagonist drugs work by interfering with the H_2 receptors and blocking the secretion of hydrochloric acid. They lower the acidity of the stomach and thereby relieve heartburn, GERD, and some kinds of ulcers. Popular H_2 receptor antagonist drugs are Zantac, Tagamet, Pepcid, and Axid.

H_2 receptor antagonist drugs were discovered by accident. The *H* in H_2 stands for histamine. At one time, the drugs were used as antihistamines, but physicians soon realized that the people who took these antihistamines for hay fever also had fewer problems with their ulcers.

Food has only so much time to be broken down by hydrochloric acid, turned into chyme, and sent into the digestive tract. The problem with these drugs is that they deprive the stomach of the hydrochloric acid it needs to digest food, especially proteins and vitamin B_{12}. Undigested food that has not been broken down properly can ferment in the gut and feed the "bad" intestinal flora. This can cause bloating, gas, and cramping. Peristaltic action, the rhythmic contractions by which food is pushed through the digestive tract, may come to a halt.

These days, physicians choose proton pump inhibitors (see page 57) over H_2 receptor antagonist drugs for the treatment of GERD. The inhibitors are considered more effective than the antagonists and they cost only slightly more.

Imuran and 6 MP

Imuran (azathioprine) and 6-mercaptopurine (6 MP) are immunosuppressants. Sometimes they are prescribed so that patients can stop taking or can take lower doses of steroids. Imuran and 6 MP are more potent than the 5-ASA family of drugs. They quiet the activity of the immune system and in so doing lower the inflammatory response.

In moderate doses, these drugs are very effective in easing inflammation in people who have ulcerative colitis and Crohn's disease. In high doses, the drugs are prescribed for leukemia and preventing the rejection of transplanted organs. (No one knows quite why Imuran and 6 MP aid in inflammatory bowel disease, but one theory holds that IBD is the body rejecting its own tissues, and that Imuran and 6 MP work against IBD for the same reason they encourage the body to accept transplanted organs.) Chemically, Imuran and 6 MP are similar. Imuran is converted into 6 MP in the digestive tract.

At low doses, most patients can take Imuran and 6 MP with minimal, of any, complications. Although controversial, some physicians even believe it is safe for women to become pregnant and bear children while taking the drug. At one point, physicians feared that these immunosuppressant drugs would increase the risk of contracting certain kinds of cancers, especially lymphomas, but those fears appear to be unfounded. Because Imuran and 6 MP lower white blood cell counts, patients are more vulnerable to infectious diseases. However, no reports have appeared of horrendous, opportunistic infections in people who have taken this drug to control inflammatory bowel disease.

To make these drugs safer, patients can take a blood test that assesses the liver metabolism of Imuran and 6 MP. These tests measure the toxic by-products of the drugs. Doctors can monitor patients to be sure that they are getting the right dose with the minimal amount of toxins.

At face value, Imuran and 6 MP appear to be relatively safe. However, to return to a theme of this chapter, we do not know the long-term consequences of taking these drugs. These drugs alter the immune system. In consideration of the law of unintended consequences, it may take years or decades to really understand the long-term side effects of taking Imuran or 6 MP.

Laxatives and Other Anticonstipation Drugs

By definition, constipation is the passing of dry, pellet-like stools up to three times per week. Most people become constipated from time to time, usually from eating a low-fiber diet, a lack of exercise, or not drinking enough liquids. Constipation is the most common gastrointestinal complaint. Women and people over the age of sixty-five are the most likely to be constipated. Constipation occurs when the feces move too slowly through the colon. Normally, the colon reabsorbs a certain amount of water from passing feces. If the feces remain too long in the colon, more water than usual is taken, and the feces become dry and hard.

Over-the-counter laxatives fall into these categories:

- *Stimulant laxatives.* Irritate the lining of the large intestine and cause it to contract and expel the feces. Brand names include Ex-Lax, Dulcolax, Senokot, Correctol, Purge, and Feen-A-Mint.
- *Bulk-forming laxatives.* Introduce fiber into the colon that absorbs water and makes the stools softer. Brand names include Metamucil, Citrucel, and Serutan.
- *Osmotic laxatives.* Draw water from the surrounding tissues into the colon to increase the weight of the stools. Product names include milk of magnesia, Haley's M-O, Epsom salts, and Miralax.
- *Lubricant laxatives.* Coat the walls of the intestines and the feces to make for easier passage. Mineral oil is an example of a lubricant laxative.

For chronic constipation, most physicians do not recommend over-the-counter preparations. They prefer osmotic agents such as sorbitol or lactulose. These disaccharide sugars are not absorbed in the small intestine. Much like saline laxatives, they draw water into the intestines to moisten the stools. As sugars, however, they encourage fermentation in the gut. They can cause bloating and gas.

Laxatives can be habit forming. If you use laxatives too often, your colon will begin to rely on them to expel the feces. Eventually, the muscles in your abdomen whose job it is to push out the feces will grow lazy and flabby, a condition called "colonic inertia." The regular use of enemas can also bring about colonic inertia. Do not under any circumstances use laxatives as a means of losing weight.

Methotrexate

Patients who do not respond to or are intolerant of Imuran or 6 MP are sometimes given methotrexate. Like Imuran and 6 MP, methotrexate is an immunosuppressant. It prevents painful inflammation of the bowel by quieting the immune system.

Unlike Imuran and 6 MP, methotrexate can have dangerous side effects. It has been known to cause scarring of the liver and cirrhosis when taken over long periods of time. Pregnant women should not take this drug because it can have hazardous consequences for the fetus. Methotrexate can also be prescribed for rheumatoid arthritis and psoriasis. It is also used to induce miscarriage in patients with ectopic pregnancy.

Metoclopramide

The old standby metoclopramide, also known by the brand name Reglan, is sometimes prescribed for delayed gastric emptying, GERD, and nausea. Although this drug is helpful for some patients, its role is often limited by its side effects. These days, the drug only has a niche role in the treatment of gastrointestinal disorders.

Metoclopramide strengthens the esophageal sphincter, the ring of muscles that separates the esophagus from the stomach. If this muscle is weak, acid from the stomach can rise into the esophagus and cause GERD, heartburn, and damage to the esophagus. As another defense against GERD, metoclopramide encourages the stomach to empty its contents. The drug has been known to cause anxiety and jitteriness. Because it hinders the brain's dopamine receptors, it is helpful against nausea.

Metronidazole

Metronidazole, also known by the brand names Flagyl and Protostat, is an antibiotic. It fights or prevents bacterial infections. The drug is sometimes prescribed for patients with Crohn's disease, and is specific for the treatment of pseudomembranous colitis (PMC).

PMC usually occurs as a consequence of antibiotic therapy and the overgrowth of the bacteria *Clostridum difficile*. Metronidazole is often used as part of a general antiparasite regimen.

As Chapter 5 points out, a problem with antibiotics is that they upset the delicate balance between "good" and "bad" bacteria in the colon. Antibiotics kill all bacteria, including "good" bacteria. These bacteria aid the immune system, make the colon function better, and most importantly, keep the "bad" bacteria in check. Metronidazole is an antibiotic. As such, people who suffer from inflammatory bowel disease or irritable bowel syndrome should consult their doctors carefully before taking the drug.

Side effects of metronidazole include cramping, diarrhea, nausea, and headaches. In extreme cases, often when prolonged or high dosages are administered, seizures and numbness in the arms and legs occur. Be careful not to drink alcoholic beverages when taking the drug or you may experience headaches, cramps, and nausea. Unless it is absolutely necessary, pregnant woman should not take this drug. If you suspect that you are pregnant, be sure to alert your doctor.

Prednisone

Prednisone, a corticosteroid, decreases the swelling and inflammation of body tissues. The drug is the synthetic version of cortisone, a hormone that the body manufactures. Swelling and inflammation are a natural reaction of the immune system to wounds, bacteria, viruses, and foreign substances. When you sprain an ankle, for example, it quickly swells. However, the pain caused by inflammation can be difficult to bear, especially for people with inflammatory bowel disease. Prednisone works by suppressing the immune system and thereby suppressing its inflammatory activity.

Most doctors have a lot of respect for, and in some cases a fear of, prednisone. The drug is indeed powerful. Usually, GI patients are prescribed prednisone when other treatments have failed or had no effect. The drug dosage usually depends on the type and severity of the disease being treated. An initial high dosage is usually pre-scribed and then tapered over a course of weeks or months. Because it suppresses the immune system, prednisone increases susceptibility to infections. The long-term use of high doses of prednisone may cause hypertension (high blood pressure), osteoporosis, weight gain, acne, and hirsutism (the excessive growth of body hair). The drug can also have a psychosomatic effect. It can cause mood swings, depression, and insomnia. Coauthor Jordan Rubin experienced hal-lucinations when he took large doses of oral prednisone for his Crohn's disease.

Prostaglandins

Prostaglandins are hormone-like substances that occur naturally in the body. In the stomach, their job is to protect the stomach lining from the burning effects of hydrochloric acid. Doctors prescribe a synthetic prostaglandin called misoprostol (Cytotec) to patients who are taking nonsteroidal anti-inflammatory drugs (NSAIDs). These patients are at risk for getting ulcers because NSAIDs inhibit the production of prostaglandins in the stomach. The synthetic prostaglandin misoprostol is designed so that patients can take NSAIDs without developing stomach ulcers. Misoprostal is another "niche" drug. At present it is not used with great frequency in the United States.

In the short term, some people experience diarrhea and stomach cramps with misoprostol. The drug can cause a miscarriage (it has been used irresponsibly to induce labor). If you believe you are pregnant, be sure to alert your doctor before taking this drug.

Proton Pump Inhibitors

Proton pump inhibitor medications have become the drug of choice for treating ulcers, GERD, peptic ulcer disease, and a rare condition known as Zollinger-Ellison syndrome. These drugs shut down 90 percent of the stomach's ability to produce hydrochloric acid. Proton pump inhibitors are sometimes called the "zole" drugs because their names all end in *zole:* lansoprazole, omeprazole, pantoprazole, esomeprazole, rabeprazole. The medications work by hampering an enzyme in the wall of the stomach, which causes the parietal cells in the stomach to secrete less hydrochloric acid.

The proton pump inhibitors work better than the H_2 receptor antagonists and they have won favor with the medical community for that reason. However, the proton pump inhibitors have all the drawbacks of the H_2 receptor antagonists, including depriving the stomach of the hydrochloric acid it needs to break down proteins and kill bacteria. Because food isn't digested as thoroughly, it may remain in the gut to ferment and cause cramping, gas, and bloating. Common side effects of these drugs are headaches, abdominal pain, diarrhea, and nausea.

Generally speaking, the H_2 blockers and the proton pump inhibitors are effective drugs. They do what they say they will do. With modest side effects, they control acid secretion and reduce the symptoms associated with GERD and other peptic disorders. However, the long-term consequences of effectively "turning off" hydrochloric-acid secretion for weeks, months, and years are not known.

Sucralfate

Sucralfate (Carafate) is prescribed to treat ulcers in the stomach and small intestine, as well as to prevent the recurrence of ulcers that have healed. The drug is a sucrose aluminum hydroxide compound. It works on the lining of the stomach and the upper portion of the small intestine (the duodenum). Sucralfate forms a gel-like coating over ulcerated tissue—in effect, it works like a bandage—so that the tissue can heal without being subjected to hydrochloric acid and other caustic substances. Besides coating ulcers, the drug inhibits the pepsin enzyme in hydrochloric acid and protects the stomach against bile acids.

Sucralfate works very well and has remarkably few side effects. Of concern, however, is the aluminum in sucralfate. Aluminum is a toxin. It dries the mucosal lining of the intestine and can lead to constipation. It has been implicated in Alzheimer's disease. Antacids can interfere with the effect of sucralfate. If you take antacids, take them a half hour before or after sucralfate. The drug also decreases the absorption of some medications, including tetracycline, digoxin, and certain antibiotics.

❖ 3 ❖

The Primitive Diet

This chapter looks at the primitive diet with an eye toward highlighting the differences between it and the typical modern diet. We believe that the primitive diet is the superior of the two diets. We as humans are genetically programmed to eat a primitive diet like the one our ancestors ate. The primitive diet consists of simple nutrient-dense foods that are rich in vitamins, minerals, fiber, protein, and essential fats. Yes, you read that correctly: Fat is an essential part of a healthy diet. By contrast to the modern diet, the primitive diet is moderately low in carbohydrates.

The primitive diet is in many ways the polar opposite of our modern diet. The modern diet is rich in calories, depleted of nutrients, and overburdened with unhealthy kinds of fat. It includes an unprecedented amount of carbohydrates, mostly in the form of simple sugars. The modern diet is the proverbial "recipe for disaster." It is the foundation of many modern illnesses, including digestive diseases.

This chapter examines different components of the primitive diet—carbohydrates, fats, proteins, dairy products, fiber, and others—to see what makes this diet so healthy. Along the way, we explain the damaging effects of our present diet. We explain why hydrogenated oils are so dangerous to your health, for example, and why consuming too many carbohydrates can lead to heart disease and obesity. Thirty or more centuries ago, humans ceased being hunter-gatherers and took to the agrarian way of life. It was the beginning of civilization as we know it and it was a constructive development (although some may argue this point). From the point of view of the body's physiology and biochemistry, however, the agrarian way of life has been an utter catastrophe. The gastrointestinal tract still yearns for the food it used to eat. The stomach grumbles because it wants the lean meat of wild game rather than white bread and sugary snacks.

How Healthy Were Primitive Humans?

Conventional wisdom says that primitive humans were undernourished and plagued by illness. They died young, if not by violent death then by infectious disease. They were dirty and infested with lice. The Neanderthal hovering by the fire in his sooty, smoke-filled cave, his body wracked by disease, is a stock figure in popular movies and the funny pages. Most people accept at face value the English social philosopher Thomas Hobbes's well-known description of primitive humans: "No arts, no letters, no society, and which is worst of all, continual fear and danger of violent death, and the life of man solitary, poor, nasty, brutish, and short."

However, Hobbes and the other social philosophers of the Enlightenment had a reason for painting such a bleak picture of primitive life. They wanted to contrast the ordered society that they envisioned to one of lawlessness and brutality. For that reason, they exaggerated the harshness of primitive life. The ancient Greeks and Romans, by contrast, celebrated the past. Their mythology told of a golden age of peace and happiness. Every year, they celebrated the feast of the Saturnalia to commemorate the Golden Age and lament its passing.

Is our view of primitive life accurate? Obviously, primitive humans didn't have the benefit of modern medical science. Infant mortality rates were higher than they are today. (The rates ranged from 20 to 30 percent!) Many more children died from infant diseases. However, taking into account the traumatic stress and accidents that befell primitive humans, a realistic assessment shows that they were physically healthy. Our pre-agricultural ancestors were in many ways healthier than we are.

We can learn about the health of primitive humans by studying people who still eat a primitive diet and lead a primitive lifestyle. We can also examine the records of anthropologists, explorers, and others who came into contact with primitive people. We can study the skeletons and teeth of primitive people for evidence of vitamin and mineral deficiencies. The evidence suggests that humans before the advent of agriculture were stronger, bigger, and healthier. Generally speaking, when hunter-gatherers took to agriculture, their health declined.

Consider this archaeological evidence to show how healthy hunter-gatherers were compared to their grain-growing descendants:

- The skeletons of pre-agricultural people are taller in stature; the bones have more density.
- Pre-agricultural people lived longer, taking into account infant mortality rates, childhood diseases, and physical trauma. Although primitive people did not live as long as modern North Americans and Europeans, their life expectancies compare favorably with the people in some twenty-first-century developing countries.
- The rates of infectious diseases were higher in agriculturalist societies (although this was due in part to the higher population densities).
- Nutritional deficiencies such as iron-deficiency anemia and pellagra were more frequent in agriculturalist humans. Pellagra is a vitamin deficiency caused by a lack of niacin.
- The number of dental caries and enamel defects was higher in agriculturalist societies.

While it is true that most hunter-gatherers did not live long enough to acquire cardiovascular disease or cancer, the major causes of death in the United States and Europe today, we know that the ones who did live long acquired these diseases infrequently. We know this because cancer and heart disease are rare among people alive today who eat a primitive, hunter-gatherer diet. Among the Kitava islanders of Papau New Guineau, for example, death from heart attacks and strokes is extremely rare. In a study of 213 Kitava islanders aged twenty to ninety-six conducted in 1991, all the adults had a low diastolic blood pressure (below 90). Instead of gaining weight after age thirty, all the adults lost weight. The islanders' diet consisted of fruit, fish, tubers, and coconuts. Rather than heart disease, the leading causes of death were infections, accidents, and complications from pregnancy and old age.

Unfortunately, the number of isolated societies that are cut off from the modern diet keeps shrinking. Only a handful of remote societies now eat the diet of our ancient ancestors. Canned food, refined sugar, and white flour are consumed nearly everywhere on Earth. Almost every society has made the transition from the primitive diet to the modern diet.

To learn about primitive health, we can look to observations made in the past. In some cases, witnesses observed societies as they made the transition from the primitive to the modern diet. These witnesses were able to see from one generation to the next how the primitive and the modern diet contrast. The picture isn't pretty. Primitive people consistently suffered the effects of ill health when they switched to the modern diet. Consider these observations about the health status of primitive people:

- The medical doctor and missionary Dr. Albert Schweitzer wrote about his 1913 stay in Gabon, Africa: "I was astonished to encounter no cases of cancer. I saw none among the natives two hundred miles from the coast. . . . I can not, of course, say positively that there was no cancer at all, but, like other frontier doctors, I can only say that, if any cases existed they must have been quite rare. This absence of cancer seemed to be due to the difference in nutrition of the natives compared to the Europeans."
- In his *Cancer: Disease of Civilization* (Hill and Wang, 1960), the explorer and anthropologist Vilhjalmur Stefansson recounts his unsuccessful search for cancer among the Inuit. His book men-

tions a whaling ship doctor named George B. Leavitt, who found but one case of cancer in his forty-nine-year career among the Inuit of Alaska and Canada. By the 1970s, after the Inuit had begun consuming a modern diet, breast cancer had become a frequent form of malignancy.

◆ In a comparison between acculturated and less-acculturated Inuit, heart disease and high blood pressure were noticeably higher in the acculturated group. In a 1958 survey of native Alaskans, the subjects reported no symptoms of hypertension, but a similar survey taken eleven years later of native Alaskan women showed that their levels of hypertension had become comparable to those of Western women.

◆ Among the Australian Aborigines, cases of diabetes were rare prior to the 1970s, but according to Professor Kerin O'Dea of Monash University, diabetes among Aborigines in the twenty-to-fifty age group is now ten times higher than that of Australians whose ancestors came from Europe.

◆ Anthropologist Wilmon Menard, writing in the 1920s, relates how the Polynesians of the Marquesas Islands took to eating canned food and sugary confections because of the prestige that these European goods brought the people who ate them. The population of 100,000 dwindled to 2,500. However, when the price of copra (the dried kernel of the coconut) dropped and the Marquesans could no longer afford imported food, they returned to their traditional diet and soon reacquired their vigorous health.

Some of our best information about the primitive diet comes from a Harvard-trained dentist named Dr. Weston A. Price. (For more information see page 68.). Dr. Price traveled to five continents in the 1930s to observe primitive people, their diet, and the state of their health. He traveled to the remote valleys of Switzerland and to the rugged Outer Hebrides islands. He lived with the Inuit of Alaska and with various Indian tribes in Peru. Dr. Price recorded the lives of the Torres Strait islanders of Melanesia, the Polynesians, the Australian Aborigines, the Maori of New Zealand, and various tribes people in east and central Africa. Wherever he went, he observed how the modern diet brought ill health and tooth decay to people who had before enjoyed excellent health with the primitive diet. Dr. Price took detailed notes about primitive dietary habits. Here are some observations from his book *Nutrition and Physical Degeneration* (McGraw Hill, 2002), originally published in 1939:

- Switzerland: "The isolated groups dependent on locally produced natural foods have nearly complete natural immunity to dental caries, and the substitution of modern dietaries for these primitive natural foods destroys this immunity."
- Outer Hebrides Islands: "I was advised that in the last fifty years the average height of Scotch men in some parts decreased four inches, and that this had been coincident with the general change from high immunity to dental caries to a loss of immunity in a great part of this general district. A study of the market places revealed that a large part of the nutrition was shipped into the district in the form of refined flours and canned goods and sugar."
- Tongan Islands: "Following the war [World War I], the price of copra went from $40.00 per ton to $400.00, which brought trading ships with white flour and sugar to exchange for the copra. The effect of this is shown clearly in the teeth. The incidence of dental caries among the isolated groups living on native foods was 0.6 percent, while for those around the port living in part on trade foods, it was 33.4 percent. Now the trader ships no longer call and this forced isolation is very clearly a blessing in disguise. Dental caries have largely ceased to be active since imported foods became scarce, for the price of copra fell to $4.00 a ton."
- Ethiopia: "In one of the most efficiently organized mission schools that we found in Africa, the principal asked me to help them solve a serious problem. He said there was no single question asked them so often by the native boys in their school as why it is that those families that have grown up in the mission or government schools were physically not so strong as those families who had never been in contact with the mission or government schools."

- New Zealand: "Whereas the original primitive Maori had reportedly the finest teeth in the world, the whites now in New Zealand are claimed to have the poorest teeth in the world."
- Australia: "The rapid degeneration of the Australian Aborigines after the adoption of the government's modern foods provides a demonstration that should be infinitely more convincing than animal experimentation. It should be a matter not only of concern but deep alarm that human beings can degenerate physically so rapidly by the use of a certain type of nutrition, particularly the dietary products used so generally by modern civilization."

At times, Dr. Price writes rhapsodically about primitive people, their endurance, their stamina, their physical strength, and their natural beauty. They did not suffer from obesity, heart disease, or cancer at the rates we do. Thanks in large part to their diet, they enjoyed a vibrant health that has been lost to modern civilization.

Why the Primitive Diet Is So Nutritious

No matter how far we have progressed socially and technologically, our bodies continue to crave the foods of our ancestors. We are literally designed to eat their foods. Our genetic constitutions and nutritional requirements were established during our prehistoric past. Our physiology and biochemistry cry out for a primitive diet.

Before the advent of agriculture, the human diet consisted mostly of fruits, vegetables, fish, and lean meat from wild animals. Primitive people were nomads. They ate a variety of foods, even by today's standards. Although our supermarkets pride themselves on offering variety, the variety of food in supermarkets doesn't hold a candle to the variety of food that our ancient ancestors ate. Our ancestors had the run of the countryside. They ate an enormous variety of animals, wild grasses, vegetables, grubs, roots, insects, nuts, seeds, and so on. Species of fruits and vegetables had yet to be bred or cultivated, so the variety within plant species in the diet was quite large. Biologist Gary Nabhan estimates that Native Americans who lived in the Southwest United States had eleven hundred plants

DR. WESTON A. PRICE

One of the keenest observers of changes in the diets of primitive people was a Harvard-trained dentist named Dr. Weston A. Price. Alarmed by the number of cavities, the crooked teeth, and the deformed dental arches he saw in his young patients, Dr. Price wondered if these abnormalities were caused by nutritional deficiencies. Price believed, and rightfully so, that dental health is a good indicator of physical health. Deformed dental arches, crooked teeth, and cavities are signs of physical degeneration and a vulnerability to disease.

In the 1930s, Dr. Price undertook a study of the primitive diets in different parts of the world to find out if the modern diet caused the physical degeneration he was observing in his patients. With his wife, Florence, he left his home in Ohio and embarked on a six-year journey that took him to primitive societies on five continents. Wherever Dr. Price went, he photographed and studied the inhabitants' teeth. He made detailed notes about the primitive people's diet, the state of their health, and their way of life. Dr. Price chose an opportune time to undertake his study. In the 1930s, the last remaining societies in the world where people ate the primitive diet were making the transformation to the modern diet. Dr. Price had a chance to compare people, sometimes in the same family or household, who had grown up with the primitive and who ate the modern diet.

Dr. Price reported his findings in an extraordinary book, *Nutrition and Physical Degeneration*. He found that the primitive people who were cut off from the modern diet had very little tooth decay and perfectly formed teeth and jaws. The photographs in the book are astonishing. The narrow faces, misshapen jaws, and crooked teeth of the people who ate the modern diet are shown in stark contrast to the wide faces, perfect teeth, and perfectly formed dental arches of their fathers, mothers, sisters, and brothers who ate a primitive diet. What accounted for the primitive people's good physical health? Their diet, Dr. Price concluded. Wherever he went, he noticed that the people who ate the modern diet suffered from physical degeneration. Dr. Price suggested, moreover, that dietary deficiencies may cause poor brain development and lead to social disorders such as juvenile delinquency and high crime rates.

In a period of history when primitive people were disparaged and sneered at, Dr. Price made the startling suggestion that modern humans could learn from the primitives. He advocated returning to the primitive diet that had made our ancestors so healthy. He said we could learn much from some of their lifestyle practices as well, especially those pertaining to child rearing and child development. In Chapter 1 of his book, "Why Seek Wisdom from Primitive Peoples?" Dr. Price wrote:

> No era in the long journey of mankind reveals in the skeletal remains such a terrible degeneration of teeth and bones as this brief modern period records. Must Nature reject our vaunted culture and call back the more obedient primitives?
>
> Many primitive races apparently have prevented the distortions which find expression in unsocial acts. If so, cannot modern society do this by studying and adopting the programs developed through centuries of experience by the primitives?

in their diet. Hunter-gatherers were always on the move. They expended a lot of energy acquiring their food. They were anything but sedentary.

Then, as the human population increased and the amount of wild game dwindled, a profound shift occurred. Humans became agriculturalists. Where previously they had eaten lean meat from a variety of animals, they now ate a less healthy meat from a limited group of domesticated animal species. Cereal grains became the primary feature of the diet. People drank cow's milk for the first time. Starchy fruit and tubers replaced tart fruit and wild grasses. The variety of food that people ate diminished because people no longer foraged for food in the wild but grew it themselves. Life became more settled and civilization as we know it began to develop and eventually flourish.

While the shift from the hunter-gatherer to the agrarian diet marked a decline in human robustness, the worst was yet to come. The next profound change in diet occurred at the beginning of the Industrial Revolution. As people moved from farms to the cities, a need arose for food that could travel long distances and be stored for long periods of time without spoiling or bruising. Moreover, with the population increases, the farmers who remained on the land had to feed many more people. This combination of more mouths to feed and the need for food that wouldn't spoil easily gave rise to new agricultural practices and food-processing techniques. Now farmers spray their crops with pesticides and herbicides to increase the crop yields. They use chemical fertilizers with high nitrogen contents. Cattle are fed antibiotics and growth hormones. Fruit is gas-ripened. The packaged food industry serves up food made with strange combinations of refined flour, hydrogenated oil, corn sweeteners, and salt. Artificial preservatives and sweeteners disguise food that would otherwise be unpalatable. Refining removes much of the nutritional value from grain. The overconsumption of sugar, largely from soda pop and sports drinks, has contributed to a rise in diabetes, osteoporosis, and tooth decay. At the same time, we have become sedentary. Whereas our primitive ancestors foraged near and far for their food, we need travel only the distance from the couch to the refrigerator.

Writing in the 1930s, nutritionist Jean Bogart remarked, "The machine age has had the effect of forcing upon the peoples of the industrial nations (especially the United States) the most gigantic human feeding experiment ever attempted." And he didn't know the half of it. Bogart did not foresee food irradiation, the genetic engineering of food, or fast food. (To primitive humans, "fast food" was an antelope.) What the outcome of this latest dietary change will be is unknown. We do know, however, that the food we eat today is profoundly different from the food we are genetically programmed to eat. We are supposed to eat the same food as our primitive ancestors. Is it any wonder that gastrointestinal diseases are on the rise, since the gastrointestinal tract is the part of the body that is forced to try to absorb and digest this newfangled food?

In the rest of this chapter, we look at different parts of the primitive diet and examine why this diet is more nutritious and better for gastrointestinal health than the modern diet. Before going into the details, however, consider these profound differences between the primitive diet and the modern diet:

- About 70 percent of the calories that the average person eats come from foods that were unavailable in primitive times. Primitive people did not eat refined sugar, large amounts of cereal grains, or starchy vegetables such as potatoes.
- The primitive diet comprised 30 to 40 percent protein, 20 to 30 percent carbohydrates, and 30 to 50 percent fat. By comparison, the modern diet in the United States comprises roughly 15 percent protein, 50 percent carbohydrates, and 35 percent fat.
- The majority of the fat in the primitive diet came from healthy omega-3 fats and saturated fats from grass-fed animals. Most of the fat in our diet comes from omega-6 fats, hydrogenated oils loaded with trans fats, and saturated fat from grain-fed animals raised with artificial hormones and antibiotics.
- Primitive people obtained their carbohydrates from fruits and vegetables, not from refined grains. Consequently, the amount of fiber in their diet was considerably higher than the amount in ours.
- No refined food is found in the primitive diet. That means no canned food, pasteurized milk products, white flour, refined sugar, or hydrogenated vegetable oils.

Carbohydrates

Two of the primary goals of the Guts and Glory Program are to restrict the consumption of carbohydrates and to encourage the wise choosing of which carbohydrates to eat. This program is thus unique in that it emphasizes both the quantity and quality of the carbohydrates consumed. Reducing your consumption of high-glycemic carbohydrates (the carbohydrates found in grains and starchy tubers) can lower blood insulin levels. Lowered levels of insulin in the blood provide many benefits, including better control of blood sugar and reduced body inflammation. Another benefit of reducing carbohydrates in the diet is an improvement in the intestinal flora. Harmful bacteria and yeasts in the intestines feed on unabsorbed carbohydrates. By restricting carbohydrates, you foster the good bacteria and thereby foster intestinal health.

What Are Carbohydrates?

Carbohydrates are composed of sugar molecules that are chained together. They provide energy for the cells in the body. Carbohydrates come in two categories: sugars and starches. Sugars are simple carbohydrates. Simple carbohydrates are sweet-tasting and can be found in fruit. Table sugar is an example of a simple carbohydrate. Starch is a complex carbohydrate. Complex carbohydrates take longer to digest. These carbohydrates are found in vegetables, bread, pasta, and rice, among other foods.

Of the three macronutrients—protein, fat, and carbohydrates—only carbohydrates are unessential to the human diet. Yes, you read that correctly. Carbohydrates are *not* strictly necessary in the human diet. Humans can exist for extraordinarily long periods of time without carbohydrates as long as their essential protein and fat needs are met.

Carbohydrates are divided into four classifications:

1. *Monosaccharides.* Single-sugar molecules that can go directly from the small intestine to the bloodstream. They do not require splitting by enzymes first. The three types of monosaccharides are glucose, fructose, and galactose. (A word ending in the letters *ose* denotes a sugar.)
2. *Disaccharide.* Two-sugar molecules. For these sugars to be digested and passed into the bloodstream, the molecules must be split into single sugars by enzymes in the lining of the small intestine. The four kinds of disaccharides are:
   - *Lactose.* Found in dairy products.
   - *Sucrose.* Found in table sugar. It is used in many kinds of

canned and processed foods. Some fruits and nuts contain
sucrose.

➤ *Maltose and Isomaltose.* Found in germinating cereal seeds.
They are many-sugar starches, but they are digested in part
by enzymes in the saliva. By the time they reach the small
intestine, they have been broken down into two-molecule
disaccharides.

3. *Polysaccharides (starch).* Many-sugar molecules chained together. They are the most difficult to digest, as enzymes must
break the complex chain of molecules. Of the two types, amylose
and amylopectin, amylose is easier to digest. In the case of amylose, the sugar molecules are chained in a linear fashion and the
digestive enzymes in the small intestine can get between the molecules more easily to break them down. In amylopectin starch,
the sugar molecules branch off from one another.

The body breaks down all carbohydrates into glucose, a single
sugar, so that the molecules can pass through the wall of the small
intestine and be absorbed. Blood carries the glucose to the cells in
the body and the cells use the glucose for energy.

The Problem of Unabsorbed Carbohydrates

Many researchers believe that unabsorbed carbohydrates are a potential source of intestinal diseases. Of the three macronutrients—
proteins, carbohydrates, and fat—carbohydrates are the most
difficult for people with digestive problems to break down. Some
undigested carbohydrates do not pass out of the body with the feces.
Instead, they remain in the small intestine, where they feed harmful
bacteria and upset the balance of the intestinal flora. When enough
unabsorbed carbohydrates find a home in the small intestine, they
attract the attention of microbes in the colon. Some of these microbes migrate to the small intestine and multiply. They consume
the undigested carbohydrates and cause bacterial fermentation. This
harmful fermentation can lead to bowel problems.

The by-products of fermentation—gas and acids—make it even

more difficult for carbohydrates to be digested. The result is a vicious cycle, as outlined by Elaine Gottschall in her book *Breaking the Vicious Cycle*. Unabsorbed carbohydrates encourage bacterial fermentation, and bacterial fermentation makes it more difficult for carbohydrates to be absorbed, with the problem continually getting worse as more unabsorbed carbohydrates are put into the equation. What's more, to protect itself against microbial toxins, acids, and unabsorbed carbohydrates, the intestine produces excess mucus. This mucus comes between the digestive enzymes on the intestinal wall and the carbohydrates to make absorbing the carbohydrates even more difficult. Enzymes that normally break down carbohydrates cannot reach the carbohydrates to do their job.

According to primitive wisdom and current science, the best carbohydrates are the monosaccharides. Fruits, vegetables, nuts, seeds, and honey are sources of monosaccharide carbohydrates. For proper intestinal and homornal health, however, limit your consumption of sweet carbohydrates such as fruit and honey. Fruit and honey are wholesome foods, but they are concentrated forms of carbohydrates. For that reason, they potentially can disrupt your insulin balance. Generally speaking, vegetables are always the best choice for carbohydrates.

If this book had a mantra, it would be this: Decrease the total amount of carbohydrates you eat and be selective about the quality of the carbohydrates you eat. By following this one piece of advice, you can achieve and maintain intestinal health and overall health as well.

How Refined Carbohydrates Cause Health Problems

Refined carbohydrates include white bread, ordinary white and brown table sugar, crackers, white rice, commercial breakfast cereal, and noodles and pasta made from white flour. When sugar beets, sugarcane, wheat, and rice are refined, their fiber is stripped away, and in the process, many of their nutrients are lost as well. Many enzymes, minerals, and vitamins are also removed in the refining process. You end up with a skeletalized food with little nutritional value.

Chemically speaking, refined carbohydrates are one step away from sugar. As soon as you eat a refined carbohydrate, your body converts it to glucose—in other words, to sugar. Eating white bread is, chemically speaking, not very different from eating candy. To metabolize refined carbohydrates, the body has to dip into its precious reserve of vitamins, minerals, and essential fats. In effect, refined carbohydrates are a concentrated food much like vitamin and mineral supplements. They have a powerful effect. Especially when they are eaten alone, without proteins or fats, they invade the body in a rush and cause a sudden surge of blood sugar—a surge that disrupts the hormonal functions and can contribute to diabetes and other health problems.

Hormones are molecules that the body produces to regulate sexual maturation, the immune systems, and other bodily functions. The hormone insulin transports glucose—that is, blood sugar—through the bloodstream and into the cells so that the sugar can be used for energy. It also coverts blood sugar to glycogen and stores the glycogen in the liver and in muscle. Insulin also facilitates the uptake of fat into the adipocyte (fat cell) as well as prevents the release of fat from the adipocyte. Because insulin is so important to the management of blood sugar, the pancreas produces large amounts of it when you eat refined carbohydrates.

One responsibility of the hormones is to help the body remain in balance. For this reason, the hormones often come in pairs, with one hormone counterbalancing the other. Insulin is an example of an anabolic hormone. These hormones help build the body structures and store energy. Other examples of anabolic hormones are the sex hormones (testosterone, estrogen, and progesterone) and growth hormone, which grows and repairs the body tissues. Insulin, an anabolic hormone, is counterbalanced by a catabolic hormone called glucagon. Catabolic hormones break down the bodily structures and release energy. Whereas insulin, an anabolic hormone, stores glycogen (converted blood sugar) in the liver and muscle, as well as fat in the adipocyte, glucagon, as a catabolic hormone, stimulates the release of energy from the liver, muscle, and fat cells. Other catabolic hormones are the thyroid hormones T_1 and T_3, which are produced by the thyroid gland, and cortisone, a glucocorticoid hormone that is produced by the adrenal glands.

Eating refined carbohydrates floods the body with blood sugar and thereby disrupts the delicate balancing act between the anabolic and the catabolic hormones. First the body produces insulin to carry the blood sugar to the cells as energy. Then, to compensate for the overproduction of insulin, an anabolic hormone, the body either suppresses the production of other anabolic hormones or it increases the production of catabolic hormones, most notably the glucocorticoids. This has many deleterious effects:

- *Decreased tissue growth and repair.* Growth hormone, an anabolic hormone, is suppressed when insulin is overproduced. As a result, tissue growth and repair are held back.
- *Altered immune function.* The overproduction of glucocorticoid hormones suppresses the immune system. This makes the body more susceptible to infection and disease.
- *Increased propensity toward inflammation.* Increased insulin causes the production of more pro-inflammatory prostaglandins.

Refined Carbohydrates and Obesity

The body's mechanism for knowing when it has eaten too much is led astray by refined carbohydrates. Normal carbohydrates with their fiber intact are bulky. You can tell when you have overeaten unrefined carbohydrates—fruits, vegetables, whole-grain bread—because they weigh on the stomach and make you feel like you have eaten a lot. But refined carbohydrates are a calorie-dense, nutrient-depleted, fiber-depleted food. As anyone who has wolfed down a bag of potato chips can attest, you can eat a lot of refined carbohydrates without feeling full. Before you know it, you have eaten too much and you feel bloated. The body's inability to regulate the intake of refined carbohydrates is directly responsible for the obesity crisis in the United States. It may be responsible as well for the epidemic rise in adult-onset diabetes.

Properly Prepared Grains

As explained earlier, our primitive ancestors did not get their carbo-hydrates from cereal grains. They ate fruits and vegetables. Most anthropologists believe that grain cultivation began when wild game started to die out and the human population increased. Our ances-tors, in their wisdom, began supplementing their diet with increas-ing amounts of vegetation, first wild grain and then cultivated grain. Our primitive ancestors always understood that grains could be eaten. However, milling grains was difficult and time-consuming. Cereal grains became a practical food source only after the invention of the mill stone and other milling technology.

Our ancestors who ate grain prepared it very carefully before baking. They sprouted (germinated), sour-leavened, or fermented it to make its nutrients more bioavailable. Sprouting grain seeds un-locks their B vitamins. Sprouting and fermenting also neutralize the phytic acid and enzyme inhibitors in grain. Phytic acid is found in the bran of all grains. In the intestinal tract, it binds to and keeps several different minerals—such as iron, calcium, and magne-sium—from being properly absorbed. Seeds contain enzyme inhibi-tors so that they don't sprout until they are safely planted in the soil, but these enzyme inhibitors can interfere with the digestive enzymes in the digestive tract. Soaking and fermenting the grain, however, neutralizes the enzyme inhibitors in the grain seeds.

Along with a lack of exposure to sunlight, the causes of the rick-ets epidemic during the Industrial Revolution may have included the phytic acid in cereal grains. In nineteenth-century England and Scotland, the urban poor were afflicted with rickets. This disease is caused by an inability to absorb calcium, vitamin D, and phosphate. It strikes infants and young children, and causes their bones to soften. All evidence of rickets is absent in the skeletons of primitive people, who sprouted and soaked their grain to remove the phytic acid. The English and Scottish of the Industrial Revolution didn't take this precaution.

If you wish to consume grains, eat only sprouted whole organic grains. When making bread, try sprouting the grain seeds overnight before baking. In the bakery or market, look for sprouted whole wheat breads or sourdough breads.

Deceived by Sugar

The body hungers for sweet foods for a very important reason. In nature, sweetness in fruits and vegetables means that a fruit or vegetable is ripe and therefore loaded with its maximum capacity of vitamins and minerals. A fruit or vegetable is never as nutritious as when it is ripe and sweet-tasting. Our genes tell us that sweet foods are nutritious, and that's where the trouble starts. Refined sugar is concentrated sugar. It is sweeter than the natural sugar found in ripe fruit. Given a choice between an apple and bottle of soda pop, many people choose the sweeter of the two, the soda pop. Their genes tell them that the soda pop, being the sweeter, is more nutritious. Refined sugar is a superb liar. It tells the body it is high in nutrition when really it is extremely unhealthy.

Our primitive ancestors did not eat sugar. The only sweet flavor they knew was that of raw wild honey. Eating honey was probably a real treat for them, since wild honey is so hard to come by. We recommend avoiding refined sugar altogether and eating ripe fruit to salve your sugar cravings. Honey is also an excellent substitute for sugar. It contains minerals and other nutrients. Raw, unheated honey has an added benefit—it contains the enzyme amylase, which helps with digestion.

Besides the problems with diabetes and obesity, excess sugar in the diet can also cause:

- *Candida infections.* Sugar feeds *Candida albicans,* the yeast that causes vaginal yeast infections and thrush.
- *Crohn's disease.* Crohn's disease patients on average have sugar-rich diets. Wrote Dr. K. W. Heaton in "Dietary Factors in the Etiology of Inflammatory Bowel Disease" in *Inflammatory Bowel Diseases* (Churchill Livingstone, 1990). "The connection between Crohn's disease and a sugar-rich diet is proved beyond reasonable doubt. Apart from smoking, this is the strongest clue to an environmental etiology of a disease."

By the way, when you shop for raw honey in the grocery or health-food store, look for the words "raw"and "unheated" on the label. The honey should be cloudy in appearance and should need to be spooned, not poured, from the jar. Most honey producers heat the honey to make it flow more easily into the jars. Producers can heat honey and still call it "raw" as long as they don't heat it above a certain temperature. Still, honey that has been heated loses its nutritional properties no matter how little it was heated. Look for raw, unheated, cloudy honey to obtain honey with the most nutritional value.

Proteins

Protein, along with carbohydrates and fat, is an essential macronutrient. Protein is the basic building material of the body. The body needs protein, and the amino acids from which it is made, to build the muscles. Unless you get enough protein, your body cannot build new cells and tissue. Enzymes, antibodies, and hormones are made primarily of protein. Protein increases the stamina and fuels most of the biochemical activities. It builds muscle strength and supports the immune system. Animal sources are the best suppliers of protein. Beef, chicken, fish, eggs, and milk are called *complete proteins* because they supply all of the essential amino acids. Vegetables and fruits are called *incomplete proteins* because they do not supply all of the essential amino acids.

Protein composed a larger part of the primitive diet than of the modern diet. Whereas our diet is roughly 15-percent protein, 30 to 40 percent of the primitive diet was made up of protein-rich food. Our primitive ancestors got most of their protein from meat, fish, and cultured dairy products. The meat was considerably healthier than today's farm-raised meat. For one thing, it was leaner in general, and the fat it contained was of a healthier type. The wild fish and game that our ancestors ate was organic in every sense of the word. Most of the dairy they consumed was raw and cultured, and therefore rich in probiotics and enzymes. It came from goats or sheep that grazed on rich pasture land. It was more nutritious than the milk from modern cows.

In his study of people who followed the primitive diet, Dr. Weston Price found that those whose diet consisted chiefly of fish were the healthiest. They had stronger bones, fewer cavities, and the best overall health. Fish is rich in vitamins A and D, as well as in zinc and iodine, two minerals that are depleted in the soil but are found in abundance in the ocean. Deep-sea fish such as tuna and salmon contain healthy omega-3 fatty acids. These fatty acids help lower the level of cholesterol in the blood. They can also lower the risk of heart disease and possibly relieve hypertension.

Red meat is also a great source of protein. Red meat is full of zinc, magnesium, and vitamins B and D. By eating grass-fed beef, buffalo, lamb, and venison, you can eat a diet similar to the primitive diet, as grass-fed animals have a similar lipid profile to that of wild game. The ratio of omega-3 to omega-6 fat in wild game is 1 to 3.5 or 4. By comparison, the ratio of omega-3 fat to omega-6 fat in grain-fed beef is about 1 to 20. Grass-fed cattle resembles wild game in that it contains higher levels of omega-3 fat. Primitive people also ate the organs, brains, eyes, glands, and gonads of wild game. Organ meats are rich in vitamins A and D. They contain healthy omega-3 fat. In the brain, for example, the ratio of omega-3 to omega-6 fat is 1 to 1.

The fish and meat that our ancestors ate was superior to ours in that it was free of antibiotics and steroids. Try to get grass-fed beef, buffalo, lamb, and venison and free-range or pastured chicken and poultry. Free-range chickens have a natural diet of grass, grass seeds, and insects. The meat from these chickens, as well as their eggs, is rich in omega-3 instead of omega-6 fatty acids. Traces of the antibiotics and other medications that are fed to cage-raised chickens remain in the eggs after they have disappeared from the chicken's blood. (For a discussion of the advantages of grass-fed beef, see page 82.)

Many people are afraid to eat red meat because of its so-called high fat content. However, meat from properly raised animals is not high in fat. Lean meat, like the kind in seafood, wild game, and grass-fed beef, is 85-percent or more protein and 15-percent or less fat by caloric content. By comparison, meat from conventionally raised animals can be as high 75-percent fat.

The researchers who promote the idea that meat is unhealthy neglect to understand two very important facts:

- *All meats are not created equal.* Many older studies did not separate the different types of meat. In other words, cured and processed meats like ham and salami were considered to be the same as a sirloin steak.
- *The fat content of grass-fed meats and grain-fed meats are as different as night and day.* Grass-fed meats are rich in omega-3 fats and low in omega-6 and saturated fats. You could say that meat and animal products derived from grass-fed livestock are "health food."

Fats

Fat is the third member of the trio of macronutrients. Fat is absolutely necessary for body maintenance. Our bodies are designed to store excess fat so we can use it later as energy if we have to go for long periods of time without food. If you burn off your fat reserves, your body draws upon your muscle tissue for energy. Fat provides structural support for the cell membranes, the material that surrounds the cells. A great deal of our nervous system as well as our brain is made up of fat. Fats are also involved in a host of metabolic processes. As everyone knows, fat makes food taste good. It is filling. It supplies fat-soluble vitamins such as A, D, and E to the body. A diet with a high percentage of fat, if it is the right kind of fat, can be better than a low-fat diet.

Our primitive ancestors knew the value of fat and ate it every chance they got. Without understanding what made fat so nutritious, they understood that eating fat was good for their health. In his studies of primitive people, Dr. Price found that all primitive people went out of their way to obtain foods high in fat, such as

❖

THE ADVANTAGES OF GRASS-FED BEEF

Most cattle in the United States that are raised for beef spend the first six to eighteen months of their lives grazing at pasture. There, they eat a healthy, varied diet composed of different types of grasses with a few tasty treats thrown in—insects, insect eggs, and soil organisms. When the grazing period is over, the cattle are shipped to feed-lots, where they are "finished," to use the terminology of the beef industry. Actually, the animals aren't as much finished as they are fattened. Cattle are sold by weight. Everything that can be done to make them fatter is done.

Cattle spend four to eight months in the feedlot. There, they are given growth-stimulant hormones and steroids to make their meat more tender. The cattle eat a feed mixture composed of (sometimes moldy) grains and other, not-as-savory foods. The feed can include ground cardboard, chicken or cattle manure, and what is known as "tankage"—the ground-up flesh, hooves, and bones of other animals. (Tankage is often the source of contamination by salmonella and other bacteria, and the prions that cause mad cow disease). Because the animals live so closely together in crowded pens, diseases are rampant, so the animals are fed antibiotics to prevent disease. The meat of grain-fed cattle can be as much as four to six times fattier than the meat of cattle raised in grass pastures.

This diet of grain feed and drugs has many deleterious effects:

◆ The content of omega-6 fat is increased. Feedlot cattle absorb unhealthy amounts of omega-6 fat from the grain in their feed.
◆ The grain in feed has usually been subjected to pesticides. These pesticides find their way into the animals' flesh and, later, into the consumer's body.
◆ About 20 million pounds of antibiotics are given to farm animals each year. Strains of bacteria develop a resistance to the antibiotics. Some evidence suggests that these bacterial superstrains may be passed to humans in meat products from cattle.

◆ Artificial hormones and toxins collect in the animals' organs, especially the liver, rendering these food products unhealthy. This is especially unfortunate because the organs are normally some of the most nutrient-rich parts of the animal.

Grass-fed animals live their lives in pastures. Grass-fed beef is leaner and therefore lower in calories. The meat is richer in healthy omega-3 fat. The cattle absorb this kind of fat from the grass blades they eat. Grass-fed beef and lamb also contain larger amounts of conjugated linoleic acid (CLA), which has been extensively studied for its positive effect on the immune system and its ability to improve the body's muscle-to-fat ratio. Grass-fed beef does not contain any toxins or antibiotics. Raising cattle in pastures is healthier for the animals and for the ranchers who raise them. (For retail sources of grass-fed beef and other healthy meats, see "Resources" on page 333.)

butter, organ meats, blubber, and fish. In a comparison of the American diet and the diet of primitive people, Dr. Price found that the primitive diet offered ten times the number of fat-soluble vitamins as the standard American diet of the early 1900s. Tests done on the standard American diet of today would prove much more disappointing.

The Different Kinds of Fat

You are not alone if you are confused by the different kinds of fat. Once upon a time, fat was fat, and it was bad for your health. Fat is still a dirty word in most places, although nutrition-savvy consumers realize that there are different types of fat, each with its own implications for health and disease. If you pay attention as you stroll the aisles of the supermarket, for example, you may notice new terms in the fat lexicon: omega-3 and omega-6, saturated and unsaturated, and monounsaturated fat. What do all these terms mean? Here is a thin glossary of fat terminology:

- *Saturated fat.* This fat is solid at room temperature. It is stable and does not go rancid even when it is heated, which makes it ideal for cooking even at high temperatures. Saturated fat is found mostly in animal and dairy products, but it can also be found in coconuts and palm kernels. Traditional foods rich in saturated fat contain appreciable amounts of other beneficial fats, including CLA, caprylic acid, lauric acid, and butyric acid. These fatty acids are extremely beneficial to the health of the immune system and digestive tract. They can supply a significant portion of our energy requirements.

- *Monounsaturated fat.* This fat is liquid at room temperature. However, because this fat retains some of the characteristics of saturated fat, it becomes solid when refrigerated. This fat does not become rancid easily and is ideal for low-temperature cooking. Olive, canola, and peanut oils are high in monounsaturated fat, as are almonds, pecans, peanuts, cashews, and avocados.

- *Polyunsaturated fat.* This fat is liquid at room temperature as well as when refrigerated. It is very unstable and can go rancid easily. It is completely inappropriate for cooking at any temperature. (Yes, you read correctly: *inappropriate.*) Examples of polyunsaturated fat are fish oils as well as most vegetable and seed oils.

Complicating the polyunsaturated picture are the two kinds of polyunsaturated fat. These fats are deemed essential because the body can't make them on its own:

- *Omega-3 fatty acids.* You can get this fatty acid from flaxseed oil, walnuts, and pumpkins seeds. The elongated forms of this fatty acid are known as eicosapentaenoic acid (EPA) and docosahexaenoic acid (DHA). These complex forms of omega-3 fats can be found in ocean fish such as salmon, tuna, and mackerel, as well as in grass-fed meats, free-range poultry, and eggs from pasture-raised hens. Studies show that the omega-3 fatty acids are helpful against blood clots, heart disease, high blood pressure, diabetes, colitis, and inflammatory diseases.

◆ *Omega-6 acid.* This fatty acid is found in vegetable oil, sunflower oil, peanut oil, and other grain, nut, and seed oils.

It is not so much that the omega-3 fats are good and the omega-6 fats are bad. What is important is balance. Consuming omega-3 and omega-6 fats in the proper ratio is what really matters. In the primitive diet, the ratio of omega-3 to omega-6 fats was between 1 to 2.5 and 1 to 4, whereas the ratio in the modern diet is between 1 to 20 and 1 to 40. Scientists speculate that a diet with a high ratio of omega-6 to omega-3 fats can lead to many health problems, including a compromised immune system, poor skin, inflammation, heart disease, diabetes, and even cancer. To get the proper balance of omega-3 to omega-6 fats, eat more of the aforementioned omega-3-rich foods and avoid seed and vegetable oils. Seed and vegetable oils are used for the production of many processed foods.

The Dangers of Trans Fats in Hydrogenated Oil

If omega-6 fat, when taken in excessive amounts, can be called "the bad," then trans fat has to be called "the ugly." Beginning in the 1950s, food manufacturers were faced with the problem of how to keep the food on shelves from spoiling. The era of the supermarket had begun. Foods had to travel long distances and sit on grocery-store shelves for long periods of time. To solve the problem, the food manufacturers invented trans fatty acids, also known as trans fats.

Trans fats are produced by a process known as partial hydrogenation. In this chemical process, polyunsaturated fat—usually in the form of liquid vegetable or soybean oil—is superheated and then subjected to pressurized hydrogen and a nickel catalyst. Partial hydrogenation causes some of the carbon atoms to lose one of their double bonds. This causes the molecule to become straight where normally it is bent or crimped. The straight configuration makes a vegetable oil that is naturally polyunsaturated more like a saturated fat. Now the oil is solid at room temperature and far less likely to spoil.

Partial hydrogenation serves the goal of people in the food industry who want their packaged baked goods to last longer on the shelf. Margarine and shortening are the best examples of trans fatty acids. These substances (and "substance" is the operative word) are stable and do not turn rancid quickly. In addition, people seem to like the consistency that shortening and margarine can give to food. The next time you are shopping for packaged food, look for "partially hydrogenated oil" or "partially hardened fats" on the label. You will find the term on four out of five items in the supermarket. Partially hydrogenated oil is now the most common food preservative. Although the oil is made from polyunsaturated vegetable oil, it has been biochemically engineered to be harder and not go rancid.

Unfortunately, partially hydrogenated oil has an insidious effect on health. Putting aside for a moment what a toxic soup partially hydrogenated oil is, the trans fats in hydrogenated oil cause trouble because the body doesn't recognize them correctly. Trans fat has been changed biochemically to make it more like a saturated fat, yet the body treats it like a more flexible polyunsaturated fat. As mentioned earlier, fat provides structural support for the cell membranes. Human cell membranes are made of a combination of fatty acids and proteins, but mostly fatty acids. Trans fats are misfits that compromise the integrity of the cell membranes. Cell membranes constructed of trans fats cannot function optimally. Their biochemical processes no longer occur at the proper rate because the trans fat acts as a jamming mechanism. Some researchers have suggested that consuming trans fat and smoking cigarettes are equally dangerous to the heart.

Here are some of the deleterious effects of the trans fat in hydrogenated oil:

◆ *It decreases insulin sensitivity.* Because the insulin receptors on the cell membranes become less sensitive, they don't respond as well to insulin. For the purposes of illustration, let's say that someone in good health needs two insulin molecules to get one molecule of glucose through the cell wall, whereas a person who is insulin-insensitive needs five insulin molecules to achieve the same end. The insulin-insensitive person's pancreas must work harder and harder to make more insulin. Eventually, the person can no longer produce enough insulin, glucose starts to build up, and adult-onset diabetes and obesity result.

- *It may promote cancer by its derangement of the cell membranes.*
- *It raises the level of low-density lipoprotein (LDL) cholesterol in the blood and lowers the level of high-density lipoprotein (HDL) cholesterol.* In other words, it increases the bad cholesterol and decreases the good cholesterol.

Hydrogenated and partially hydrogenated oils are disguised oils. They would be inedible if not for the chemical processes they undergo to disguise their true flavor and odor. To make margarine, for example, the soy, corn, cottonseed, or canola oil is mixed with nickel oxide, exposed to extreme high heat and pressure, mixed with soap-like emulsifiers and starch to improve its consistency, steam-cleaned to remove its foul odor, bleached to change its color, dyed the color of butter, injected with artificial flavors, and compressed into tubs or blocks.

Recently, the FDA started requiring food manufacturers to list the amounts of trans fat and hydrogenated oil on food labels. To qualify as "trans fat–free," a food product must contain .5 gram or less of trans fat per serving. But you can do yourself a big favor by avoiding foods with hydrogenated oil altogether. Writes Sally Fallon about hydrogenated oil in *Nourishing Traditions* (New Trends Publishing, 1999): "The popularity of partially hydrogenated margarine over butter represents a triumph of advertising duplicity over common sense. Your best defense is to avoid it like the plague."

Is Fat Responsible for Heart Disease?

Our society is fixated on fat as the cause of coronary heart disease. Starting in the 1950s with the so-called lipid hypothesis, the American public has been led to believe that heart disease is caused by high levels of saturated fat and cholesterol in the diet. The idea is that saturated fat and cholesterol promote atherosclerosis and are behind the rise in heart disease. Heart disease rates rose steadily during the previous century. By 1950, heart disease had become the leading cause of death. At present, 40 percent of Americans die of heart disease. Accordingly, we have been told to reduce our consumption of red meat, whole milk, eggs, and butter. The lipid hypothesis is almost unquestioned, but is it correct?

This evidence contradicts the lipid hypothesis:

- Studies have shown that people whose blood cholesterol is low are just as prone to atherosclerosis as people whose blood cholesterol is high.
- Heart disease was rare in the United States before 1920, yet previous to that year the American diet was high in saturated fat.
- Rates of heart disease continue to climb although the consumption of red meat, butter, and eggs has declined drastically.
- People in primitive cultures with diets that are extremely high in fat—for example, the Inuit of the Arctic Circle and the Masai of East Africa—do not suffer from atherosclerosis or heart disease.

Mary Enig, Ph.D., and others have written very persuasively that the studies done in the 1950s that formed the basis of the lipid hypothesis were flawed. The original researchers failed to distinguish between the different kinds of fat. They concluded that all fat is bad without looking into what kinds of fat—saturated, monounsaturated, or polyunsaturated—the subjects of the study ate. Could it be that partially hydrogenated oil and increased carbohydrate consumption are behind the increase in heart disease? We certainly think so.

Dairy Products

Although hunter-gatherers did not eat dairy products, primitive nomads drank the milk of their cattle, goats, sheep, and even horses. Primitive people fermented milk products as a means of preserving them. Archeologists have found Sumerian tablets dating to six thousand years ago that explain how to ferment milk to prepare cheese.

Yogurt has been a food staple of the Middle East and Caucasian Mountains for many thousands of years.

The biggest differences between our milk and the milk that primitive people drank are due to our use of drugs and pasteurization. The nonorganic milk that most people drink comes from cows that are fed hormones and antibiotics. A century ago, a Holstein produced 400 to 500 pounds of milk annually. Today, the average Holstein produces 20,000 to 30,000 pounds! This high milk production is due to growth hormones. Some research, however, has shown that hormone-treated cows produce milk that is high in a protein called insulin-like growth factor 1 (IGF-1). This protein stimulates cell growth and has been associated with certain kinds of cancer, especially prostate cancer. Cows are often raised in close quarters and are therefore subject to infectious diseases. Due to excessive milking, their udders are usually excoriated and infected. For those reasons, cows are fed antibiotics.

Most people cannot conceive of drinking milk or taking any milk product unless it has been pasteurized. Pasteurization is named for Louis Pasteur, the French scientist who invented the process. In pasteurization, milk is heat-treated to destroy any disease-causing bacteria. Some argue that stainless steel tanks and other sanitizing innovations in the milk production industry have made pasteurization unnecessary. Here are some of the drawbacks of pasteurized milk:

- *Like antibiotics, pasteurization kills good as well as harmful bacteria.* Raw milk contains lactic-acid-producing bacteria. Lactic acid can kill certain pathogens and thereby prevent disease.
- *Pasteurization kills the enzymes in milk.* The lack of these enzymes makes milk harder to digest.
- *Pasteurization lowers the potency of some of the vitamins in milk, chiefly vitamins C and B_{12}.* It also makes calcium, magnesium, phosphorus, and sulfur less bioavailable.
- *The U.S. Government Accounting Office reports that 30 percent of commercial milk samples contain measurable levels of contaminants such as pesticides and antibiotic residues.* Pasteurization

does not rid milk of these contaminants from industrial milk production.

◆ *Pasteurization makes milk more difficult to digest.* The proteins become harder and more ball-like, making it more difficult for the necessary digestive enzymes to lock on to them and digest them.

Only California and Georgia permit raw, unpasteurized milk to be sold in markets, and raw milk is rare even in those states. You can, however, sometimes buy raw milk directly from dairies. Raw milk is delicious and has a consistency closer to cream than milk. Mixed with fruit, it makes a delicious desert. If you buy raw milk from a dairy, make sure the cows are fed on grass, are free of growth hormones and antibiotics, and have been tested for tuberculosis and brucellosis. Raw milk, by the way, is fresh milk. The pasteurized milk in grocery stores may be three to four weeks old. It goes from the dairy to a processor to a wholesaler and then to the retail grocery story where it is sold. Some cheeses, especially the imported ones, are made with raw milk. Look for "raw milk" on the label.

The Health Benefits of Fermented Dairy Products

The best dairy products are the lacto-fermented kind—yogurt, kefir, hard cheeses, cream cheese, cottage cheese, and cultured cream. People who normally can't consume dairy products because they are lactose-intolerant can oftentimes tolerate fermented dairy products because the enzyme lactase is found in those products. This enzyme is produced by the friendly bacteria found in fermented products. It can break down and digest lactose, the milk sugar found in dairy products. What's more, properly prepared fermented products should contain little or no residual lactose because the bacteria feeds on this sugar during the fermentation process. In its wake, the bacteria leave galactose, an easy-to-digest monosaccharide-type sugar.

Fermentation increases the vitamin B and C content of milk. Most importantly, fermentation is good for intestinal health. It supplies beneficial bacteria to the intestinal tract and produces lactic acid, a substance that aids the absorption of calcium, copper, iron, magnesium, and manganese. By acidifying the gut, which makes it easier for proteins to be absorbed in the small intestine, the *Lactobacillus* bacteria in fermented dairy products make minerals more bioavailable. Some *Lactobacillus acidophillus* strains in fermented dairy products produce natural antibiotics that are useful against infections. Chapter 5 explains in detail how fermented dairy products contribute to intestinal health.

Got Goat's Milk?

Goat's milk is the most widely consumed dairy beverage in the world. Fully 65 percent of the world's population drinks goat's milk. Goat's milk has been a staple in much of the world since Biblical times. For people with intestinal disorders, goat's milk and goat's-milk products have the potential to heal. Whereas cow's milk requires three hours to be absorbed, goat's milk requires only twenty minutes. At half the size of those in cow's milk, the protein molecules in goat's milk have thinner, more fragile membranes. For that reason, they are easier to absorb through the wall of the small intestine. Here are some of the other advantages of drinking goat's milk:

- *It is less allergic than cow's milk because it doesn't contain the protein complexes in cow's milk that stimulate allergic reactions.* Children who have allergic reactions to cow's milk have seen their allergies improve after switching to goat's milk.
- *It doesn't as readily produce gas or bloating.* Because goat's milk is digested quickly, it doesn't remain in the small intestine and ferment. It contains 7-percent less lactose than cow's milk.
- *It is high in the medium-chain fatty acids that inhibit candida.*
- *It is not mucus forming.*
- *It is a rich source of selenium.* This mineral is believed to be an immunoregulator. It quickens a sluggish immune system but quiets an overactive one. In this way, selenium keeps the immune system tuned and balanced.
- *It doesn't contain the Mycobacterium avium subspecies paratu-*

berculosis (MAP) microorganism. This microorganism is found in 22 percent of American cattle herds, according to a study by the National Animal Health Monitoring System. Some researchers believe that MAP causes Crohn's disease. In fact, one American gastroenterologist has found MAP in more than 90 percent of his patients with Crohn's disease. Pasteurization does not kill the MAP microorganism. Researchers have noted that Crohn's disease is on the rise in the cow's-milk-drinking areas of the world.

Fiber

Fiber, which is also known as roughage, is the indigestible remnants of plant cells in food. Fiber is made chiefly of plant cellulose, but may also contain hemicellulose, pectin, lignans, gums, and mucilages. Sources of fiber include vegetables, fruits, whole grains, and beans. Fiber is necessary for regular bowel movements. It prevents constipation. Fiber increases the elimination of waste matter in the large intestine and pressures the rectum muscles to loosen and expel waste. There are two kinds of fiber. Insoluble fiber cannot be broken down at all, whereas soluble fiber dissolves in water. Most fibrous foods contain both types of fiber. Insoluble fiber is believed to reduce the risk of colon cancer. Weight-loss programs recommend fiber because it gives people the feeling that they are filled up without contributing more calories to their diet.

Primitive people ate far more fiber than we do. Although Americans are constantly being reminded to eat more fiber, the average American eats approximately 8 grams per day. In 1850, the average American ate 20 to 30 grams daily, which happens to be what the National Cancer Institute recommends eating. In pioneering studies made in the 1970s, a British missionary surgeon named Dr. Dennis Burkitt observed that rural Africans who ate high-fiber diets had far less colon cancer than people in the West. They had almost no diabetes, constipation, or irritable bowel syndrome as well. Dr. Burkitt observed that Africans who ate a Western diet suffered from these diseases. He concluded that the Africans' high fiber intake accounted for their good intestinal health.

Dr. Burkitt's studies marked the beginning of "the fiber hypothesis," the idea that eating large amounts of fiber and decreasing fat intake can prevent colon cancer as well as diverticulosis, hemor-

❖

IS FROZEN FRUIT GOOD TO EAT?

The majority of the produce in grocery stores, even organic produce, is truck ripened. Instead of being allowed to ripen on the tree, vine, or ground, produce is picked several weeks before it is ripe and allowed to ripen while it is being transported to the grocery store. People who live in Florida and the other states where citrus fruit is grown often find themselves driving behind a truck loaded with what looks to be limes. Upon closer inspection, however, the limes turn out to be oranges that have been picked early so they can ripen on their way to the store. Fruits and vegetables are sometimes harvested early and then gas-ripened with ethylene, a by-product of kerosene combustion, to make them ripen faster. Another technique is to blanch vegetables by exposing them to short bursts of heat and submerging them in boiling water to break down the fiber and make it softer.

We believe that you should eat organic fruits and vegetables that have not been grown with pesticides or chemical fertilizers. What's more, you should eat fruits and vegetables that are in season, since these food items are less likely to have been truck-ripened, gas-ripened, blanched, or boiled. However, because eating organic fruits and vegetables in season is not always an option, we endorse eating frozen produce. This produce is harvested and frozen when it is fully ripe—in other words, when it is loaded with its maximum capacity of vitamins and minerals. While it is true that freezing destroys some of the enzymes in food, frozen produce often presents the best option for getting healthy organic produce in your diet. And in the case of berries and certain fruits, the difference between fresh and frozen food is minimal.

rhoids, and colonic polyps. For thirty years, the fiber hypothesis was considered the gospel truth, but the hypothesis has been refined in recent years. Fiber is a carbohydrate. Many people eager to improve their health by eating more fiber eat high-fiber, high-carbohydrate foods such as bran, fibrous breakfast cereals, whole wheat bread, brown rice, and potatoes. However, as this book points out time and time again, high-carbohydrate foods are a primary cause of intestinal disease. The mineral-blocking phytates mentioned earlier in this chapter are found in large amounts in the bran part of the grains, and this part happens to be the highest in fiber content. You could eat a loaf of whole wheat bread with the goal of improving your fiber intake, but you will really just get more carbohydrates than fiber.

The kind of fiber that promotes colon health is found in low-carbohydrate, high-fiber food. These foods include broccoli, cauliflower, soaked or sprouted seeds and nuts, carrots, celery, and lettuce. Fruits and vegetables with edible skins are especially high in fiber. Besides providing fiber, these foods are rich in vitamins and minerals. (For a discussion of frozen fruit, see page 93.) Mucilaginous fiber decreases transit time, the amount of time that food spends in the colon before it is expelled. A lowered transit time means that the food has less time to ferment or putrefy in the colon. Toxins are quickly flushed out. Mucilaginous fiber soothes inflamed tissue in the lining of the gut. It can be found in psyllium seeds, marshmallow root, slippery elm, chia seeds, and flaxseeds.

Unfortunately, many people with gut disorders have a hard time with fiber, particularly insoluble fiber. Usually, cooking, juicing, pureeing, or fermenting vegetables and fruits is necessary before they can be eaten. We recommend going to the extra trouble to prepare vegetables. They are the best source of fiber.

Condiments

Go into most restaurants and you will see a selection of condiments—salt, pepper, ketchup, and mustard—on the table. Most people keep a small supply in their pantry or refrigerator. Condiments have been a part of the human diet for many centuries, but their purpose has been lost in modern times. Originally, condiments were digestive aids. They were meant to be taken in small amounts with a meal to encourage proper digestion. Unlike the condiments of today, almost all of the original condiments were fermented. This is because the lactic acid produced by fermentation helps digestion and improves intestinal health.

The next time you dress up your hot dog at the ballpark, consider the pedigree of ketchup. From the Chinese *ke-tsiap*, ketchup started out as a fermented fish-brine sauce. Sailors brought it from China to England, where the locals added pickled cucumbers, kidney beans, and oysters to the mix. New Englanders made tomatoes the chief feature of ketchup in the late 1700s. Today's ketchup is loaded with sugar and corn syrup, and is no longer fermented.

Lacto-fermentation is difficult to achieve on an industrial scale. For that reason, the makers of modern condiments use vinegar in the brine. This makes the condiments more acidic. Worse, many condiments are pasteurized. Pasteurization kills the beneficial lactic acid in condiments. Condiments have ceased to be aids to digestion. They are used to dress up prepared food and give it a little more tang. Ironically, dieticians recommend cutting back on condiments, the foods that people ate originally to promote good health

Most people put more salt on their food than any other condiment. Salt is one of the oldest food additives. Even people who lived far from the ocean obtained salt by burning sodium-rich grasses and mixing the ash into their food. Although some have argued that salt raises the blood pressure, this controversial idea is still open to debate. Salt provides chloride for the manufacturing of hydrochloric acid, the stomach acid that breaks down food. It stimulates salivation. It is an enzyme activator. And of course, it makes food taste better.

Conventional table salt like the kind you buy in most stores is processed. Aluminum compounds are added to keep the salt dry. The trace minerals and iodine salts that occur naturally in sea salt are removed during processing. To make the salt a pristine white, it is exposed to bleaching agents.

We recommend a natural, unrefined salt called Celtic sea salt. This light-gray salt comes from Brittany in France, where it is gathered in clay-lined ponds as part of a two-thousand-year-old tradition. Celtic sea salt is high in organic iodine from plants and the tiny skeletons of ancient marine life. It includes many trace minerals, including sodium chloride and magnesium salts. (To purchase Celtic sea salt, see "Resources" on page 333.)

Enzymes

Enzymes are proteins that act as catalysts for chemical reactions in the body. They are the labor force of the body. They speed up the rate of chemical reactions. They initiate chemical reactions but are not themselves changed by those reactions. Enzymes take the food we eat and turn it into chemical structures that are able to pass through the cell membranes of the small intestine and into the bloodstream. Enzymes are found in all living organisms.

Raw food contains enzymes that assist with digestion. As soon as you put raw food in your mouth, the enzymes begin digesting it, and they continue to do so in the cardia (upper) portion of the stomach after the food is swallowed. These digestive enzymes—*proteases* to digest protein, *amylases* to digest carbohydrates, and *lipases* to digest fat—break down food so it can be absorbed in the small intestine.

Our primitive ancestors knew the value of raw food to digestion. Not only did primitive people eat raw fruits and vegetables, they ate raw meat. The Inuit, for example, ate raw fat from seals, whale blubber, and raw fish. These foods contain an abundance of the enzyme lipase. (The Inuit were formerly known as the Eskimo, a derogatory term from the Cree language that means "he eats it raw.") Some Pygmies devouring the decomposing carcass of a dead elephant in equatorial Africa, when asked how they tolerated such unsavory food, replied that they were eating the meat of the elephant, not its odor. Does eating raw meat seem repulsive to you? In genteel Victorian London, physicians prescribed sandwiches made from raw thyroid glands to help rejuvenate aging patients.

Prolonged heat over 118 degrees Fahrenheit kills all enzymes. Therefore, cooking destroys the digestive enzymes in raw food. Heat processing also destroys enzymes, as does pasteurization. Since as most people eat cooked food, processed food, or pasteurized food, the modern diet is empty of vital enzymes. Raw food, you could say, is alive. Unless you make a point of eating more raw food, you lose the benefits of live food and its digestive enzymes.

In his classic *Enzyme Nutrition* (Avery Publishing Group, 1985), Dr. Edward Howell proposed the idea that everyone is born with a finite store of enzymes. Enzymes, he noted, fall into three classes: metabolic enzymes that direct body functions; digestive enzymes secreted by the pancreas that help digest food; and enzymes found in raw food that assist with digestion. Two of these classes are found in the body. Dr. Howell believed that eating too much cooked food depletes the body's store of finite enzymes. To digest cooked food, the body must draw upon its own enzymes, and that leaves fewer enzymes for other functions—for operating the brain, muscles, organs, and tissues. Dr. Howell believed in eating raw food to keep the body's store of enzymes from being depleted. He wrote:

> A certain amount of raw, uncooked food in the diet is indispensable to the highest degree of health. Assuming that the proteins, fats, carbohydrates, minerals, and vitamins are equally available for nutrition in raw and cooked food, any demonstrable nutritional superiority of raw food must then be ascribed to the "live" quality of raw food, and when this live quality is subjected to analysis, it is shown to consist of . . . no other property than that possessed by enzymes.

The enzymes in fruits and vegetables fully develop when the fruits and vegetables are ripe. A ripe banana, for example, has far more digestive enzymes than a green banana. For this reason, you should try to eat ripe fruits and vegetables that have not been truck-ripened or gas-ripened. What's more, some seeds and nuts contain enzymes inhibitors. These substances prevent seeds and nuts from sprouting until they are nestled deeply enough in the soil. Enzyme inhibitors serve an important role in nature, but they also make the enzymes in fruits and nuts unavailable. You can, however, free the enzymes in seeds and nuts by soaking them before eating.

Besides obtaining digestive enzymes from raw food, you can get them from health supplements. In our experience, digestive enzyme supplements have helped patients with gastrointestinal disorders immensely. The supplements aid digestion and also reduce inflammation in the colon.

Fermented Vegetables and Fruits

Primitive people knew the value of fermented food. They fermented vegetables and milk not only to preserve those items, but to take advantage of the health benefits of fermentation. As explained earlier, our ancient ancestors consumed yogurt and kefir. They seemed to know instinctively that foods cultured with lactic-acid microorganisms strengthen the helpful flora in the gut and promote intestinal health. Fermented vegetables and fruits have the same effect.

Fermented vegetables and fruits are some of the oldest foods on the planet. The Romans ate sauerkraut, a dish made from fermented cabbage. Sauerkraut, which contains vitamin C, was valued by the English navy as a means of preventing scurvy. It was kept in barrels aboard ship. In Asia, fermented soybean products—miso, natto, tamari, and shoyu—have been consumed for centuries. The Indians eat various chutneys made from fermented fruit. In nearly every culture, fermented food is part of the diet, usually in the form of a condiment or side dish to be eaten along with the meal. Lacto-fermented beverages also have a long history. Wine, beer, ginger beer, kvass (a beverage made in Russia from stale rye bread), tea and vinegar concoctions, and pulque (an alcoholic beverage made in Mexico from fermented sap) are examples of lacto-fermented beverages.

The lactobacilli in fermented vegetables and fruits contain digestive enzymes that help break down food. Lactobacilli make the vitamins in food more potent and increase the digestibility of food. By acidifying the gut, they make proteins and minerals more bioavailable. Natural, lactic-acid-fermented drinks contain small amounts of sugar and healthy minerals in ionized form. These drinks are thirst-quenching. Research indicates that they are absorbed faster than water. In traditional societies, these mildly alcoholic beverages are consumed in the field to keep thirst at bay.

Stocks, Broths, and Gelatin

Unfortunately for our health, stocks, broths, and gelatins, which require several hours of careful simmering, are no longer an important part of the modern diet. People believe they are too busy to makes these foods, yet these are some of the most nutritious foods you can eat. "Good broth resurrects the dead," according to a South American proverb. Stocks, broths, and gelatins are folk remedies for colds and the flu in almost every culture.

Stocks, broths, and gelatin are especially beneficial for people who have intestinal diseases because they are very high in nutrients and the gastrointestinal tract can absorb them without having to do a lot of work. Gelatin, the odorless, tasteless substance extracted by boiling bones, animal tissues, and hoofs, is especially easy to digest. Broth from meat and animal bones is an excellent source of many important minerals, including iodine, chloride, sodium, magnesium, and potassium. Iodine is especially plentiful in stock made from fish bones and heads.

Dr. Francis Pottenger believed that stocks, broths, and gelatin are easy to digest because they contain hydrophilic colloids. Colloids are large molecules. Hydrophilic means "water loving." Normally, the colloids in cooked food are the opposite of hydrophilic—they are hydrophobic. They don't attract liquids. But stocks, broths, and gelatins, although they have been cooked, attract digestive liquids. This explains why they are easier to digest than other cooked food.

Beverages

The modern diet is insufficient in water, and the beverages that are in the diet are often more harmful than healthy. In most cases, our primitive ancestors were able to obtain drinking water straight from the source—from a river, creek, or spring. Natural water is extremely healthy. This water is mineral-rich and "structured"—that is, the water has a strong electrical charge and low surface tension. It is not as dense as conventional tap water. No one knows precisely why people in some cultures live on average longer than others, but many attribute longevity to healthy drinking water. For sources of structured drinking water, also known as clustered water, see "Resources" on page 348.

Soda pop is marketed aggressively to the young. Soda pop has been rightfully called a "sweet poison." The ubiquitous vending machine that sells soda pop can even be found in schools. In a year 2000 study conducted at the University of Saskatchewan, researchers found that girls in their early teens who often drink soda pop have an increased risk of fractures and osteoporosis. The culprit is probably the phosphoric acid in soda pop, which impedes the absorption of magnesium and calcium. Soda pop represents yet another inroad made by sugar into the American diet. It is often blamed for the increase in obesity among children. Americans drink twice the amount of soda pop as they did twenty-five years ago.

To avoid the calories imparted by sugar, many pop drinkers are turning to sugar-free beverages. However, aspartame, the artificial sweetener found in most sugar-free soda pop brands, may be worse than sugar. Aspartame has been implicated in seizures, depression, and neurological disorders such as dizziness and muscle aches. It may also cause weight gain. In an American Cancer Society study of 78,000 women, those who consumed artificially sweetened foods gained more weight over a one-year period than those who consumed sugar-sweetened products. The researchers speculated that the sugar substitutes may have stimulated the women's appetites and encouraged them to eat more.

The other beverage that has gained in popularity in recent years is coffee. This substance injures the stomach and esophagus. It relaxes the sphincter muscle that controls the passage of food from the esophagus to the stomach and may permit hydrochloric acid from the stomach to splash into the esophagus and cause heartburn. On account of its caffeine content, coffee can tax the adrenal glands and can lead to adrenal gland exhaustion, a condition in which the adrenal glands fail to release adrenaline. Some believe that adrenal gland exhaustion weakens the immune system and makes the body more susceptible to disease and infection.

Concentrated fruit juices and sports drinks are also better avoided. They contain copious amounts of sugar. These drinks present all the problems that a diet high in sugar presents. They cause a sudden surge of blood sugar that disrupts hormonal functions and can contribute to diabetes and other health problems.

Almost as important as what to drink is when to drink. We think you should avoid drinking liquids with meals because the fluid may dilute the digestive enzymes. Drink between meals instead. Avoid ice-cold beverages as well. Traditional societies simply did not drink ice-cold beverages. The body must use enzymes to raise the temperature of an ice-cold beverage before it can absorb it. Ice-cold drinks may shock the system and temporarily shut down digestion. In Asian cultures, cold drinks are almost never consumed.

❖ 4 ❖

The Primitive Lifestyle

This chapter picks up where Chapter 3 left off, only instead of explaining how we can learn from the diet and eating habits of our primitive ancestors, this chapter explains how we can learn from the way they lived. In many respects, primitive humans lived much healthier lives than we do. Their environment was cleaner. They spent more time outdoors. They led more vigorous lives. In this chapter, we look at the lifestyle techniques of primitive people that we can put to use in modern times for the benefit of our health.

Exercise

Primitive hunter-gatherers had no conception of exercise. The idea of going for a jog around the lake or along the beach was unknown to them. They didn't have time to exercise because they were too busy moving around. Their very survival depended on hunting and foraging. By contrast, we live in the most sedentary time in human history. The farm has been mechanized and machines such as leaf blowers have taken the sting out of manual labor. Our bodies, however, were made for vigorous activity, which in our day means exercise.

The notion that you should exercise for health dates back to the time of Hippocrates in 400 B.C. Exercising tones the muscles and improves cardiovascular function. It increases your stamina and gives you a feeling of well-being. It is one of the best ways to alleviate stress. Exercise is even an effective antidepressant. Recent studies have demonstrated that moderate exercise is equivalent to drug therapy in the treatment of mild to moderate depression.

Exercising also stimulates peristalsis, the rhythmic expanding and contracting of the intestinal walls that forces evacuation. Improper diet is usually cited as the cause of constipation, but a sedentary lifestyle can also be a major contributing factor. The intestinal tract is similar to a long muscle in the way it pushes everything downward. Exercising tones and strengthens this muscle. It makes the intestinal tract stronger. Exercising also helps prevent hemorrhoids. Sitting for long periods of time can swell and stretch the blood vessels around the anus, causing hemorrhoids, but exercising gets you off the couch and increases the flow of blood.

Remember if you are new to exercising to start gradually and pick up the pace over a period of weeks. Even professional athletes start slow when they are recovering from an injury or starting a new season. Understandably, most people who are extremely ill cannot exercise. If you are ill, start with short outdoor walks. Staying indoors not only contributes to the weakening of muscles and their atrophy, but keeps you from getting the sunshine and fresh air you need for health. Set exercise goals for yourself—small ones at first and more ambitious ones later. Eventually you will feel stronger and happier.

Mental Health

The digestive system seems to register emotional states, especially stress, more acutely than any other part of the body. You can have butterflies in your stomach, for example. Stress alters nerve impulses and hormone signals. Heartburn, constipation, ulcers, and irritable bowel syndrome have all been associated with stress.

Keeping a good mental outlook is often easier said than done, of course. Sometimes climbing out of the doldrums seems impossible. But good mental health almost always accompanies good physical health. Coauthor Jordan Rubin credits his recovery from Crohn's disease to his persistent faith. Even in his darkest hour, Jordan believed that his health would one day be restored. Keeping a positive outlook and believing in your heart that an answer to your health problem exists are crucial.

Chewing Slowly

Digestion starts with chewing. As you chew, saliva enters your mouth and digestive enzymes such as amylase in the saliva start to break down the carbohydrates in the food. Meanwhile, the movement of your jaw causes the parotid glands behind your ears to send a signal to the thymus gland to produce T-cells. These white blood cells fight infection. They are produced as a precaution in case the food you are chewing contains toxins or pathogens. As you chew, you increase the surface area of the food. If you chew the food carefully and thoroughly, it arrives, not in chunks, but in liquid form in your stomach.

The need to chew food thoroughly seems hardly worth explaining, but the number of people who do not chew their food adequately is surprising. People eat while they drive their cars. They eat standing up. They inhale their food and wash it down with juice or coffee. Food eaten these ways, especially if it contains fiber or carbohydrates, is much more difficult to digest. Inadequate chewing may contribute to intestinal disease. Coauthor Jordan Rubin believes that years of "scarfing down" his food contributed to his development of Crohn's disease. Besides giving you an opportunity to savor your food, eating slowly and carefully is a good method of losing weight. In a study of the chewing habits of obese people, it was discovered that the obese take smaller bites of food but chew fewer times than nonobese people.

Slow eaters feel full and satisfied without overeating. There appears to be a lag time between the stomach's recognition and the brain's recognition that you have had enough to eat. The brain, it appears, gets the message to stop eating after the stomach. Eating slowly allows the two organs to be in better synch with each other.

In other words, eating slowly permits the brain to understand when the stomach is full. Just by eating slowly, you can control your weight and cure many mild gastrointestinal maladies as well.

Here are the golden rules of chewing and eating:

◆ Chew each bite between twenty-five and a hundred times.
◆ Always sit down when eating.
◆ Do not eat when you are angry or upset. Doing so obstructs digestion.
◆ Do not eat while you are working or in the middle of another activity that requires your concentration. (If you are eating while reading this book, please put down the book and enjoy your food. We'll be here for you later!) Eating should be a leisurely activity.

Chewing thoroughly was a fad at the turn of the last century. The fad was started by a New England Yankee named Horace Fletcher, who believed that thorough chewing was the key to good health and longevity. "Nature will castigate those who don't masticate," he warned. Followers of Fletcherism (as it was known) included John D. Rockefeller, Upton Sinclair, and Henry James. Fletcher believed in chewing each bite thirty-two times, once for each tooth.

Our primitive ancestors probably ate their food slowly. They had a spiritual relationship with food and probably savored it for that reason. In many primitive cultures, animals are believed to have spirits, and eating an animal means consuming its spirit as well as its body. For this reason, eating may have been a slow, slightly solemn occasion. Some primitive cultures believe that sharing a meal forges a bond between people because the diners eat the spirit of the same animal. Something of this belief has come down to us and can be seen in the sharing of food on Thanksgiving and other feast days.

Proper Bowel Alignment

Primitive people squatted to relieve themselves. This custom is still followed in much of the world today. Infants adopt the squatting posture instinctively. Although squatting is uncomfortable for the average person, it aligns the colon properly for elimination and empties the colon more completely. At the end of the rectum is a 90-degree bend known as the anorectal angle that is designed to prevent incontinence. In the squatting position, the 90-degree bend is straightened out and elimination is more complete. Squatting also relieves some of the straining that can cause hemorrhoids.

Simply bending at the waist while you are sitting on the toilet does not provide the benefits of squatting. To adopt the Western toilet to squatting, several companies offer elimination benches that fit around the toilet. To obtain one of these benches, see "Resources" on page 350.

Sleeping Habits

Before electricity and electric lighting, before kerosene lamps and tallow candles, people went to sleep at sunset and awoke at dawn. Nature imposed a healthy sleeping regimen on primitive people. The amount of sleep people get on average has dropped over the past century. In 1910, when the majority of Americans still lived on farms, the average person slept for nine hours each night. Since then, factory regimentation and nine-to-five job schedules have disrupted people's sleeping habits, and people in industrialized countries now sleep an average of 7.5 hours per night.

How much sleep you need depends on a number of factors, including your gender, the speed of your body metabolism, the quality of the sleep you get, and your age. Newborns require twenty hours of sleep and the elderly only six or seven hours. What goes on in the body during sleep is still rather mysterious, but researchers agree that getting enough sleep is essential for optimum health. Lack of a good night's sleep impairs the nervous system, clouds memory, encumbers physical performance, and makes concentrating more difficult. According to the U.S. National Highway Safety Administration, drowsiness at the wheel now causes more automobile accidents than alcohol. Current research has even linked sleep deprivation to impaired sugar control, a weakened immune system, and an increased risk of developing cancer.

Some researchers believe that each hour of sleep you get before midnight is worth two or more hours of sleep after midnight. These researchers believe that the body's Circadian rhythms are attuned to sunlight. When the sun sets, drowsiness follows because the body wants you to sleep. Benjamin Franklin was right, these researchers believe. Early to bed and early to rise, makes a man healthy, wealthy, and wise.

Short Fasts

Primitive people did not eat three square meals a day. The notion of eating breakfast, lunch, and dinner at the same time each day was foreign to them. They would go five, six, or seven hours without food. Short fasts are healthy because they make the body draw upon its glycogen reserves. They also make the body more sensitive to insulin. When you eat food, especially carbohydrates, insulin in your body converts glucose—that is, blood sugar—to glycogen and stores the glycogen in the liver and in the muscle. Excess sugar is also turned into triglycerides, which are eventually stored as fat in the fat cells. Glycogen and fat are preserved energy. When you fast, your body cannot get energy from food, so it initially releases its glycogen reserves and subsequently releases its fat. While you fast, the pancreas gets a rest because it doesn't have to produce the digestive enzymes or insulin needed to process foods and ultimately control blood sugar. Short fasts prevent obesity because they make you leaner. They also give the body a much needed respite from the digestive process. Studies done on Islamic people observing the holy month of Ramadan, who fast during daylight and gorge themselves with a large evening meal, have shown that the blood lipids (cholesterol and triglycerides) are improved during the fasting period.

Psychologically, short fasts reacquaint you with hunger. Hunger is the body's signal to eat, yet most people don't experience this very basic sensation because they eat throughout the day and are always sated. Short fasts put you in touch with your body's craving for food and help you understand when it is truly necessary to eat. We don't recommend fasts that last longer than eighteen hours a day, but eating during only a six-hour period each day is a great way to enhance digestion and regeneration.

Proper Breathing

As anyone who has taken singing lessons knows, most people don't breathe correctly. They don't breathe with their abdomen, but rather with their chest, taking short, shallow breaths. The proper breathing technique is to gently push out your abdomen while inhaling through your nose. Inhale slowly until your lungs fill with air and then slowly exhale. This way, you breathe into the bottom of your lungs. If you see your chest, not your abdomen, rising and falling as you breathe, you are breathing incorrectly. Sometimes proper breathing is called "belly breathing" because it causes the abdomen to rise and fall. Infants are belly breathers. We learn to breathe incorrectly when we are told to "puff out your chest and look sharp." If you want a lesson in how to breathe correctly, watch an infant breathe.

Proper breathing relieves stress and lowers the blood pressure. It delivers life-giving oxygen to the seven trillion cells in the body. Through a chemical process called oxidation, it permits the body to eliminate toxins and to convert nutrients to energy. You cannot breathe correctly if your clothes are too tight. You may have to loosen your belt or wear more comfortable clothes to breathe properly. Try setting aside five or ten minutes a day to practice deep breathing. Take a slow, deep breath through your nose as you count to 5, and then quickly exhale through your mouth. Repeat this for five to ten minutes. You may feel light-headed because you are increasing your intake of oxygen.

Dry Heat Baths

Many cultures use a dry heat bath of some kind. The sweat lodge was an institution among some Native American tribes. As well as bathing in their *bania*, the Russians held wedding services and child-births there. The best-known dry heat bath, the sauna, originated in Finland. Most Roman bath houses included a sauna. When the Roman Empire receded, the Arabs modified the Roman bath house and created a smaller dry heat bath called the *hammam* (the word means "spreader of warmth" in Arabic). Mohammed enthusiastically supported the *hammam*. Some mosques included a *hammam* to help the faithful comply with the Islamic laws of hygiene. In 1850, the travel writer David Urquart extolled the *hammam* in his *The Pillars of Hercules*. Urquart coined the term "Turkish bath" to describe the *hammam*. Thanks to Urquart's book, the Turkish bath enjoyed a huge surge in popularity in England and Germany in the nineteenth century. Mail order houses and traveling salesman in America and England sold what they called "Turkish baths for the home" (they were actually small steam cabinets that could be tucked in a corner). Technology has made it possible to build a sauna into a residential home fairly inexpensively. For sources of these at-home saunas, see "Resources" on page 350.

Sweating provides the health benefits of a fever without the fever itself. The body kills pathogens and cancer cells when its temperature is raised. The average person emits a quart of sweat during fifteen minutes in a sauna. Sweating clears out fat-soluble toxins, heavy metals, pesticides, and herbicides. Dry heat is an excellent way to relieve stress.

In traditional cultures, dry heat baths have a spiritual element. *Loyly*, the Finnish word for the steam that is released when water is poured onto the sauna rocks, means "spirit." The sweat lodge was and still is a means of spiritual cleansing for Native Americans. For primitive hunters, the sweat lodge had an added benefit—it sweated out the hunter's body odor and made it possible for him to sneak up on his prey without being detected.

Hydrotherapies

Hydrotherapy is the use of water for the treatment of disease and the promotion of well-being. Hydrotherapies include hot-water and cold-water baths, clay baths, bathing with essential oils, bathing in mineral springs, mud wraps, seaweed wraps, whirlpools, Jacuzzis, sitz baths, and compresses. Most hydrotherapies fall into the "folk medicine" category. According to their practitioners, they work either by relaxing the body, in the case of warm baths, or by invigorating it, in the case of cold ones. The hot and cold water are supposed to shock the immune system and make it hardier. Whatever the merits of hydrotherapy really are, everyone agrees that bathing is a relaxing activity. The ancient Greeks advocated bathing for health. In nineteenth-century Europe, popular mineral spas where visitors could "take the waters" sprang up across Germany and France. In our time the hot tub, a kind of mini-spa, has become a feature of some suburban homes.

Light

Most of the vitamin D you obtain comes from sunlight. It is synthesized by your skin when you are exposed to the sun. Vitamin D encourages calcium absorption, and calcium, in turn, makes for stronger bones and teeth. For this reason, we believe that you should expose yourself to the sun for twenty minutes a day. If your follow the Guts and Glory Program, you will get the fat-soluble vitamins A and D and sunburn will not be a problem. Vitamins A and D regenerate tissue and prevent sunburn. The ability to synthesize vitamin D diminishes as you grow older. For that reason, people older than fifty need to spend more time in the sun, especially if they live in the northern climates, which get less sunlight.

Some researchers believe that full-spectrum indoor lighting is necessary for good health. Photobiologist John Nash Ott coined the term "malillumination" to describe what happens to your health when you are exposed to fluorescent lighting or other lighting that doesn't emanate a full spectrum of color. As malnutrition describes the effects of an improper diet, malillumination describes what happens to your health when you live and work under lighting that does not emanate a full spectrum of color. According to Ott, headaches, eyestrain, depression, and diseases such as cancer and arthritis can be attributed to poor lighting. Ott's controversial theories credit the rise in cancer and other diseases to a lack of time spent outdoors. About 90 percent of people work indoors. No one denies that seasonal affective disorder (SAD) is caused by a lack of sunlight. Five million Americans suffer from this malady, according to the National Institutes of Health. For sources of full-spectrum lighting that you can use in your home, see "Resources" on page 350.

On a side note, John Nash Ott has a small place in baseball history. He was responsible for changing the color of the underside of the visors on the caps that the players wear. In the early 1970s, Ott suggested to a Cincinnati Reds scout that the players would be able to see the ball better if the undersides of their cap visors were gray instead of green. The Reds took his suggestion and won the National League pennant. Soon most Major League baseball teams made the switch from green to gray.

Air Quality

Primitive people did not have the problems with air pollution that we have. These problems are well documented. Diesel fuel, nitrogen oxide, and sulfur dioxide particulates—the "fine particulate matter" that causes air pollution—cloud the air above many cities. In a study conducted by the New York School of Medicine, researchers determined that lung cancer death rates in cities increase by 8 percent for every increase of 10 micrograms of fine particulate matter per cubic meter. In other words, there is a direct correlation between air pollution and lung cancer.

Less studied than the air quality above cities is the air quality indoors. To preserve energy, buildings are better insulated than ever before, but this has a downside in that fresh air cannot penetrate the buildings as easily. Breathing lifeless, recirculated air, especially the kind found in large office buildings, is not good for your health. Primitive people spent most of their time outdoors, which greatly enhances health. Volatile organic chemicals from office equipment, building materials, carpeting, and paint, as well as molds circulating in buildings' ventilation and heating systems, have been known to cause headaches, dizziness, and in some cases damage to nerves. If you can, open a window to let in the fresh air, and sleep with a window open as well. Keeping green plants indoors is another great way to improve air quality. For commercially available air filters that are designed to improve the quality of indoor air, see "Resources" on page 350.

Water Quality

Primitive people drank vibrant, mineral-rich water straight from the source—from a river, creek, or spring. The water had a strong electric charge and low surface tension. It was thinner and livelier than conventional tap water. Some researchers have suggested that the quality of drinking water more so than any other factor is the reason why people in some cultures live on average to a very old age. For sources of structured drinking water, the water that is similar to what primitive people drank, see "Resources" on page 348.

One way to ensure that the water you drink is healthy is to avoid chlorinated water. Water is chlorinated to kill microorganisms, but the chlorine also kills the healthy probiotic bacteria in the intestines. (Chapter 5 explains why this bacteria is so important to good health.) Chlorine also destroys the natural acidity of the skin, which is the first barrier against disease. For all these reasons, you should avoid drinking, bathing in, and swimming in chlorinated water.

Clothing

Primitive people did not have the tailoring skills to make tight clothing and they were better off because of it. Tight clothing isn't good for your health. It impairs breathing and movement. Tight clothing, belts, and waistbands can cause heartburn. They put pressure on the stomach and can force stomach acid into the esophagus. Loose clothing permits the body to breath and perspiration to evaporate. If perspiration doesn't evaporate, bacteria on the skin can invade the perspiration and cause offensive body odors, especially in the underarms, in the groin, and on the feet.

Natural fabrics permit the body to breath better than synthetic fabrics. They absorb twice as much moisture. Natural fabrics are easier to clean, which means you don't have to resort to phosphate detergents to wash them. Cotton, wool, cashmere, silk, and linen are natural fabrics. Synthetic fabrics include acetate, acrylic, nylon, polyester, rayon, and spandex. Most of these fabrics are derivatives of petroleum products. They do not breathe, which makes them cold in the winter and hot in the summer. Wrinkle-free and permanent-press fabrics are chemically treated with formaldehyde resins and can cause allergic reactions.

Electromagnetic Influences

Electromagnetic fields are all around us. Electric substations, transformers, power lines, fluorescent lights, microwave ovens, computers, cell phones, and wiring in the home all create electromagnetic fields. Unfortunately, no comprehensive studies about electromagnetic influences have been published and some people are quite shrill on the subject of the harm they allegedly cause. No one really knows what the long-term effects of exposure to electromagnetic fields are. We are in the midst of a vast experiment on the effects of electromagnetism on human health.

Some have suggested that electromagnetic fields interfere with cell growth and brain waves, suppress the production of melatonin, trigger childhood leukemia, and cause multiple sclerosis. The good news is you can reduce your exposure to electromagnetic fields by making sure the buildings in which you live and work are properly wired. In a 1996 study by the Canada Mortgage and Housing Corporation, researchers found that 90 percent of exposure to electromagnetic fields resulted from faulty wiring in homes and offices. Powerlines and electrical devices accounted for a mere 10 percent.

One school of thought says that direct physical contact with the Earth—being "grounded"—is necessary for good health. This school says that the body stores harmful static electricity and currents from electromagnetic fields because the body is insulated from contact with the ground. Physical contact with the ground, however, dispels the stored electricity much as a ground wire carries away excessive electrical current. For a grounding device that may replicate walking on the Earth with bare feet, see "Resources" on page 351.

Chemicals

Our world is awash in chemicals. Deodorants and makeup, hair coloring products, air fresheners, household cleaners, and detergents all contain chemicals that are potentially harmful. The skin is good at absorbing these chemicals. To give you an idea how absorptive the skin is, you can step on a garlic clove in bare feet and smell garlic on your breath within two minutes. Finding safe alternatives to chemical-laden products is necessary for good health, especially in light of the fact that most people don't sweat enough or wear clothes that breathe properly. Chemically safe products are also good for the environment.

We recommend reading *The Safe Shopper's Bible* by Dr. Samuel Epstein and David Steinman (John Wiley and Sons, 1995). It offers advice for obtaining household, cosmetic, and other products that are chemically safe.

Cooking with the Proper Utensils

Aluminum cookware is popular because it is inexpensive and it conducts heat well. However, the aluminum can leach into food while the food is being cooked. If you cook with aluminum pots and pans, you run the risk of getting aluminum in your food, and aluminum has been implicated in Alzheimer's disease. Stainless steel and cast iron are preferable to aluminum cookware. Avoid Teflon because the coating tends to flake and may come off in food.

In a microwave oven, the water molecules in food are vibrated forcefully. This creates friction between the molecules and heats the food from the inside out. In the process, the molecules are deformed into radiolytic compounds. Cooking also creates these compounds, but on a smaller scale. In Switzerland, researchers conducted experiments to see what effect eating microwaved food has on the blood. They discovered a decrease in white blood cells and hemoglobin, the material that delivers oxygen to the body tissues. Until more is known about microwave cooking, we recommend cooking the conventional way.

❖ 5 ❖

The Jungle in Your Gut

D on't look now, but one hundred trillion bacteria and other microorganisms are currently living in your intestinal tract. In fact, there are more bacterial cells in your gut than there are cells in your entire body. The total weight of this microbial zoo is estimated to be three to five pounds! Your gut is a jungle where good, bad, and indifferent bacteria and microbes fight it out. "Jungle in Your Gut"—it sounds like the title of a B movie, but the bacteria and microbes that live in your gut are essential to your health and well-being. They help the immune system. They increase or decrease your risk of being infected by disease. They synthesize valuable nutrients, including essential B vitamins. Beneficial microorganisms in your gut also play a major role in the digestion of food.

This chapter explains how the microorganisms in the gut function. It describes the health benefits of friendly microbes and explains how you can increase the amount of friendly microbes in your gut with fermented foods and probiotic supplements. This chapter looks at ways in which these microscopic friends aid the immune system. Finally, Chapter 5 goes beyond probiotics and describes homeostatic soil organisms (HSOs), a special kind of probiotic that is obtained from the soil.

The Bacteria and Microbes in Your Gut

To most people, "bacteria" and "disease" are synonymous terms. But some of the bacteria that live in the intestinal tract are very good for you. As the saying goes, "The enemy of my enemy is my friend." Friendly bacteria in the gut—also known as intestinal flora, probiotic bacteria, or simply probiotics—keep harmful bacteria in check. (These days, the term "probiotics" usually refers to whole foods or supplements that strengthen the intestinal flora.) Inside the colon and small intestine, a turf war is raging, with each kind of bacteria striving to colonize the intestinal walls. And this war is a good one. Because the bacteria have to compete with one another, no single bacteria can gain the upper hand and wreak havoc—at least in a healthy intestinal tract.

Intestinal flora are the beneficial bacteria that keep salmonella, giardia, *Helicobacter pylori,* and other disease-causing microorganisms and parasites from proliferating on the intestinal walls. Many pathogenic microorganisms must attach themselves to the lining of the intestinal tract to cause disease. Intestinal flora occupy space on the intestinal walls and thereby prevent the absorption of these pathogens into the bloodstream. The intestinal flora secrete acids (acetic, formic, and lactic acids), hydrogen peroxide, and natural antibiotics that exclude harmful bacteria from the colon and send them scurrying down the intestinal tract, where they are eventually expelled in the feces. Feces are composed of two-thirds indigestible plant fiber and one-third live and dead bacteria that have been expelled. Intestinal flora help maintain a clean, well-balanced intestinal environment where pathogens don't have room to flourish.

How do the bacteria get into our intestines? A fetus, which obtains all its nourishment from its mother, has a sterile intestinal tract. However, bacterial microbes start colonizing the body from the moment the fetus begins its journey through the birth canal. Soon more bacteria are introduced via the breast milk and formula. Bacteria enter the intestinal tract in the air we breathe and the food we eat. Besides the intestinal tract, bacteria colonize the skin, mouth, throat, and vaginal mucosa of women. We ingest and expel a few ounces of bacteria every day.

From 400 to 500 different types of bacteria live in the colon and the ileum, the lower portion of the small intestine. That number of bacteria may seem overwhelming, but 20 species make up three-quarters of the total. The most prominent bacterial species in the colon are *Bacteroides, Bifidobacteria, Pepto streptococcus, Fusobacteria, Rheumanococcus, Lactobacillus, Clostridia,* and *Escherichia coli,* better known as *E. coli.* Do any of these names ring a bell? *Lactobacillus* is the bacteria that is used to culture milk and create yogurt. Most people know *E. coli* as the bacterium that causes severe food poisoning and sometimes death. However, *E. coli* represents a whole family of bacteria. Only a few wayward members can cause severe intestinal disease in humans.

Enemies of Intestinal Flora

Later in this chapter, we describe the foods you can eat and the supplements you can take to strengthen the intestinal flora. Meanwhile, you should know about the enemies of the intestinal flora. Antibiotics, some drugs, and oral contraceptives take their toll on the intestinal flora. Diet has an effect as well. Stress can also be a factor. Here is a list of enemies of the intestinal flora:

- ◆ *Antibiotics.* Antibiotics cause most of the bacteria in the intestines—good, bad, and indifferent—to die off. That leaves room for powerful antibiotic-resistant bacteria, yeast, and fungi to seize new ground in the gut and proliferate.
- ◆ *Antacids and acid-blocking medications.* Hydrochloric acid destroys the harmful bacteria in the stomach and keeps it from reaching the intestines. Antacids, however, neutralize hydrochloric acid. This permits harmful bacteria to pass through the stomach to the intestines.
- ◆ *Laxatives.* Peristaltic action, the rhythmic contraction of the intestinal walls, expels harmful bacteria in the feces. The continual use of laxatives can slow peristaltic action because the body grows lazy and relies on the laxative instead of its own muscle action to expel feces. In a lazy gut, harmful bacteria aren't expelled as readily from the colon. They remain in the colon longer.

- *Stress.* Long-term stress also slows peristaltic action and permits harmful bacteria to remain longer in the colon. Stress decreases the production of digestive enzymes, the effect of which is to allow undigested food to feed harmful bacteria in the colon.

- *Excessive carbohydrates.* Evidence shows that many carbohydrates are not digested, but remain in the colon. These unabsorbed carbohydrates may attract pathogenic microbes into the colon, which arrive to consume the undigested carbohydrates. The result is bacterial fermentation. This fermentation process creates intestinal gas and can injure the lining of the intestinal tract. An injured intestinal tract may eventually cause a host of gastrointestinal maladies.

- *Oral contraceptives.* Birth control pills alter the pH of the intestines, making it less acidic and more alkaline. An alkaline environment encourages the growth of pathogenic bacteria and yeasts such as *Candida albicans.*

- *Chlorinated water.* Drinking water is quite commonly disinfected with chlorine to kill microorganisms such as bacteria and viruses. Like antibiotics, however, the chlorine in drinking water kills the bacteria in the gut—the helpful as well as the harmful variety.

- *Steroids.* Besides suppressing the immune system, these drugs—including prednisone, hydrocortisone, and other corticosteroids—create an ideal environment for the proliferation of *Candida albicans* and other fungi.

- *Nonsteroidal anti-inflammatory agents (NSAIDs).* Drugs such as aspirin and ibuprofen keep the prostaglandins from doing their work. The hormone-like prostaglandins are responsible for many tasks, including repairing the intestinal wall. NSAIDs, therefore, contribute to leaky gut syndrome and other ailments in which the intestinal wall is permeated.

- *Anal intercourse.* This sexual activity introduces bacteria, viruses, protozoa, and yeast into the colon. These invaders can overpower the intestinal flora and disturb the ecological balance of the large intestine.

A Look at the Friendly Bacteria

General speaking, the so-called friendly bacteria improve digestive health by acidifying the colon and helping it maintain a proper pH level. In an acidic colon, harmful bacteria have a more difficult time growing and thriving. The acidity of the intestines is measured on the pH (potential hydrogen) scale, a logarithmic scale from 0 to 14. The higher numbers indicate that a substance is more alkaline; the lower numbers indicate it is more acidic. Ideally, the intestines should have a low pH, since harmful bacteria thrive in an alkaline environment, not in an acidic one.

Bacteria fall into two categories: aerobic and anaerobic. Aerobic bacteria require oxygen to survive; anaerobic bacteria do not need oxygen. There is no oxygen in the dank, musty large intestine, so aerobic bacteria cannot live there. Some kinds of aerobic bacteria are oxygen guzzlers. They drive harmful bacteria out of the small intestine by using up much of the oxygen.

Besides acidifying the colon, friendly bacteria assist the immune system by preventing infection. They manufacture important B-complex vitamins and increase the absorption of the protein in food. They make minerals more bioavailable and increase our resistance to food poisoning. Most friendly bacteria are members of the lactobacillus family or the bifidobacterium family.

The Lactobacillus Family

The lactobacillus family of friendly bacteria includes *Lactobacillus acidophillus, Lactobacillus bulgaricus, Lactobacillus plantarum,* and *Lactobacillus casei. Lacto* is Latin for "milk." These bacteria are found in cultured milk products such as yogurt and kefir, and in properly prepared sauerkraut. They were discovered in the early 1900s by Russian biologist Dr. Elie Metchnikoff. (For the story of their discovery, see page 124.) They reside mostly in the small intestine.

Probiotics in the lactobacillus family produce lactic acid, a substance that helps to acidify the gut. Lactic acid also helps with the absorption of calcium, copper, iron, magnesium, and manganese. By acidifying the gut, making it easier for proteins to be absorbed in the small intestine, lactobacillus makes the aforementioned minerals more bioavailable.

Some *L. acidophillus* strains produce natural antibiotics—*acidolin, acidophilin, lactobacilin, lactocidin,* and *bulgarican*—that are useful against streptococcus and staph infections. The advantage of these substances over synthetic antibiotics is that the natural ones target selected bacteria, not all the bacteria in the gut. They are not toxic to lactobacilli or to human cells. They are especially potent enemies of salmonella, Clostridium botulinum, and *E. coli.* Some strains of *L. acidophillus* produce hydrogen peroxide, which can kill *Candida albicans* directly and thereby prevent thrush caused by the overgrowth of candida.

L. acidophillus is very effective against chronic diarrhea because it inhibits the growth of so many kinds of harmful bacteria. So-called sticker strains of *L. acidophillus* are known for vigorously attaching themselves to the intestinal wall and keeping harmful bacteria from finding a place there.

In general, viruses are harder to kill than bacteria. There are very few specific antiviral agents in the current drug armamentarium. Some evidence, however, suggests that probiotics may be effective against viruses. In one experiment, acidolin, the antibiotic produced by *L. acidophilus,* demonstrated the ability to disintegrate polio and vaccine cells. In another experiment, 95 percent of herpes patients who were given *L. acidophilus* and *L. bulgaricus* tablets saw their genital herpes completely disappear. Dr. D. J. Weekes, who conducted the experiment, wrote that the high degree of acidity produced by the lactobacilli may have been responsible for deactivating the herpes simplex virus. In an *in vitro* study conducted at the University of Washington on HIV, the virus that causes acquired immune deficiency syndrome (AIDS), researchers found that "the likelihood of transmission may be influenced" by hydrogen peroxide–producing lactobacilli. The researchers were careful not to make any claims, since their study was conducted in a Petri dish, but it holds out hope for future experiments pertaining to HIV and probiotics.

Luncheon meats, hot dogs, bacon, ham, sausage, and other meats are cured using nitrates and nitrites. These chemicals preserve meat, make it look redder and more appetizing, and prevent the formation of botulism bacteria. In the body, however, nitrates and nitrites are turned into a cancer-causing agent called nitrosamine. Some strains of *L. acidophilus* can neutralize nitrosamine and thereby help prevent colon, stomach, and esophageal cancer.

Finally, all bacteria in the Lactobacilli family produce the enzyme lactase. This enzyme is needed to break down and digest lactose, the milk-sugar found in milk products. People who are lactose-intolerant cannot digest milk because their bodies don't make the lactase enzyme. People with lactose intolerance can, however, usually eat cultured milk products—yogurt and kefir—because the lactose has been broken down by the lactic-acid bacteria contained in the cultured dairy product.

The Bifidobacteria Family

Bacteria in the bifidobacteria family include *Bifidobacteria bifidum*, *Bifidobacteria longum*, and *Bifidobacteria infantis*. These bacteria are found mostly in the colon. They are the most common resident bacteria in the large intestine. Like the lactobacillus bacteria, they are good at adhering to the intestinal walls and crowding out harmful bacteria. They also secrete lactic acid to help acidify the colon.

Bifidobacteria manufacture B-complex vitamins—B_3, B_5, B_9, B_{12} (although there is some debate as to whether these vitamins are produced too deep in the gut to be absorbed). Bifidobacteria may also play a role in reducing cholesterol.

Bifidobacterium infantis is found in mother's milk. Babies obtain this important probiotic from their mothers. This illustrates yet again why breastfeeding is so important to babies' health.

Getting More Probiotics in Your Diet

One of the best ways to improve your intestinal health is to strengthen your intestinal flora by including probiotics in your diet.

DR. ELIE METCHNIKOFF AND THE
DISCOVERY OF LACTOBACILLUS

The health benefits of probiotics were discovered in the early 1900s by a Russian biologist named Dr. Elie Metchnikoff. Dr. Metchnikoff is credited with bringing yogurt to the attention of the West. From 1888 until his death in 1916, he was director of the Pasteur Institute in Paris. In 1908, he shared the Nobel Price in Medicine with Paul Ehrlich for the discovery of phagocytes, the large white blood cells of the immune system that destroy toxins and bacteria.

In the last decade of his life, Dr. Metchnikoff studied longevity. His interest in why some people live longer than others led him to examine the Bulgarian tribes of the Caucasus Mountains. These people still live on average well into their nineties. The primary reason for the Bulgarian's good health, Dr. Metchnikoff concluded, was the yogurt they ate. He argued that the bacteria in yogurt is healthy because it acidifies the gut and keeps putrefactive bacteria in check. In honor of the Bulgarians, Dr. Metchnikoff named one of the bacteria isolates he discovered in yogurt *Lactobacillus bulgaricus*.

To prove his hypothesis, Dr. Metchnikoff attempted to isolate the *Lactobacillus bulgaricus* from the cultured milk product being consumed by the Bulgarians and orally and rectally implant the bacteria in the gastrointestinal tract of the subjects of his experiment. The experiment ultimately failed because the isolated strain of bacteria did not implant. Nevertheless, when the cultured yogurt–type dairy food was consumed intact with its naturally occurring friendly microorganisms, it was able to impart health and longevity to its users. Dr. Metchnikoff's experiments support one of this book's basic premises—that the best way to enhance the health of the gastrointestinal tract is to consume lacto-fermented foods and probiotics in a base of lacto-fermented foods.

Dr. Metchnikoff was one of the first scientists to propose a connection between disease and harmful bacteria in the intestines. He hypothesized that poisons produced in the bowel might be the cause of some diseases—a hypothesis that proved correct. Dr. Metchnikoff held out great hope that "beneficial" bacteria could be used medicinally to combat deleterious bacteria. However, before Dr. Metchnikoff's ideas could be tested or realized, antibiotics came along. They became the preferred method of antimicrobial therapy. In our present state of ever-increasing antibiotic resistance, Dr. Metchnikoff's work is being revisited. The best way to combat some of these bugs may turn out to be with beneficial bacteria.

Throughout his life, Dr. Metchnikoff shared his discoveries enthusiastically with colleagues. By 1910, he had his fellow scientists at the Pasteur Institute eating yogurt. In 1919, the first industrial production of yogurt was begun in Barcelona, Spain, using bacterial cultures obtained from the Pasteur Institute. The distinctive sour taste of yogurt put off many people, but by the 1950s, the dairy industry began mixing fruit syrups with yogurt and the food gradually achieved a degree of popularity. Today, yogurt is found in every supermarket.

Probiotics keep harmful bacteria in check. They work hand in hand with the immune system to prevent dangerous pathogens from entering the body. Probiotics are a natural medicine. Humankind has been taking probiotics for many thousands of years in the form of cultured, lacto-fermented food. Fermentation with lactic-acid microorganisms adds probiotics to food and makes the food easier to digest. It increases the beneficial flora in the intestines as well.

The two ways to increase your consumption of probiotics are to get them in probiotic supplements or fermented whole foods. Probiotic supplements are friendly bacterial strains that have been cultured, isolated, and placed into powders, pills, or refrigerated dairy products. Unfortunately, only a handful of probiotic supplements are worth taking, in our opinion. Most probiotic supplements do not contain the valuable cofactors—the enzymes, minerals, and other components—found in whole foods. Sometimes suspect bacterial strains are used in supplements. Often the probiotic bacteria die before they can be of any benefit. By contrast, probiotic whole foods combine lactic acid and various other organic acids, vitamins, minerals, proteins, and enzymes—all working together to form that magic stuff we call food. Later in this chapter we discuss a probiotic compound that combines the valuable lactobacilli and bifidobacteria with powerful strains of microbes from the soil, all cultured in a whole-food medium.

A Mouth-Watering Survey of Fermented Foods

Our ancient ancestors seemed to know instinctively that lacto-fermented foods—that is, foods cultured with lactic-acid microorganisms—were good for them. They fermented food to preserve it. But they also relished fermented food for its nutritional value and delicious flavor. Fermented foods, which are rich in probiotics, are some of the oldest foods known to humankind.

Surveying the fermented foods that our ancestors have handed down to us is a mouth-watering proposition. Sauerkraut, made from fermented cabbage, was a mainstay of the Roman army and is still savored in Germany and elsewhere. Koreans eat their own form of sauerkraut, called *kim-chee*, which they make from many kinds of vegetables as well as cabbage. In the United States, pickled cucumber and pickled relish are favorites. In India, a variety of chutneys are made from different kinds of fruit. The French delight in the cornichon, a small crisp pickle made from the gherkin cucumber.

The best-known lacto-fermented foods, yogurt and cheese, are made from cow's and goat's milk. Kefir, another milk product, has been a staple of the Caucasus Mountains since time immemorial. The Mongols of Genghis Khan's time drank kumiss, a drink fermented from mare's milk. Icelanders drank syra, a beverage made from fermented whey.

Lacto-fermented beverages are consumed in almost every culture. In Mexico, people drink pulque, the fermented juice of the agave cactus (tequila is distilled pulque). Mead, a fermented honey drink, was a favorite of the Saxons, Celts, Vikings, and other free-wheeling Northern European tribes. Kvass, a lacto-fermented beverage made from stale rye bread, is sold in carts to this day on the streets of Moscow. "You know what a peasant's food is—bread, kvass, onions," wrote Leo Tolstoy in "The Kreutzer Sonata," a short story. "With this frugal nourishment he lives, he is alert, he makes light work in the fields." Munkoyo, a sweet beverage also known as sorghum beer, is consumed in southeast Africa. Beer made from fermented rice has long been drunk in India, China, and Japan.

Before the introduction of commercial brewer's yeast, many breads were made from fermented grain. Americans on the Western frontier made sourdough bread and biscuits. Ethiopian injera pancakes are made from fermented teff. Pozol, the Mexican cornbread, is also a fermented product.

In Asia, fermented soybean products—miso, natto, tamari, and shoyu—are used as condiments. These foods are slowly but surely finding their way into the American diet.

Whole-Food Probiotics

As we explained earlier, the best way to get probiotics is to consume them in whole foods, not to obtain them from isolated probiotic supplements. In Chapter 9, as well as in "Resources," we list sources for high-quality, therapeutic, lacto-fermented foods and probiotics. Adding these products to your daily diet can improve your health and longevity. Who knows? Maybe you will live and thrive well into your nineties like the Bulgarians.

Probiotic Supplements

As we stated earlier, most probiotic products are isolated from their culture medium. For that reason, they lack the valuable cofactors that are present in whole-food probiotics. They are bacterial isolates, and as such, the body cannot absorb them easily and sometimes cannot even recognize them.

In the short run, some supplements may work like antibiotics and destroy harmful bacteria in the gut. Two such supplements, one composed of eight beneficial bacteria and the other composed of fourteen strains of friendly microorganisms, have proven valuable in clinical studies. The second of the two above-mentioned probiotic preparations behaves much like a fermented food. It contains HSOs, which appear to be hardier than standard probiotics and can withstand stomach acidity better. (HSOs are explained later in this chapter.) In the long run, you are better off getting probiotics from live fermented foods or from whole-food probiotic supplements.

To make sure the bacteria reach the intestines, most manufacturers stuff their products with many more microorganisms than are found in fermented whole foods. One such product, for example, contains a hundred thousand times more bacterial microorganisms than can be found in a normal serving of fermented food. Bacteria have a very high attrition rate. They die off in the container as well as in the acidic environment of the stomach. The die-off rate of bacteria can be compared to that of a sea turtle's eggs. A sea turtle lays thousands of eggs in the hope that two or three young turtles will make it to the water and survive into adulthood. In the case of fermented probiotic products that contain HSOs, the number of friendly microorganisms may be much less, but they are hardier strains and have an easier time making the safe journey from the mouth to the intestinal tract. In the intestinal tract, lactobacilli and other friendly microorganisms with a good source of food multiply approximately every twenty minutes under the right conditions. And that brings up another advantage of whole-food lacto-fermented probiotics: They contain within their substrate the nutrients they need to survive and multiply in the gastrointestinal tract.

Check the expiration date carefully, but even if the probiotic supplement you are considering is within its expiration date, the number of "live cells" is probably significantly lower than the number on the label. Research has shown that as little as 20 percent of the bacteria in probiotic supplements are still alive when the capsule or powder is ready for consumption. What's more, the large number of microorganisms in probiotic supplements can trigger an immune-system response that kills off the 20 percent of bacteria that actually makes it to the small intestine. When the tens of billions of bacteria enter the body, the body may assume it is being invaded by foreign pathogens. Probiotics are, after all, bacteria. Gerald Tannock, writing in *Probiotics: A Critical Review* (Horizon Scientific Press, 1999), states that the immune system may kill off many probiotic bacteria.

Most probiotic supplements are processed by centrifugation or ultrafiltration. These processes concentrate the cell biomass. In centrifugation, the cultured cell biomass is hurled around a centrifuge with tremendous force. This injures the structure of the cells such that they cannot withstand the acidic rigors of the gastrointestinal tract. In ultrafiltration, the cells are squeezed through an industrial sieve, a less damaging process but one that nevertheless weakens the cells. In centrifugation and ultrafiltration, the bacteria are separated from the supernatant, the culturing medium in which the bacteria are grown, and the supernatant is discarded. The supernatant, however, may be as important as the bacteria themselves. The supernatant is food for the bacteria. It contains enzymes and antimicrobials that help bacteria withstand stomach acid.

The best processing technique for probiotic supplements duplicates the natural process of lacto-fermentation. Producers grow probiotics in whole, nutrient-dense foods that contain the proper growth media for the microbes. When the growing process is complete, the microbes are dried quickly at low temperatures. Including the substrate in the product is extremely important because the substrate may be the key that helps the product aid human health.

To test the viability of a probiotic supplement, drop a few caplets into two to four ounces of milk and let the milk sit at room temperature for twenty-four to forty-eight hours. This test measures the ability of the probiotic to produce enzymes that break down or predigest food. If the probiotic supplement is viable, the milk will curdle to a thick yogurt-like consistency. Any probiotic that cannot pass this simple test is probably not capable of doing its job in your body.

(Another type of product that has become popular in recent years but that we recommend avoiding is the prebiotic supplement. For a discussion of prebiotics, see page 130.)

❖

PROBIOTICS VERSUS PREBIOTICS

Besides getting probiotics in foods or supplements, some people recommend feeding the friendly bacteria in the gut by taking *prebiotics*. A prebiotic is a nondigestible fiber. One such product, fructo-oligosaccharides (FOS), which is found naturally in artichokes, onions, chicory, garlic, and leeks, is supposed to selectively stimulate the friendly bacteria in the gut and thereby make it proliferate. The problem with prebiotics is that selectively feeding bacteria in the gut is not a realistic proposition. Instead of selectively feeding intestinal flora, prebiotics most likely feed all the bacteria, friendly and unfriendly.

Popular prebiotic supplements include FOS and inulin. In our experience, these supplements do not help patients, but instead cause them to develop bloating and gas. We have seen patients become significantly worse by taking FOS and inulin. The foods and supplements recommended in the Guts and Glory Program, lacto-fermented foods, and whole-food probiotic products serve as excellent probiotics and prebiotics in their own right. You don't need prebiotic supplements.

The Gastrointestinal Tract, the Immune System, and Leaky Gut Syndrome

Here is a novel idea: You are hollow. Your gastrointestinal tract, from your mouth at one end to your anus at the other, is a hollow opening through the middle of your body. And no part of your body is more intimate with the outside world than your gastrointestinal tract. Your skin is exposed to moisture and sunlight, but compared to your gastrointestinal tract, your skin is an iron-clad fortress. Food, bacteria, viruses, and toxins enter your gastrointestinal tract. Your GI tract must extract what it needs and expel the rest. It must literally absorb parts of the outside world for nourishment.

It appears that the intestinal flora and the human body have a symbiotic relationship. The body permits the friendly bacteria to live in the intestinal tract. In return, the friendly bacteria form the first line of defense against bacterial disease, viruses, toxins, and parasites. The friendly bacteria coat the walls of the intestinal tract, protecting it against harmful invaders. In this way, they take some of the burden off the immune system.

The gastrointestinal tract, in fact, plays an extremely important role in the immune system. At birth, about 70 percent of immune system cells are associated with the intestines. In adulthood, the figure is 40 to 50 percent. The gut-associated lymphatic tissue (GALT) secretes special "killer" cells into the mucosa of the intestines to fight bacteria, viruses, and toxins. These cells include macrophages, natural killer cells, mast cells, and intraepithelial lymphocytes. Their job is to identify and destroy dangerous substances to keep them from permeating the walls of the intestines and poisoning the body. The intestinal tract is the first line of defense against disease.

Because so much of the immune system is associated with the intestines, bowel diseases do double harm. They not only disrupt digestion and absorption, they also interfere with vital immune-system functions. When the immune system in the intestines fails, toxins and bacteria are able to permeate the intestinal lining and poison the body. This condition has been referred to as leaky gut syndrome.

In a leaky gut, so the theory goes, bacteria, parasites and their toxins, undigested protein, and fungi that would otherwise be destroyed are allowed to pass through the space that exists between the cells of the intestinal wall. These substances can then cause inappropriate stimulation of the immune system. The immune system, thinking that these large molecules are foreign substances, starts producing antibodies against them. The antibodies, in turn, get into various tissues and can cause an inflammatory reaction. Antibodies that attack the gut lining may cause Crohn's disease or colitis. These antibodies also damage the mucosal coating of the intestinal walls such that the immune-system cells found in the mucosal coating can no longer do their jobs as well. As a result, bacteria, parasites, and viruses that would otherwise be destroyed can enter unharmed into the bloodstream. Once in the blood, they can potentially infect almost any body organ or tissue.

Researchers speculate that leaky gut syndrome (or some hybrid of it) can lead to a variety of medical maladies. Leaky gut has been implicated in a variety of disorders ranging from autism to chronic fatigue syndrome, edema, and allergies. A potential root cause of many of these disorders, it seems, is unbalanced intestinal flora. Promoting friendly bacteria in the gut with the use of probiotics, therefore, is an excellent defense against a variety of conditions.

Beyond Probiotics

The first half of this chapter described the friendly bacteria in your intestines and the many different ways that these bacteria contribute to good health. Friendly bacteria assist the immune system. The microorganisms coat the lining of the intestines and prevent harmful bacteria from gaining a foothold. Like antibiotics, some friendly bacteria secrete substances that destroy harmful microorganisms such as yeast, bacteria, viruses, and parasites. The first part of this chapter explained how to strengthen the friendly bacteria in your gut by eating fermented foods and taking probiotic supplements.

What the first part of this chapter didn't explain is that friendly bacterial organisms can be obtained from the soil as well as from fermented foods. In fact, our ancient ancestors, who weren't as conscientious about cleaning their food as we are, ate these friendly bacterial organisms along with their food. For that matter, our not-so-ancient ancestors ate them as well when they lived and worked close to the soil on farms. These friendly microorganisms may be superior to normal probiotics in many ways. They are called HSOs, or homeostatic soil organisms.

What Are HSOs?

Homeostatic soil organisms are tiny bacterial microorganisms that live in the soil. In nature, HSOs provide the soil and plants with nutrients. They make the soil more lush and fertile. They release enzymes into the soil that kill off yeasts, molds, and other materials that hinder plants from growing. HSOs sterilize the soil of organisms that cause rot. Through the root system, they feed their nutrients to the plants. HSOs also produce growth hormones that encourage seeds to sprout and mature. As a plant grows, soil organisms increase in number to nourish the plant. They are absorbed through the roots and become part of the plant's cellulous fiber. HSOs do to the gut what they do to the soil—they destroy viruses, yeasts, molds, and fungi. In the gastrointestinal tract, they help maintain a state of homeostasis. They do that by keeping the GI tract free of harmful pathogens and by increasing the absorption of food as it passes through the intestinal lining.

In times past, HSOs were abundant in the human diet. People consumed HSOs along with their fruits and vegetables. To preserve meat, certain native cultures buried it in the ground. Once there, it became saturated with HSOs, which our ancestors consumed when they dug up the meat and ate it. In some cultures, fruits and vegetables were buried in the soil. Ancient humans understood that buried produce was healthier, although they didn't understand why. Dogs may well bury bones for the same reason that our ancient ancestors did—to get the benefits of HSOs.

In the nineteenth century, when the term "farm-fresh produce" was more than an advertising slogan, Americans regularly ate fruits and vegetables straight from the soil of their farms and gardens. When the so-called sod-buster got hungry, he simply pulled a carrot out of the ground, brushed it off, and ate it, dirt and all. Without knowing it, these farmers made sure their gastrointestinal tracts functioned well by consuming extracurricular HSOs. Some have suggested that a lack of HSOs in the diet may be at the bottom of Dr. David Strachan's famous "hygiene hypothesis," in which he suggests that incidences of asthma, hay fever, and eczema are rising in children because our environment isn't dirty enough.

HSOs are bacterial microorganisms. Like any bacteria, they are alive. Agricultural practices that are meant to kill harmful bacteria and parasites kill healthful HSOs as well. Pesticides, germicides, and fungicides deplete the soil of HSOs. HSOs that survive the harvest are killed off by pasteurization and heat-based food-processing techniques. Compared to our ancestors, we ingest very few HSOs, and the ones we do ingest are not as vital as the ones our ancestors consumed. The health benefits that HSOs provide to the intestines, the nutrients and hormones that they provide to the body, have been virtually eliminated from the modern diet.

The good news, however, is that you can make HSOs a part of your diet. You can do that by taking health supplements that contain HSOs.

Discovery of HSOs

A recent *Business Week* article called "Down in the Dirt, Wonders Beckon" described how scientists are isolating and cloning microorganisms in the soil with an eye toward making use of these organisms to promote health. These soil-based microorganisms are still something of a mystery. But scientists are very excited about them. The hope is that they can be made to function like antibiotics and fight disease. As the *Business Week* article points out, 1 gram of soil can contain 10,000 microorganisms. HSOs are an example of these microorganisms being used to improve health—in this case, human gastrointestinal health.

Homeostatic soil organisms were discovered and developed by a scientist named Peter W. Daubner, Ph.D. As a young man, Dr. Daubner was intrigued by an idea he got from a colleague and mentor by the name of Emil Tiger, Ph.D. Dr. Tiger believed that the cure for every disease is found in nature. Many pharmaceutical drugs are compounds that have been isolated from natural ingredients. What if, instead of isolating compounds from known quantities, scientists searched for natural materials with which to make medicines? In other words, instead of mining known quantities for compounds, what if scientists searched far and wide for new material with which to work? The search, Drs. Tiger and Daubner believed, would always yield rewards if it were true that the cure for every disease is found in nature.

Keeping in mind Dr. Tiger's idea, Dr. Daubner happened to be hiking in a rainforest in the late 1970s when he came upon an unusual piece of ground. (Dr. Daubner prefers not to say where he obtained his first samples.) The ground was decomposed, soft, and mushy. The leaves on the plants that grew in the ground were five times larger than the leaves of similar plants that grew elsewhere in the rainforest. Dr. Daubner reasoned that the soil contained concentrated nutrients worth studying. He gathered a sample of the soil and put it in a sock.

Upon his return to the United States, however, he discovered that the bacterial microorganisms in the soil had died. Still, what he saw under his microscope captivated him, and he made four more trips to the special place in the rainforest. At last, on his fourth trip, he returned home with a living sample. The bacterial microorganisms in the soil, the ones from which homeostatic soil organisms were bred, had arrived safely. Dr. Daubner soon learned how to keep the organisms alive, induce a dormant state of hibernation, and bring the organisms out of dormancy when he wanted to experiment with them. The twenty-three-year-old knew he was on to something and that his life would never be the same. He thought the microorganisms he discovered in the rainforest might hold the key to wellness from disease. The microorganisms Dr. Daubner captured seemed to be as old as the Earth itself.

Dr. Daubner spent the next decade selectively breeding superior strains of the bacteria and trying to find out what these microorganisms could do. Taking advantage of his connection to the University of California and its biological databases, he identified the different microorganism strains in the soil sample. To find out if they were toxic, he fed them to fingerling fish. The fish showed no signs of ill health. To the contrary, the fish that ate the bacterial microorganisms grew faster and larger than the other fish. Laboratory rats that ate the microorganisms also thrived. The scientist applied the bacteria to open wounds on his own skin and, encouraged by the results, ingested them himself.

Throughout his experiments with HSOs, Dr. Daubner also worked on perfecting a substrate for the bacteria to grow on. The substrate is to bacteria what the soil is to a plant or food is to a human or animal. The substrate feeds the bacteria. Unless the substrate is a nourishing one, the bacteria can't grow adequately or remain vital. Dr. Daubner experimented with ionic minerals, the skeletal remains of plants, single-cell phytoplanktons, and other macro- and micronutrients that originated in different places on the Earth. Slowly but surely, he devised a substrate in which the microorganisms could grow and thrive. Incorporated into the substrate was a delivery system that protected the microorganisms on their journey from the mouth through the digestive tract and ensured proper colonization. When he at last devised an ideal substrate, it was as though the microorganisms had come home again, he reported. Dr. Daubner had fashioned a substrate from ancient materials for the ancient bacterial microorganisms he had discovered in the rainforest. Today, consuming HSOs is like eating an ancient plant that was grown in pure, unpolluted soil.

How HSOs Differ from Conventional Probiotics

HSOs are probiotics. Like the Lactobacillus and Bifidobacterium families described in the first half of this chapter, they help balance the intestinal flora and bring good health to the small and large intestines. They secrete lactic acid, hydrogen peroxide, and acetic acid to help acidify the intestines. However, HSOs offer health benefits above and beyond conventional probiotics.

For one thing, HSOs appear to be heartier than their conventional cousins. They are better able to survive the acidic environment of the stomach and arrive safely in the small intestine. Most probiotic supplements contain hundreds or thousands of times more colony-forming units (CFUs) than can be found in a normal serving of fermented food. The high numbers ensure that some of the bacterial microorganisms make it through the acidic environment of the stomach and into the intestines. With HSOs, however, it isn't necessary to inflate the numbers because HSO microorganisms can pass through the stomach intact. Humans have been eating them for many thousands of years. The body, so to speak, recognizes them as food.

What really distinguishes HSOs from ordinary probiotics is their resilience. No matter what the pH of the intestines is, HSOs can find a home there. Like bacteria of the Lactobacillus and Bifidobacterium families, HSOs occupy and colonize the walls of the intestines and in so doing displace the harmful bacteria that are lodged there. But HSOs also dislodge accumulated decay on the walls of the intestines and flush it out as waste. They clean decay from the intestinal walls and thereby allow more nutrients to pass through the walls and be absorbed. They are very aggressive against molds, yeasts, fungi, bacteria, and even viruses.

More Health Benefits of HSOs

Coauthor Jordan Rubin gives HSOs much of the credit for his victory in the battle against Crohn's disease. After taking HSOs for a month, he began to feel more energetic. His appetite returned. Week by week, he put on more weight and gained more muscle mass. How exactly do HSOs benefit the intestinal tract? These pages explain the dirty details.

HSOs can feed on the hydrocarbons found in food. As such, they can break down food into its most basic elements. Food that has been split this way can pass more easily through the walls of the small intestine and be absorbed. This is why people who take HSOs often feel more energetic and strong.

HSOs stimulate the production of a protein called alpha-interferon. Genetically engineered alpha-interferon is used to treat viral hepatitis, Kaposi's sarcoma, genital warts, and non-Hodgkins lymphoma. Alpha-interferon increases the body's production of cytokines, the messengers of the immune system. Cytokines alert the immune system to the presence of an invader and induce healthy cells to produce enzymes that counter infections. In some cases, they also kill foreign cells. So far, genetically engineered alpha-interferon has been a disappointment. The drug is prohibitively expensive, must be delivered in high doses, can be toxic, and does not stimulate the immune system adequately. What's more, it appears that the body manufactures numerous subspecies of alpha-interferon for different viruses and antigens. The beauty of HSOs is that they stimulate the body's own natural alpha-interferon production. In so doing, they enhance the immune system's ability to fight off disease.

HSOs produce proteins that rouse the immune system. In effect, these proteins trick the body into thinking it is being attacked by a bacterium, virus, parasite, or other antigen. To respond to what it thinks is an attack, the immune system produces huge pools of uncoded antibodies. Uncoded antibodies are not preprogrammed to attack specific antigens. They are freelancers and can roam and attack wherever they are needed. Now the body has these extra antibodies at its disposal to ward off diseases and infections. The result is a stronger immune system and an enhanced ability of fight off diseases that have already been contracted.

HSOs can also help with the absorption of iron. HSOs stimulate the body to produce a protein called lactoferrin. This protein binds to and surrounds iron particles so that harmful bacteria or parasites can't get at them. What's more, lactoferrin carries iron particles through the acidic gastric environment to the small intestine where they can be absorbed. In unpublished research, Peter Rothschild, M.D., Ph.D., reported that iron particles carried by lactoferrin are 95 percent bioavailable, far above the 7 percent average.

In addition to the wonderful health benefits provided by using HSOs, agriculture is now reaping the benefits of these very same microorganisms in crop production. Using HSOs, one farmer in Asia was able to increase crop yield of a certain type of melon by 80 percent and increase the brix rating (sugar and nutrient content) from 14 to 16.5 all without the use of synthetic chemicals and pesticides. This is truly groundbreaking when you learn that melons typically require fourteen to sixteen pesticide and herbicide spray cycles.

Studies on HSOs

Studies are currently being conducted using HSOs in a multiple of disease states. While the "official verdict" may not be in, we endorse

HSOs as an important component of regaining GI health, given their enormous potential benefit and essentially nonexistent side effect profile. Coauthor Jordan Rubin continues to attribute a great deal of his success over Crohn's disease to these remarkable organisms.

❖ 6 ❖

A Plethora of
Problematic Programs

---

eople with serious illnesses are at a highly vulnerable point in
their lives. They desperately want to get well and very often
grasp at straws to achieve this end. A plan or step-by-step program with inflated guarantees of success can carry great appeal for
these individuals. They just want to plug into some kind of system
whose only demand is that they follow along.

This chapter looks at problematic diets and programs to which
people with gastrointestinal disorders are naturally drawn. Coauthor Jordan Rubin experienced most of these diets and programs
firsthand when he was ill with Crohn's disease. Coauthor Dr. Joseph
Brasco has personally toyed with some of these programs and has
consulted with many patients who have also tried them.

Problematic Diets

The first half of this chapter looks at a handful of popular diets. To
be specific, it looks at (take a deep breath before reading the rest of
this sentence) vegetarian diets, the raw food diet, the food-combining diet, the Specific Carbohydrate Diet, the gluten-free diet, the
anticandida diet, the macrobiotic diet, the balanced macronutrient
ratios diet (Zone diet), the ketogenic diet (Dr. Atkins New Diet

Revolution), the elimination/detoxification diet, the rotation diet, the R-diet, and of course, the standard American diet.

Most people start the day with a doughnut or muffin, coffee, and orange juice. At mid-morning, they eat a bagel with cream cheese. At lunch it's a turkey sandwich with some chips and a soft drink. The afternoon finds them going to a vending machine for a candy bar. For dinner they eat meat, potatoes, a roll with margarine, some green beans, and ice cream for dessert. Unfortunately, by current U.S. standards the diet we just described is considered a balanced, healthy diet. However, this diet is woefully inadequate if you want to achieve optimal health through nutrition. Anyone who moves away from this kind of diet is bound to be healthier and lose weight. For that reason, most of the diets described in this chapter work to a greater or lesser degree. They work by default, which is a sad testimony to how poor the standard American diet is (this diet is sometimes known by its acronym, SAD).

Embarking on a healthy eating regimen and lifestyle in and of itself can be beneficial. It makes you pause and think about what you are eating and how the food you eat affects your health. Most people simply eat what their parents or friends eat without considering whether their diet is truly a healthy one. But being on a diet makes you conscious of what you eat. Before you bite into the old-fashioned doughnut or dig into the mashed potatoes, you ask yourself whether eating the doughnut or potatoes is good for you and how it will affect your weight and overall health.

All of these diets provide some benefits in the short run, especially for those who previously ate a standard American diet. The problem is that the initial benefits are not sustained. In the long run, these diets may in fact be deleterious to optimal health.

Vegetarian Diets

Most people (including the authors of this book) have either turned to vegetarianism or flirted with the idea of being a vegetarian at one time or another. On the surface, vegetarianism seems to be a healthy diet. Vegetarians do not eat meat, fish, or fowl. Sometimes the distinction is made between "lacto-ovo vegetarians," who eat dairy products and eggs; "lacto-vegetarians," who eat dairy products; and "vegans," who do not eat any animal products whatsoever. The rule among vegans is never to eat the product of any animal or thing that has a face. Following this rule, vegans do not even eat honey, which is made by bees.

Vegetarianism plays into all the food phobias that are so prevalent in our society. Vegetarians believe that every ill known to humankind can be ascribed to the raising of livestock and the consumption of meat, animal fat, and animal products. Vegetarians believe that health can be achieved only through the elimination of animal foods. In general, the benefits of the vegetarian diet can be boiled down to this: The diet is detoxifying. It can clean out your system. By increasing the consumption of plant food, particularly fruits and vegetables, the body's overall toxic burden is lowered. This improves overall health. After the period of detoxification is over, however, the initial benefits of the diet start to wane. Specifically, the vegetarian diet is lacking in quality protein, certain vitamins (most notably B_{12}), minerals, and essential fatty acids.

The many failings of the vegetarian diet are discussed at length throughout this book. An important point to emphasize at this time is the issue of vitamin B_{12}. Health-food store propaganda to the contrary, the bottom line is that vegetarians do not get enough vitamin B_{12}. This important vitamin can be attained *only* from animal products, especially eggs and organ meats. A deficiency in vitamin B_{12} can cause anemia, fatigue, and neurological disorders. The vitamin is essential for cell division, energy, and the formation of red blood cells. Many vegetarians believe erroneously that their vitamin B_{12} needs can be met by tempeh (fermented bean cake), spirulina (a type of algae), and brewer's yeast. But these foods do not really contain vitamin B_{12}. They contain compounds called B_{12} analogs that are structurally similar to vitamin B_{12}. Some researchers believe that spirulina actually depletes vitamin B_{12} because the B_{12} analogs compete with vitamin B_{12} and inhibit the metabolism of the vitamin.

The argument that vegetarians can get vitamin B_{12} from fermenting bacteria in their intestines is only half true. While vitamin

B_{12} can be synthesized from intestinal bacteria, this primarily occurs in the large intestine. Because vitamin B_{12} is exclusively absorbed in a section of the small bowel known as the ileum, the body cannot utilize it. It is expelled with the feces. Studies of vegans living in underdeveloped countries have shown that these vegans get their vitamin B_{12} from eating unwashed vegetables that were fertilized with human manure—manure rich in vitamin B_{12}. In underdeveloped societies where pesticides are not used, vegans also get vitamin B_{12} from insects and insect larvae on the plants they eat.

Besides lacking in certain kinds of foods, the vegetarian diet poses another problem—the type of foods in the diet. Most vegetarians eat a lot of processed carbohydrates and soy products to compensate for not eating meat. These days, soy is made into everything from ersatz tuna to ice cream. But nonfermented soy and many grains are very high in phytic acid, a substance that inhibits the body from assimilating calcium, magnesium, iron, and zinc. This is why vegetarians may suffer from mineral deficiencies. Moreover, the producers of soy milk, tofu, and other soy substitutes extract the soy from the beans with alkali solutions. This practice changes the molecular structure of the protein in the beans and makes the protein difficult to digest. To complicate this problem even further, soybeans lack vitamins A and D, both of which are needed to absorb the protein in soybeans.

Perhaps the biggest fallacy of the vegetarian diet is that some vegetarians mistakenly believe that they can eat anything and still be healthy as long as they don't eat meat or meat products. Nobody argues with the consumption of fruits and vegetables, but one of the greatest ills of vegetarianism is probably the unabashed, wholesale consumption of all types of carbohydrates. In fact, if you were to study the dietary practices of most vegetarians, you would discover that most vegetarians are really "grainetarians" or "starchetarians." This excessive consumption of carbohydrates can drive up insulin levels and jeopardize overall health, as discussed in Chapter 3.

Thousands of years of conditioning have trained the human body to want animal products and saturated fats. Ignoring this historical and genetic fact exposes vegetarians to the health problems typically associated with vegetarianism: anemia, pallor, listlessness, and poor resistance to infection. Perhaps the best argument against vegetarianism is posed by the great comedian Jackie Mason, who asked, "Have you ever seen the people that work in health food stores who load themselves up with alfalfa sprouts and carrot juice? They all look sick and emaciated. None of them look healthy. In fact, the only healthy person in the entire health food store is the owner sitting in the back stuffing his face with a pastrami on rye."

The Raw Food Diet

The advocates of the raw food diet look to the animals for guidance in the correct way to eat. They point out that no animal on the planet save human beings cooks food before eating it. Cooking spoils the vitality of food, they say. Contact with heat and immersion in boiling water undermine the potency of vitamins and minerals. Cooking destroys the enzymes in food. Potentially, it can introduce toxins into the diet.

Adherents of the raw food diet say that the diet revitalizes them, makes them feel more alive, and allows them to live longer. Variations of the diet include the fruitarian diet, whose practitioners eat only fruit, and the Hallelujah and Genesis 1:29 diets, whose followers seek nutritional guidance from the Bible and believe that God's instructions to Adam and Eve in Genesis 1:29 are in fact a command to eat raw fruits and vegetables instead of meat ("And God said, Behold, I have given you every herb bearing seed, which is upon the face of all the earth, and every tree, in the which is the fruit of a tree yielding seed; to you it shall be for meat"). One version of the raw foods diet suggests eating raw meat as well as raw fruits and vegetables.

Cooking destroys the enzymes in food. These enzymes can help with digestion. The premise behind the raw food diet is that preserving the enzymes in food is of the utmost importance because the enzymes are necessary for the proper digestion of the food and the assimilation of its nutrients. The body is entirely capable of producing enzymes, but by preserving the enzymes that are innate in our foods, you lower the body's overall metabolic stress. Raw food advocates also maintain that lessening the digestive burden allows the body to utilize enzymes in other vital capacities. For example, the enzymes that the body doesn't have to devote to digestion can be put to use lowering inflammation, protecting against cancer, and improving elimination.

Like the vegetarian diet, the raw food diet has all the advantages that come with eating plenty of organic fruits, vegetables, and nuts. Vegetables and fruits contain an abundance of antioxidants, the substances that prevent free radicals from damaging body tissue (the best known antioxidants are vitamin C, vitamin E, and beta-carotene). Fruits and vegetables contain precursors to many different vitamins (a *precursor* is any natural substance that the body converts into something it needs). Leafy vegetables contain the B vitamins (except B_{12}), calcium, and other minerals. Cruciferous vegetables such as broccoli and cauliflower contain chemicals that prevent tumors in the digestive tract.

The problem with the raw food diet, however, is that it has all the drawbacks of the vegetarian diet. Obtaining the nutrients you need to stay healthy without eating meat or animal fat is impossible. Like the vegetarian diet, the raw food diet is notoriously lacking in quality protein, minerals, vitamins (most notably vitamins A, D, and B_{12}), and essential fatty acids.

Some raw food advocates, realizing the limitations of a vegetarian-type diet, believe in consuming raw animal products in addition to fruits and vegetables. Their diet includes unpasteurized dairy products, raw eggs, and uncooked meats, poultry, and fish. Eating raw fish and meat appears barbaric by modern standards, but it certainly has precedence among primitive cultures. A combination of raw plant and animal products is in many ways a nutritionally superior diet, but not in this day and age. Agribusiness and the transcontinental and international shipping of food have raised the risk of exposure to food contamination. That being the case, the risks of eating raw meat and fish usually outweigh the health benefits.

Another reason to question the raw food diet is that some foods are easier to digest, and their nutrients are therefore easier to absorb, when cooked. There are very good reasons to cook some kinds of vegetables. Raw broccoli, cauliflower, Brussels sprouts, and kale, for example, can irritate the mouth and bother the intestinal tract if they are not cooked. Unless spinach and chard are steamed or stir-fried, the oxalic acid in these vegetables will prevent calcium and iron from being absorbed. Cooking destroys some toxins in foods and is therefore advantageous.

Many people with gastrointestinal illnesses simply cannot tolerate a predominantly raw food diet. In people with GI disorders, raw foods are incompletely digested. They can tax the intestinal tract and become too difficult to absorb. Some people with bowel disorders cannot even handle a simple green salad. One reason why raw foods give GI patients such trouble is that, although raw foods contain enzymes, the fiber and certain sugars in raw foods are nearly impossible to break down completely. Humans lack the enzyme cellulase, which is necessary for digesting plant fibers. Intestinal bacteria can ferment undigested sugar and fiber. This fermentation may produce gas, inflammation, and the subsequent pain that accompanies them.

It is also worth noting that our ancestors' consumption of fruits and vegetables was quite different from ours. The array of fruits and vegetables that they ate differed greatly from our present-day fare. They got their greens from leaves and wild grasses. The fruits they ate were small and tart. Botanically speaking, our fruits and vegetables represent the culmination of thousands of years of selective breeding on the part of horticulturalists. What they ate was much simpler. Our fruits and vegetables are much more complex than theirs and thus they tax the digestive system far more.

If you are one who wholeheartedly believes in the all raw food diet, we suggest consuming a fair amount of raw avocado, soaked almonds, pumpkin seeds, and raw coconut. These foods supply an excellent concentration of high-quality fats and other important nutrients. Although controversial, we can recommend including raw diary products with the caveat that they be obtained from a reputable, preferably local, farmer. The same admonitions apply to lightly cooked or raw meats and poultry. Make sure the animals were organically raised. Whether or not you are on a raw food diet, the abovementioned foods are a great addition to your diet.

The Food-Combining Diet

The idea behind the food-combining diet is that certain foods cannot be digested properly if they are eaten at the same time as other foods. Starches, for example, shouldn't be eaten at the same time as protein. Melons should always be eaten alone. Food combiners believe that enzymes in the digestive tract are capable of canceling each other out. The enzymes that help digest starch, for example, can cancel out the enzymes that help digest protein. Therefore, starches and protein are not digested properly if they are eaten at the same time. The undigested food remains in the gut, where it ferments, putrefies, and leaks dangerous toxins into the bloodstream. One version of the food-combining diet says that the toxins are stored in the fat tissue, which makes people who combine foods incorrectly become bloated and gain weight.

Food combiners are especially solicitous of the fruit in their diet. Fruit has to be eaten alone in most cases. Vegetables, meanwhile, can be eaten with protein or with starch, but not with both at the same time. In some food-combining diets, the rules get progressively more arcane. Certain fruits can only be combined with certain other fruits. For example, sour fruits cannot be combined with sweet fruits. One version of the diet says that only fruit can be eaten in the morning and vegetables in the afternoon.

A variation of the food-combining diet is the acid-alkaline diet. In this diet, food is divided into two categories, alkaline forming and acid forming, and the goal is to eat 80-percent alkaline-forming foods and 20-percent acid-forming foods. Grains, meats, and certain kinds of nuts are acid forming. Most fruits and vegetables are alkaline forming. Advocates of the diet believe that alkaline-forming foods are essential because humankind evolved from the alkaline environment of the ocean. Straying from the 80–20 percent alkaline-acid formula, they maintain, causes biochemical and metabolic imbalances and the health problems associated with them—gout and arthritis. Followers of the diet keep tabs on the type of foods they eat and combine alkaline-forming and acid-forming foods accordingly. Of all the food-combining principles, the balancing of acid and alkaline foods is perhaps the most prudent and actually has some element of physiologic validity.

The problem with the food-combining diet is that most of its suppositions are not based on scientific fact or historical evidence. Nothing suggests that enzymes in different types of food cancel each other out. What's more, some of the theories behind food combining are contradictory. For example, food that is not completely absorbed cannot turn into fat, as food combiners contend. Unabsorbed foods exit the body in the feces. Because food-combining diets usually emphasize eating fruits and vegetables, the diets have the same shortcomings as the vegetarian and raw food diets.

People with digestive problems may be sensitive to various combinations of foods. A general rule is to keep meals simple, limit the variety of foods you consume at any one time, and eat small meals. After you have begun following a healthy diet, your body will tell you which food combinations are good for your health.

The Specific Carbohydrate Diet

The Specific Carbohydrate Diet was designed by Elaine Gottschall and described in her pioneering book *Breaking the Vicious Cycle*. Building on the work of Drs. Sidney V. and Merrill P. Haas, Ms. Gottschall constructed her diet around the premise that undigested carbohydrates can compromise the body's health and immunity. When carbohydrates are not properly digested, they do not pass harmlessly through the small intestine and colon. Instead, the undigested carbohydrates remain in the gut, where they can potentially feed harmful microbes. The result is an overgrowth of fermenting bacteria, yeasts, and parasites in the digestive tract. As the bacteria become more plentiful, the intestinal wall is damaged, and digestion becomes even more impaired. Now the bacteria have still more undigested carbohydrates to feed on. The "vicious cycle" in the title of

Ms. Gotschall's book continues as the bacteria becomes more plentiful, digestion becomes more impaired, and the bacteria keep getting stronger as they have more undigested carbohydrates to feed on.

The Specific Carbohydrate Diet is designed to put an end to the vicious cycle. The idea is to qualitatively change the type of carbohydrates in the diet to those that are easier to digest (primarily monosaccharides, the single-sugar carbohydrates) and thus reduce the amount of undigested material in the gastrointestinal tract. Theoretically, this in turn will reduce the available substrate for the intestinal bacteria and thereby reduce the total number of bacteria. Eventually, the harmful bacteria in the gut will be "starved" and digestion will return to normal.

To feed the dieter but starve the harmful bacteria in the dieter's intestines, the diet virtually eliminates the consumption of starches and disaccharides (two monosaccharides that are bonded together). Instead of disaccharides, Ms. Gotschall has the dieter eat single-sugar monosaccharides. This type of single-molecule carbohydrate can be absorbed through the lining of the small intestine without having to be broken down first. Monosaccharides are easier to digest and can be found in raw honey, most vegetables, natural cheeses, properly fermented yogurts, and several kinds of nuts. Processed foods, grains (especially processed grains), soy products, potatoes, and corn are strictly forbidden on the Specific Carbohydrate Diet, as are white sugar (actually the disaccharide sucrose), canned vegetables and meats, and most commercially produced dairy products. The diet does not permit carbohydrates that fall into the disaccharide (double-sugar) or polysaccharide (multiple-sugar) category. In other words, starch is not permitted.

While the Specific Carbohydrate Diet is designed to limit the growth of potentially harmful intestinal bacteria, the other major goal of the diet is to encourage the growth of beneficial microflora. To achieve this end, the diet encourages the consumption of probiotics as well as fermented foods, especially properly made yogurt. (Most commercially available yogurt is not allowed to ferment long enough. For this reason, the finished product contains large amounts of the disaccharide lactose. By contrast, the predominate carbohydrate in properly fermented yogurt is galactose, a monosaccharide.)

We endorse the Specific Carbohydrate Diet. It has helped thousands. Elaine Gottschall was one of the first to popularize the concept that the modern diet with its preponderance of nonfermented grains, dairy products, and sugar has shifted the balance of the native human microflora. This shift of bacterial populations in susceptible individuals may be the root cause of minor and serious intestinal disorders.

The coauthors of this book have achieved personal and clinical success with the Specific Carbohydrate Diet. Nevertheless, the diet has weak points that can be improved upon. The diet is excellent at restricting the types of carbohydrates that are consumed, but it has no provisions for restricting the quantity of carbohydrates consumed. This is the diet's major flaw. We firmly believe that addressing carbohydrate consumption from a quantitative as well as qualitative perspective is vital for optimal health.

Another major drawback of the Specific Carbohydrate Diet is its lack of direction in regard to fat consumption. If you follow the diet in its standard "you're over your crisis" maintenance mode, it has a very high omega-6 to omega-3 fat ratio. Consuming the omega-6 fats out of proportion to their omega-3 counterparts can promote total body inflammation, and inflammation can have devastating consequences for individuals with an active bowel disease. It is widely believed by nutritional researchers that the proper ratio of omega-6 fatty acids to omega-3 fatty acids is somewhere between one to one and four to one. The omega-3 fatty acids come from grass-fed animal foods, eggs from properly raised chickens and ducks, and certain nuts and seeds. The omega-6 fatty acids occur in conventional butter and grains, nuts, and foods from animals fed mostly grain instead of grass.

The Specific Carbohydrate Diet also makes little or no provision for the quality of the food that is consumed. The importance of eating organic produce and grass-fed animal products is emphasized throughout this book. The consumption of grass-fed animal products is of particular importance because animal products make up a significant part of the diet's caloric intake. To the uninitiated, eating grass-fed animal products may appear to be an esoteric consideration, but these animal products are an essential source of the omega-3 fats and CLAs. Foods that are high in the omega-3 fats are highly anti-inflammatory. They are crucial to the healing process.

Overall, however, Elaine Gottschall's dietary recommendations for starving the bacterial microbes in the gut and improving the intestinal health are sound. The diet has helped numerous people with ulcerative colitis, Crohn's disease, celiac disease, and irritable bowel syndrome. Gottschall deserves a lot of credit for calling people's attention to the harmful effects that eating processed starches can have on the intestines. She was one of the first to get the message out that starch and disaccharides, not just the gluten in grain, are among the major promoters of bowel disease.

The Gluten-Free Diet

Gluten is a protein constituent of wheat, rye, oats, spelt, and barley. People who can't tolerate gluten in their diet may have celiac disease, also known as gluten intolerance or gluten sensitive enteropathy. The symptoms of this disease vary greatly. They can be mild with just some intestinal bloating and cramping. At their worst, they can include severe intestinal cramps, voluminous diarrhea, weight loss, and malnutrition. However, some people have celiac disease without experiencing the gastrointestinal symptoms. For example, iron deficiency anemia, osteopenia (from calcium and vitamin D malabsorption), amenorrhea, infertility, and various skin lesions are symptoms of celiac disease that are not experienced in the gastrointestinal tract. The disorder may be far more prevalent than most healthcare professionals realize. Celiac disease appears to have a genetic component and is most common among people of northern European ancestry. It has been known to appear in adolescents but its symptoms can appear at any stage of life.

Celiac disease is caused by some type of interaction between gluten and the lining of the small intestine that results in the body's inability to properly digest and absorb nutrients. Despite a great deal of research, no one is certain how gluten harms the intestines. For many years, physicians believed that celiac disease was caused by an enzyme deficiency, but recent research attributes the disease to a malfunction of the immune system. It is believed that a fraction of the gluten molecule called *gliadin* burrows into the intestinal cell membrane, reaches the white blood cells underneath, and triggers a response on the part of the immune system. The immune system sends antibodies to the spot on the intestinal wall where the gliadin did its damage, and the antibodies damage the cells on the intestinal wall. This reaction results in the classic microscopic picture of small intestinal wall flattening—that is, loss of the villi. However, current research warns that this condition may be present even in the absence of this classic microscopic picture. Perhaps the anti-endomysial antibody blood test is the most certain way to diagnose celiac disease. You can get this test at any physician's office.

Given the prevalence of celiac disease, *anybody* with any type of chronic gastrointestinal disorder—in fact, anyone with a chronic condition—should give the gluten-free diet a try. The Guts and Glory Program is a low-gluten diet. It can easily be modified to exclude gluten altogether.

The Anti-Candida Diet

The disease candidiasis, also known as candida, is caused by a yeast fungus called *Candida albicans.* As a yeast, *Candida albicans* is found in the throat, mouth, digestive tract, and vaginal tract, and on the skin. The yeast has many functions inside the digestive tract, one of which is to recognize and destroy harmful bacteria. Normally, the yeast is kept in check by the other bacteria in the intestine, but if it grows out of control, it can turn from a harmless yeast into an aggressive fungus and cause intestinal problems, vaginal infections, and an infection of the mouth and throat called thrush.

An overgrowth of candida in the intestines is thought to cause constipation, diarrhea, gas, bloating, and abdominal pain. Candida is an especially opportunistic fungus. It can grow into the walls of the intestine, effectively breaching the walls and allowing food particles, toxic waste, and yeast waste products to seep into the blood-stream, a condition called leaky gut syndrome.

Many cases of candida occur after taking antibiotics. Antibiotics kill all bacteria, friendly and unfriendly, in the gut. Because candida microbes are oblivious to antibiotics, they remain when the bacteria die, and being opportunistic, they quickly seize the empty ground and proliferate. A diet high in sugar is another potential cause, especially in susceptible individuals. Diabetes, the hormonal changes brought on by the menstrual cycle, oral contraceptives, and pregnancy can also cause a candida infection.

The object of the anticandida diet is to starve the candida fungus of the kinds of foods it prefers. First and foremost, the diet bans sugar, all foods that contain sugar, and sugary drinks. As all bakers know, yeast feeds on sugar, and the *Candida albicans* yeast is no exception. Fresh fruit and fruit juices are prohibited in the diet because the fungus feeds on natural sugars. Fermented foods such as soy sauce, beer, vinegar, sauerkraut, and pickles are not permitted. Anticandida diets vary, but all put an emphasis on not eating sugar and on avoiding fermented foods containing vinegar.

Candidiasis is not recognized as a condition by the standard medical community. Despite this fact, a "diagnosis" of candidiasis is the darling of just about every type of alternative medicine practitioner. The problem with the anticandida diet (and the concept of candidiasis in general) is that it looks specifically at yeast as the be-all and end-all of the problem. Actually, the problem is not so much *Candida albicans* as it is a lack of balance in the gut flora. The *Candida albicans* yeast is opportunistic and is found in everybody's gastrointestinal tract. The difference between candida sufferers and others is that, in healthy people's gastrointestinal tracts, the bad bacteria are kept in check by the beneficial bacteria. By reinoculating the gut with the enzyme- and probiotics-rich fermented foods in the Guts and Glory Program, you can promote the beneficial bacteria and in so doing produce an environment in the gut that is unfavorable to the growth of candida.

One friendly bacteria in the gut, *Lactobacillus acidophillus*, is especially effective against candida. Some strains of *Lactobacillus* produce hydrogen peroxide, and this chemical, in turn, kills *Candida albicans*. What's more, *Lactobacillus acidophillus* creates a more acidic environment in the intestinal tract—an environment that discourages candida growth. You can obtain *Lactobacillus acidophillus* from probiotic health supplements or by consuming yogurt, kefir, or breast milk (admittedly, this extremely healthy substance isn't available to everyone). Far from being harmful, naturally fermented foods such as real kefir, sauerkraut, and miso can be helpful against candida. Vinegar and foods that contain vinegar are not naturally fermented and thus should be avoided.

The Macrobiotic Diet

The macrobiotic diet is a mostly vegetarian, low-fat, high-fiber diet with an emphasis on whole grains and cooked vegetables. The diet is touted as a way to prevent heart disease and certain types of cancer. It is supposed to produce a feeling of well-being in people who follow it. Dieters eat whole food. Processed foods are forbidden, as are meat, poultry, and all dairy products.

The diet is based on ideas from Taoist Chinese philosophy. The Taoists believe that the universe is animated by the interplay of two primal life forces, yin and yang. Yin and yang complement and counterbalance each other. The purpose of the macrobiotic diet is to bring yin and yang into balance. Some foods fall in the yin and some in the yang category. Because brown rice and whole grains are considered the most "balancing" foods, they constitute the bulk of the diet. Foods that are "too yin" or "too yang" are prohibited. Warm drinks, for example, are considered "too yang." Meat and dairy products also fall into the "too yang" category. Alcohol, sugary foods, coffee, and strong spices are considered "too yin" and are forbidden.

The diet lays down strict guidelines as to how much of each type of food can be eaten. The guidelines are as follows: 50 percent whole cereal grains, 25 percent vegetables, 15 percent beans and sea vegetables, and 10 percent soups and miscellaneous foods.

People who follow the macrobiotic diet run the same long-term health risks as vegans, the vegetarians who do not eat eggs or dairy products. The macrobiotic diet is deficient in vitamin B_{12}, vitamin D, calcium, zinc, magnesium, and riboflavin. Studies have shown that infants who consume the macrobiotic diet suffer from anemia, iron deficiencies, and growth retardation. In infants, the diet has also been linked to rickets, a disease of skeletal deformities and weakened bones that is associated with calcium and vitamin D deficiencies.

From the point of view of gastrointestinal health, the problem with the macrobiotic diet is its recommendation that 50 percent of food come from grains. In other words, 50 percent of the diet comprises starch. As we emphasize time and time again in this book, starch is deleterious to optimal gastrointestinal health.

The Balanced Macronutrient Ratios Diet

The balanced macronutrient ratios, or Zone, diet advocates eating the macronutrients—carbohydrates, protein, and fat—in a 40-30-30 percent ratio. The goal is to get 40 percent of your calories from carbohydrate, 30 percent from protein, and 30 percent from fat. (By contrast, the food pyramid recommends a diet of 10 to15 percent protein, 55 to 60 percent carbohydrates, and the remainder of the calories from fat. By the way, livestock farmers also use these ratios as a formula for fattening swine!) Promoters of the balanced macronutrient ratios diet claim that you will lose weight, live longer, and lower your chances of getting heart disease. The diet is sometimes called the 40-30-30 diet or the Zone Diet. The diet was created by Dr. Barry Sears and promoted in his popular "Zone" books.

The premise of the diet is that reducing one's carbohydate intake to 40 percent and increasing one's protein intake to 30 percent produces a more balanced biochemical state in the body. Dr. Sears's diet focuses specifically on two hormones: insulin, the fat-storing hormone; and glucagon, the fat-releasing hormone. The diet focuses as well on a group of short-acting bioactive chemicals known as eicosanoids. Eicosanoids are involved in a multitude of bodily functions. Insulin levels and the types of fat in the diet have a strong influence on the production of eicosanoids.

The Zone books are important because they were the first to sound the alarm about the danger of carbohydrate overconsumption. Like other dietary programs, however, the Zone Diet doesn't address the quality of the food you eat. As long as you eat in the proper 40-30-30 proportions, it doesn't matter whether you eat a bagel with lox and cream cheese or a grilled free-range steak with green beans and a large salad on the side. In other words, the diet is about quantity, not quality. In fact, the diet's critics argue that people lose weight on the diet not because of the 40-30-30 ratios, but because they eat less than they did before.

Another issue with the Zone Diet is Dr. Sears's recommendation of soy protein isolates. In no uncertain terms, the authors of the book you are reading abhor soy protein isolates. Soy is a highly allergenic, inferior protein source. Soy also contains high levels of phytic acid, a substance that can bind to minerals such as calcium, magnesium, and iron and make them impossible for the body to absorb. Soy also inhibits digestive enzymes from doing their job. In so doing, it impairs overall digestion and nutrient absorption. As we emphasize throughout this book, the best way to obtain protein is through traditional high-quality sources. In other words, get your protein from meat, poultry, fish, eggs, and fermented dairy products.

A corollary to the Zone's soy protein recommendation is Dr. Sears' passionate avoidance of foods that contain arachidonic acid. This acid is a naturally occurring substance. It is found in high concentrations in many animal products, including butter, egg yolks, beef, and organ meats. Arachidonic acid can also be made by the body. The body ultimately uses arachidonic acid to form a group of eicosanoids, the short-acting biochemicals that promote inflammation. Dr. Sears's theory goes like this: Avoiding dietary arachidonic acid lowers the level of inflammatory eicosanoids in the body, which promotes better health. Avoiding arachidonic acid is the main reason why the Zone Diet is such a big proponent of soy protein. Soy protein does not contain arachodonic acid. Lowering the inflammatory eicosanoids in the body is an essential goal, especially for people with active bowel disease, but no evidence suggests that avoiding dietary arachodonic acid will achieve this goal. The best way to manage the biological levels of arachadonic acid is to reduce the levels of insulin. As Chapter 3 explained, you can do that by restricting the amount of carbohydrates you eat and correctly balancing the omega-6 and omega-3 essential fatty acids in your diet. Moreover, some arachadonic acid in the diet is vital for essential bodily functions, including the health of the brain.

The Blood Type Diet

The blood type diet is actually four different diets. The diet is based on the premise that the majority of your nutritional needs are predetermined by your blood type classification (O, A, B, or AB). While diets based on blood type, metabolic type, cultural origins, and so on have existed in the alternative health community for years, few diets have had the popular success of the blood type diet. The diet was promoted by Peter D'Adamo, N.D., and popularized in his best-selling book *Eat Right for Your Type* (Putnam, 1997).

The theory behind the diet goes something like this: The earliest humans, who all had type O blood, ate a diet composed mostly of animal foods, especially the meat of large herbivorous mammals. They ate very little or no grain. Modern people with type O blood are the descendants of these initial cavemen and they require large amounts of meat in their diets. Type O's, like the hunters from whom they descend, must exercise vigorously to burn off fat. People with type A blood are the descendants of agrarian humans who appeared after the cavemen. These more docile people do well on a diet of vegetables and fruit and require moderate exercise to maintain their health. Type A's don't produce enough hydrochloric acid in their stomachs, so they are advised to avoid meat and dairy products. Type B's are the descendants of nomadic herders who walked the earth sampling different diets as they went along. Type B's thrive on dairy products—their ancestors were herders after all—and require only moderate exercise. Last come people with type AB blood.

They do not handle meat well and instead should eat fish, grains, and soy-based foods.

The blood type diet places a lot of emphasis on substances known as lectins. Lectins are specialized proteins found on the surface of grains, cereals, and especially beans. In the test tube, lectins can cause some types of cells and molecules to stick together and agglutinate. In blood banks, one of the procedures for determining blood type is to combine purified lectins with a blood sample and observe whether cells agglutinate. Advocates of the blood type diet believe that certain lectins are incompatible with certain blood types. The diet blames lectins for many ailments, including kidney failure, arthrosclerosis, and food allergies.

The scientific community along with many nutritionists in alternative circles has been very critical of this fad diet. The diet's thesis that blood types evolved based on nutritional needs is completely unfounded. No anthropological evidence backs up the thesis. The origin of blood type differentiation is not known, but many theorize that differences in blood types occurred in response to resistance against certain types of infectious diseases.

The role of lectins in the diet has also come under fire from the scientific community. While it is true that lectins cause blood to agglutinate in test tubes, what happens to lectins in the human body is another story. Very few lectins are absorbed intact into the digestive system because, by the time they arrive in the digestive system, they have been broken down and can no longer function as lectins. Cooking food also breaks down proteins, lectins included.

In defense of the blood type diet, however, it could be said that the diet is the proverbial right train on the wrong track. Mounting scientific evidence indicates that certain lectins may be deleterious to your health. The lectins found in beans and legumes have been linked to rheumatoid arthritis in certain genetically susceptible individuals. However, the genetic link between lectins and arthritis is very complex and goes well beyond the matter of simple blood type. Avoiding certain dietary lectins appears to be evolving as an important nutritional approach for reducing bodily inflammation. However, basing these dietary avoidances on blood type appears to be without merit.

What accounts for the success of the blood type diet in many people's eyes? The blood type diet is essentially a low-calorie, healthy diet. People who take in fewer calories naturally lose weight. And like all the diets critiqued in this chapter, the blood type diet urges its devotees to lay off junk food, sugar, and white flour. Lay off those items, get a little exercise, and you are bound to lose weight and feel healthier.

The Ketogenic Diet

The Atkins, Scarsdale, and Protein Power diets are examples of ketogenic diets. These diets call for eating little or no carbohydrates. Like fasting (and starving, for that matter), not eating carbohydrates induces a physical state called *ketosis* in which the body's metabolism slows down and hunger urges are suppressed. In ketosis, the body is starved of glucose from carbohydrates, so it resorts to fat reserves for energy. To be exact, it resorts to *ketones,* the chemicals that the body produces from fat. Between hunger suppression, consuming fewer calories, and burning fat reserves, people on the ketogenic diet lose weight. Some promoters of the diet even claim that you can eat all the fat you want and still lose weight thanks to the effects of ketosis. Needless to say, being able to eat all the fat you want and still lose weight is a seemingly attractive proposition to most people.

In prehistoric times, humans often ate ketogenic diets during periods of starvation and in the wintertime when plant food was scarce and they had to subsist on animal fats and their own fat reserves. More modern people of the northern latitudes, such as the Inuit, have done the same. So the diet isn't unprecedented and the body is capable of being on the ketogenic diet without substantial harm for certain periods of time. Under the supervision of a knowledgeable physician, a ketogenic diet can be used to manage a host of illnesses, including obesity, GI disorders, childhood epilepsy, and certain types of brain tumors.

The problem with the popular version of the ketogenic diet is that it caters to current taste and whim and is not discriminate enough in its food choices. In general, ketogenic diets are not as much high-protein as they are high-fat diets. Thus, care must be taken to keep the all-important omega-6 to omega-3 ratio in balance. This is virtually impossible given the dietary suggestions of many of these books.

Also, some of the dietary suggestions are downright appalling. For example, in *Dr. Atkins New Diet Revolution*, Dr. Robert C. Atkins suggests that dieters treat themselves to a heaping helping of pork rinds! He writes: "At the other end of the spectrum is a convenience food that sounds terrible fatty, but in fact, contains nearly none. Those are the maximizers of crispness—fried pork rinds—the zero carbohydrate consolation prize for corn or potato chip addicts. Virtually all the fat has been rendered off, leaving you with the protein matrix that held the pork fat together. Your paté, sour-cream based dips and guacamole find an exceedingly crisp and comfortable home atop a fried pork rind."

The Elimination/Detoxification Diet

The object of the elimination/detoxification diet is to cleanse the body of toxic substances. Promoters of the diet claim that it improves digestion, induces a feeling of calm, and increases vitality and stamina. To cleanse the body, dieters do the following:

- Eat "clean" foods, which do not introduce new toxins or produce allergic reactions.
- Eat foods that encourage regular bowel movements. Apart from sweating, the body "eliminates" toxins in the feces and the urine.
- Eat foods that promote better blood circulation. Enhanced blood circulation hastens the metabolism and absorption of food.
- Eat foods that boost the function of the liver. The liver is the most important organ for detoxification.

The diet is sometimes a prelude to food-sensitivity testing. After dieters follow the elimination/detoxification diet for one or two weeks, the foods to which they may be allergic are gradually introduced. In this way, starting from a clean slate, dieters can find out to which foods they are allergic.

The elimination/detoxification diets vary, but all recommend the avoidance of foods that are rich in protein. Dieters eat fruits, vegetables, and foods such as onions and garlic, which are helpful to the liver. Rice and fortified rice products are often offered as a main "protein" source. Of course, the diet calls for people to drink water and sugar-free beverages to encourage the elimination of toxins by way of the urine.

The elimination/detoxification diet is very old. The ancient Greeks practiced it as part of their religious rituals. Prior to consulting an oracle, a pilgrim would purify himself by fasting and drinking water for several days. Among the upper classes of Europe in the nineteenth century, it was fashionable to visit spas, where bathers drank mineral water and ate cleansing food.

There are an inordinate number of variations of the elimination/detoxification diet and to comment on them all would be impractical. In general, they can be said to be of some benefit in the short run, but to be deleterious if adopted for any length of time. Also, as should be clear by now, we are very unimpressed with any diet plan that emphasizes nonanimal sources of protein.

The Rotation Diet

The rotation diet, also called the rotary diversified diet, is a diagnostic tool for finding out to which foods you are allergic or sensitive. The diet is for people who suspect they are allergic or sensitive to more than one food. Food allergies can be mysterious. Stress and a lack of sleep can make an allergic reaction worse than it would otherwise be. There is also an element of paranoia in food allergies. As every doctor who treats gastrointestinal ailments can tell you, some patients claim to be allergic to every type of food.

In the typical rotation diet, rotations occur every four days. For example, on Monday you eat a certain type of flour, vegetable, starch, fruit, and oil. On Tuesday it's a different flour, vegetable, starch, fruit, and oil. Same goes for Wednesday and Thursday. On Friday, a new cycle begins, and you eat the same flour, vegetable, starch, fruit, and oil that you ate on Monday. By rotating foods this way, you know precisely what you ate and you can gauge your reaction to each kind of food. You can find out to which foods you are sensitive or allergic.

The rotation diet is fine as far as it goes, but it doesn't address the underlying problem. Are your symptoms due to a true food allergy or to poor digestion, bacterial fermentation, leaky gut, or something similar? We believe that the Guts and Glory Program can strengthen your body so that you can overcome allergies by bringing your intestinal flora into the proper balance, healing your gastrointestinal tract, and strengthening your immune system. Having been allergic to more than fifty different foods, coauthor Jordan Rubin is living proof that bringing your intestinal flora into balance prevents food allergies.

The R-Diet

The R-diet is given to patients in hospitals. We describe it here for readers who have gastrointestinal disorders and have been admitted to the hospital. The diet is called the R-diet because hospital diets are formulated by registered dieticians (the diet could just as well be called the vicious cycle diet or the nonspecific carbohydrate diet). The diet is high in sugar and low in fiber. Most of the food is white—white bread, English muffins, pasta, cream of wheat, and the like. The R-diet is high in carbohydrates, especially in disaccharides, the two-sugar-molecule carbohydrate that is difficult to digest.

If you have spent any time with this book, you know that the R-diet is the opposite of the Guts and Glory Program. Whereas the diet that we advocate is low in calories and higher in nutrients, the R-diet is high in calories and low in nutrients. The very same foods that the R-diet prescribes are the ones that cause the gastrointestinal tract to become upset. From the standpoint of gastrointestinal health, the R-diet poses many problems:

- The disaccharides in starchy foods are difficult to digest. They remain in the gut, where they feed the unfriendly bacteria that cause intestinal disease.
- Because many patients who are hospitalized due to bowel disease are underweight or at risk of losing weight, the diet is high in sugar and fat. But sugar can ferment in the gut and feed the unfriendly bacteria. What's more, sugar dulls the immune system. It keeps the immune system from being wide awake.
- The R-diet is low in fiber to keep food from getting hung up in the intestinal tract. But the right kind of fiber can be good for people with gastrointestinal disorders, particularly people with constipation.

The R-diet is especially damaging in light of the fact that many hospital patients are on some kind of antibiotic. Antibiotics kill all bacteria in the gut, including the friendly bacteria that are necessary for intestinal health. An ideal hospital diet would provide properly fermented yogurt and probiotic supplements to help reinoculate the gut with healthy bacteria. The R-diet does no such thing. GI patients, some of whom are on prednisone, run an even greater risk from the R-diet. Prednisone promotes an alkaline pH in the bowel, which encourages the growth of unfriendly bacteria and fungi, including *Candida albicans.*

What can you do if you find yourself in a hospital room and you are being force-fed the R-diet? Talk to your doctor about going on a diet that promotes intestinal health and have food brought in from outside the hospital.

More Problematic Programs

So far, this chapter has looked at problematic diets. But diets aren't the only way to treat digestive illnesses. The rest of this chapter looks at problematic programs, unusual therapies, and a couple of contraptions that are supposed to improve your health.

Overall, our objection to these programs has to do with the fact that they are new and relatively untested. One of the theses of this book is that we can learn from our ancestors. By adopting their diet, we can regain our health. By trying insofar as we can to adopt the primitive lifestyle, we can restore our vigor and strength. We believe that historically based, commonsense nutrition is the key to good health, not newfangled medicines or procedures. The programs we introduce here have worked for some people. We do not deny that. But unlike the dietary principles we espouse in this book, these programs have not been tested by the fullness of time.

IV and Injectable Vitamin and Mineral Therapies

The purpose of vitamin and mineral IVs and injections is to deliver large amounts of nutrients to the body and to do so by bypassing the digestive tract. As part of his treatment for Crohn's disease, co-author Jordan Rubin took upwards of 20 grams a day of vitamin C intravenously. Jordan also injected adrenal cortical extract, or ACE, a substance derived from the adrenal glands of cows and sheep. ACE is supposed to prevent allergies, treat adrenal insufficiency, and be an anti-inflammatory agent. (In 1978, the FDA warned that ACE is obsolete and ineffective.)

As a therapy for bowel disease, IV and injectable vitamin and mineral treatments don't have much to offer. IV treatments are necessary in extreme cases for rehydration, but they can't heal your gut. In fact, ascorbic acid (vitamin C) in large doses seems to destroy intestinal flora and wreck havoc on the bowels. In theory, ascorbic acid shouldn't destroy intestinal flora when it is taken intravenously or by injection because it doesn't pass through the digestive tract. In practice, however, large doses of ascorbic acid seem to damage the intestinal flora no matter how they are delivered.

Moreover, large doses of vitamins and minerals may be dangerous. When vitamins are delivered in food, the body takes only the vitamins it needs, but when vitamins are injected, delivered intravenously, or taken orally, the body is force-fed the vitamins and minerals. What happens when the body is bombarded with vitamins and minerals is not well understood. Nobody really knows the long-term consequences of taking large doses of vitamins.

Some scientists argue that synthetic or fractionated vitamins and minerals made in the laboratory are a far cry from the natural nutrients in food. These scientists believe that vitamins and other nutrients cannot be properly absorbed except in their natural form. Writes Judith DeCava in her *The Real Truth About Vitamins and Antioxidants* (A Printery, 1997): "The human body cannot use, in a nutritional manner, chemically pure, synthetic, mirror-image vitamins as it does the natural vitamin complexes which readily find their way into the normal chemical actions and changes (biochemistry) essential to energy, growth, repair, function, and sustenance of life. Therefore, a synthetic vitamin can only be used for a drug effect: it can mask or cover over symptoms, but does not alleviate the cause of the illness, disease, insult, or injury."

To correct underlying nutritional deficiencies, the authors of this book advocate consuming nutrient-dense whole foods along with whole-food supplements such as green superfoods. By eating the foods that are highlighted in the Guts and Glory Program (see Chapter 9), you are assured of getting optimal amounts of the essential nutrients.

Oxygenation Therapies

The oxygenation therapies include ozone therapy and hydrogen peroxide therapy. The idea behind these therapies is that diseases are brought about when body tissues do not get enough oxygen. Cells that are deprived of oxygen may degenerate or become cancerous. In oxygenation therapy, the patient is bombarded with oxygen. The therapies are based on the work of Otto Warburg, the winner of the 1931 Nobel Prize in Medicine, who noticed that cancer cells and microbes cannot live in an oxygen-rich environment.

In ozone therapy, patients take medical ozone, or triatomic oxygen, a more concentrated form of oxygen. Ozone—the same stuff found in the upper atmosphere—is created in the laboratory. Using ultraviolet light, the molecules of oxygen (O_2) are converted into ozone (O_3). Promoters of the therapy are fond of calling their ozone "activated oxygen" or "charged oxygen." They claim that ozone therapy strengthens the immune system, improves the blood circulation, and delivers healing oxygen to the organs and tissues. In ozone therapy, patients breath ozone, take ozone saunas and baths, drink ozone in their water, take ozone enemas, or wear ozone body suits.

Similar to ozone therapy, hydrogen peroxide therapy is a way of delivering healing oxygen to the body. Hydrogen peroxide (H_2O_2) gives off oxygen as it decomposes. Most people know hydrogen peroxide as a disinfectant for treating cuts. Promoters of hydrogen peroxide therapy believe it can kill viruses, fungi, and bacteria in the body. People take hydrogen peroxide by drinking it, bathing in it, gargling with it, or injecting it intravenously. The hydrogen peroxide used in oxygenation therapy is not the same kind that is found in medicine cabinets. If you are interested in this therapy, be sure to consult a physician.

The oxygenation therapies fall decidedly in the alternative category. They are experimental. Whether oxygen prevents or inhibits the growth of cancer cells is open to debate. Some people argue that a negligible amount of oxygen is delivered during a therapy session, so it doesn't matter at all whether oxygenation therapy works. By the way, promoters of oxygenation therapy sometimes claim that it is sanctioned in Germany, where the therapy is fairly popular. However, the therapy is not sanctioned in Germany by any governmental body.

Photoluminescence

Photoluminesence is also known as ultraviolet blood irradiation and photo-oxidation therapy. In this treatment, the patient's blood is drawn into a cuvette and exposed to ultraviolet light. Among other things, the promoters of the therapy claim that it stimulates the immune system, has anti-inflammatory effects, and helps the body metabolize cholesterol. The ultraviolet rays are supposed to kill bacteria, viruses, and fungi. Photoluminesence has been approved by the FDA for the treatment of cutaneous T-cell lymphoma. It has been practiced since the 1930s. In his book *Into the Light* (Second

Opinion Publishing, 1996), Dr. William Campbell Douglas explains the treatment in detail.

Whatever its merits, photoluminescence is not meant for people who suffer from bowel disorders. We do not recommend it. Furthermore, a fair amount of expertise is needed to conduct the procedure. The equipment must be sterilized. If you decide to try this therapy, make sure you do so under the care of a licensed practitioner.

Frequency Therapy

Frequency therapy was invented in the 1930s by a maverick scientist from San Diego named Royal Raymond Rife. Rife believed that radio waves set to the right frequency could destroy different kinds of viruses and bacteria in much the same way that opera singers can shatter glass with their singing voices. Rife determined which radio frequencies—he called them mortal oscillatory rates, or MORs—could kill which disease-causing organisms. By tuning a machine he invented called the Rife Frequency Generator to the right frequency, Rife believed he could target and kill different bacteria and viruses. According to Barry Lynes's *The Cancer Cure That Worked: Fifty Years of Suppression* (Marcus Books, 1987), government agents destroyed Rife's records on behalf of the medical establishment in the 1950s!

Royal Raymond Rife and the Rife ray treatment (as frequency therapy is sometimes known) have all the trappings of an *X-Files* episode, but a handful of people in alternative medicine consider Rife a misunderstood genius. Several clinics offer frequency therapy. Rife frequency generators are marketed under a bunch of different names: the TINS machine, the Zapper, and others. The machine can be purchased over the Internet and used by patients in their homes.

Frequency therapy is difficult to administer. No procedure for administering it has been established. We include it in this book as a sort of benchmark. If you are riding the hamster wheel of alternative medicine and you have begun to consider frequency therapy, we respectfully suggest that your journey has taken you to the far fringes of alternative medicine and perhaps it is time to follow ET's example and "come home." Whatever its merits in the eyes of some people, the Rife Frequency Generator has not demonstrated any large-scale efficacy against gastrointestinal disorders.

DMSO

Dimethyl sulfoxide, or DMSO as it is better known, is an antioxidant. An antioxidant is a substance that slows the decay of tissues by oxygen. Antioxidants do their work by hunting down and destroying free radicals, the molecules that cause oxidation. Natural antioxidants include vitamin C and beta-carotene. Besides being an antioxidant, DMSO is a topical painkiller. It is used on strains and cuts. It has been used to treat swelling, arthritis, skin ulcers, and burns. In one double-blind, randomized study, it was used to successfully treat patients with ulcerative colitis.

More than ten thousand articles about DMSO have been published in scientific journals. In the United States, the FDA has approved DMSO for preserving transplant organs and for treating interstitial cystitis and bladder disease. Many physicians argue that DMSO should be used more widely. However, the drug's rotten-egg odor more so than opposition from the FDA may be the reason why it is not widely used. DMSO smells disagreeably of sulfur. Whether patients take it orally or topically, their breath soon smells of sulfur. Interestingly, the powerful odor has made experimenting with DMSO difficult. In double-blind studies, patients are given a drug or a placebo without knowing which they have been given. In the case of DMSO, patients always know whether they are getting the drug or the placebo. The odor of DMSO is pungent and unmistakable.

Without resorting to DMSO, you can obtain sulfur in your diet by eating high-protein foods such as meat, eggs, and poultry. Sulfur is plentiful in egg yolks. You can also obtain sulfur from onions, garlic, cabbage, Brussels sprouts, turnips, and kale.

Colon Therapy

Colon therapy refers to the cleansing of the colon by repeatedly and gently flushing it with water. The therapy goes by many different names: colonic, colon lavage, colon irrigation, high colonic, and colon hydrotherapy. Waste material that remains in the colon can putrefy and become toxic. It can leak through the intestinal wall into the bloodstream. A buildup of waste matter on the wall of the colon can also inhibit peristalsis, the rhythmic flexing of the intestinal muscles by which the feces are expelled. The object of colon therapy is to clean the colon, detoxify it, and restore it to good health.

For severe constipation, we recommend colon therapy. The therapy can also be beneficial for people who have functional bowel disorders or weak intestinal muscles and cannot expel feces. People who are flaring or have inflammatory bowel disease, however, should not undergo colon therapy because they run the risk of perforating the colon wall. In fact, anyone with an acute bowel disorder should forgo colon therapy. Make sure that the person from whom you're getting the colon therapy is a member of the International Association of Colon Therapists (IACT), or is otherwise certified to give the procedure.

Another form of colon therapy is the coffee enema. This therapy is designed to detoxify the liver. Caffeine in the form of coffee travels up the hemorrhoidal vein to the portal vein and from there to the liver. It stimulates the liver and gall bladder to discharge bile. Coffee, it seems, enhances the liver's ability to detoxify. Until 1972, the prestigious *Merck Manual,* the handbook for doctors in the United States, included a description of coffee enemas. The rules about colon therapy also apply to enemas and coffee enemas. If you are flaring or have inflammatory bowel disease, you should avoid enemas.

❖ 7 ❖

Troublesome Tests and Tenuous Techniques

T his chapter is for people who have digestive problems and must
sort through the various therapies and diagnostic techniques.
In this chapter, you will find our assessments of a dozen or
more troublesome tests and tenuous techniques. Some of these tests
and techniques are more troublesome and tenuous than others.
They are described here to help you, along with your physician,
decide what the best course of treatment is.

Applied Kinesiology

Applied kinesiology (AK) is a muscle-testing therapy technique. It
is popular with some chiropractors in the United States. AK borrows ideas from traditional Chinese medicine. Practitioners believe
that a life-energy called Qi (pronounced CHEE) moves through
channels called meridians in the body. If the Qi is blocked or congested, a disease, allergy, or other untoward consequence can result.
Acupuncturists stick needles in the meridian points to unlock and
redirect the flow of Qi.

In applied kinesiology, the practitioner applies gentle pressure
to an identifier muscle and notes the result. Practitioners are trained
to isolate different muscles and muscle groups for testing. If the
muscle is spongy and yields easily, the meridian to which it is linked

may be blocked or congested, and this can signal a problem in an organ or gland. AK practitioners believe that weakness in each muscle is associated with a certain disease or organ dysfunction. After the initial diagnosis, the AK practitioner may massage the acupuncture meridians to unblock the Qi. Some practitioners prescribe nutrients and health supplements. Applied kinesiology was developed by a chiropractor named George J. Goodheart, Jr. in the 1960s. It is sometimes called bio-kinesiology, behavioral kinesiology, or just kinesiology.

Applied kinesiology is not an exact science. Putting aside the question of whether the meridians exist and whether Qi influences the functioning of the organs and glands, muscle testing by itself is a tenuous activity. Muscle fatigue on the part of the patient, the amount of leverage and force used by the practitioner, and a host of other variables make AK unreliable. In our experience, AK provides very subjective results. Different practitioners get different test results. AK cannot be universally learned or applied accurately. For these reasons, AK should not be relied on as a valid form of diagnosis.

By the way, kinesiology is the study of physical activity. Kinesiologists study muscular mechanics as they relate to the movement of the human body. Applied kinesiology is something else altogether.

Biological Terrain Assessment

In biological terrain assessment (BTA), urine, blood, and saliva specimens are analyzed using the BTA S-2000 computer software program with an eye toward understanding the patient's biochemistry. The idea behind BTA is to look for the underlying causes of disease by examining a patient's health on the biochemical level. BTA practitioners claim that the tests can detect diseases in the early stages long before the patients exhibit outward signs. Practitioners say they can monitor a patient's biochemical environment and in so doing are able to prescribe treatments that truly help the patient.

Urine, blood, and saliva are measured for their reduction oxidation (redox) values, pH balance, and resistivity:

- *Redox values.* The number of electrons. Electrons are needed to combat oxidative stress, the damage that free radicals do to body tissue. They also play a role in creating and storing energy in the form of adenosine triphosphate (ATP).
- *pH balance.* Acidity versus alkalinity. This measurement tells whether nutrients are being properly absorbed and enzymes are functioning properly.
- *Resistivity.* The body's resistance to the flow of electrical current, a measure of mineral concentrations. A high concentration of minerals can mean that the body is dehydrated. A low concentration may indicate the onset of osteoporosis.

The critics of BTA argue that the tests aren't as sophisticated as their promoters make them out to be. They contend that standard blood and urine analyses can accomplish more than the BTA tests. The only advantage of the BTA tests, the critics insist, is the sophisticated computer readouts and charts which make it easier for the doctor and patient to examine the test results.

Comprehensive Digestive Stool Analysis

Many laboratories, including the Great Smokies Diagnostic Laboratory of Asheville, North Carolina, offer a comprehensive digestive stool analysis (CDSA) that consists of eighteen different tests. The analysis is very popular with complementary and alternative practitioners. It measures absorption, the intestinal environment, digestion, and intestinal function. For an extra fee, the analysis also tests for parasites. The analysis is meant to help physicians identify and treat gastrointestinal diseases. The CDSA includes tests in these broad categories:

- *Absorption.* Tests for cholesterol, long-chain fatty acids, and total short-chain fatty acids.
- *Intestinal environment.* Tests for dysbiosis, friendly bacteria (lactobacillus, bifidobacterium, and others) and unfriendly bacteria (salmonella, vibrio, and others), as well as yeasts.
- *Digestion (or maldigestion).* Tests for triglycerides (a dietary fat),

undigested meat and vegetable fibers, pH, and fecal chymotrypsin (a measure of pancreatic insufficiency).

◆ *Intestinal function.* Tests for fecal color, mucus, blood, and imbalanced intestinal flora.

The CDSA can be a useful analysis, but it is expensive and not covered by most insurance policies. From the standpoint of the primitive diet, our quarrel with this test has to do with its definition of "normal." We believe that a diet high in carbohydrates from grains is unhealthy and therefore not normal. The microbial population in the gut of a person who consumes the foods recommended in the Guts and Glory Program is very different from the microbial population that the CDSA considers healthy or normal. What's more, we do not share the CDSA's ideas about which bacteria are friendly and which are unfriendly. In our experience, the analysis often doesn't correlate with the symptoms our patients and clients report. Patients who suffer from gas and bloating sometimes get a good CDSA, for example, and patients who report minor GI problems sometimes get a terrible CDSA. Finally, the environment of the gut is constantly changing. Tests like the CDSA should always be considered in light of the fact that stool sample analyses can measure only gut health at a particular moment in time. These tests can never be entirely conclusive.

Contact Reflex Analysis

Contact reflex analysis (CRA) advertises itself as a way of identifying the nutritional deficiencies that cause illness. After a diagnosis, patients are almost invariably given a nutritional product made by a Wisconsin-based company called Standard Process Labs. The majority of people who practice CRA are chiropractors.

Dick A. Versendaal, D.C., the developer and chief promoter of CRA, compares the nervous system to a computer with thousands of miles of electrical wires. The wires connect every organ, gland, and body tissue. The wires also connect with each other at "fuses" or "breaker switches" that he calls reflex points. By testing one of the eighty reflex points that Versendaal has identified, a CRA practitioner can monitor the health of a particular part of the body. To conduct a test, the practitioner places one finger on a reflex point and pulls on the patient's outstretched arm. If the arm can be pulled down, the disease corresponding to the reflex point in question is present. Writes Versendaal, "By contacting these reflexes, using the body's muscular system as an indicator, we are able to monitor the function of body systems."

CRA is one of those testing procedures that gives alternative medicine a hokey, bad name. In general, we recommend avoiding contact reflex analysis as a primary tool for dispensing dietary and supplement advice.

Electrodermal Screening

Electrodermal screening, or EDS, is an East-meets-West technique for measuring the energy flow in the meridians of the body and for diagnosing a patient's health. The term *meridian* comes from traditional Chinese medicine. The life energy Qi flows through the body's meridian channels, according to traditional Chinese medicine. Acupuncturists examine the body's meridian points—the places where the Qi is concentrated—in their diagnoses. If they discover that the Qi is congested or needs redirecting, they insert a needle in the proper meridian point. Because the meridians carry the Qi to and from the internal organs, acupuncturists can heal the internal organs by inserting needles in the correct meridian points.

Electrodermal screening was invented in the 1950s by a German acupuncturist named Dr. Reinhardt Voll. Dr. Voll was engaged in mapping the acupuncture points electronically when he became interested in measuring the electrical resistance and the polarization of the different acupuncture points and meridians. The doctor created a metering machine called the Dermatron for measuring the electrical resistance. Using the machine, he devised a system for examining the different organs by means of their meridians. A reading of 50 on the Dermatron showed that the internal organ associated with a meridian was healthy. But a reading below 45 indicated "organ stagnation and degeneration," while a reading above 55 meant that the organ associated with the meridian being measured was inflamed.

Since Dr. Voll's initial studies, the Dermatron has been refined. Present-day Dermatrons—including the Computron, the Listen System, and the Biotron—are capable of detailed computer analyses of different aspects of health. Electrodermal screening also goes by the name electro-acupuncture (Dr. Voll's name for the procedure), bio-energy regulatory technique (BER), bio-energetic testing, and bio-resonance therapy (BRT).

Coauthor Jordan Rubin underwent electrodermal screening with ten different practitioners. EDS is not an exact science. One practitioner told Jordan he was allergic to one thing and another said he was allergic to something else. Each practitioner, it seemed, performed electrodermal screening in a different way. Once again, EDS appears to be a very subjective method of screening. While many respected physicians use EDS as a helpful tool in determining the etiology of a disease, we recommend avoiding it as a primary diagnostic tool.

Enzyme Potentiated Desensitization

Enzyme potentiated desensitization (EPD) is a technique for relieving allergies and chemical sensitivities. It has also been used to treat eczema, asthma, rhinitis, and other inflammatory diseases. To become desensitized to the foods to which they are allergic, patients are given skin injections with very small amounts of an allergen mixed with the enzyme beta-glucuronidase. Through repeat exposure to small amounts of the allergen, the patient's sensitivity is gradually reduced. The beta-glucuronidase enzyme is injected along with the allergen because this enzyme is released in the tissues during an allergic reaction.

In the immune system, helper T-cells, a type of white blood cell, mark the bacteria, toxins, and other invaders so they can be destroyed. An allergic reaction to food occurs because helper T-cells mistakenly mark a certain type of food as an invader. According to its backers, EPD works by reeducating the helper T-cells. During the treatment, white blood cells called T-suppressor cells disable the miscoded helper T-cells to keep them from instigating an allergic reaction.

In England, where allergy shots are responsible for twenty-five to thirty deaths per year, EPD has become the preferred treatment for relieving allergies. Still, the treatment is tenuous and not enough is known about it at this time to recommend it. EPD is sometimes called low dose immunotherapy (LDI).

Food Allergy Tests

All allergies, food allergies included, are caused by an autoimmune reaction. *Autoimmune* describes when the immune system is over-stimulated and attacks the body. Food allergies are brought on when the immune system thinks mistakenly that a certain kind of food is harmful. When the allergic person eats the food, his or her immune system manufactures immunoglobulin E (IgE) antibodies. These antibodies, in turn, react to the food and cause the immune system to release large amounts of histamines and mediator chemicals to protect the body. The result is an allergic reaction—difficulty breathing, rashes, pruritus, joint pain, vomiting, a swelling of the throat, and an increased heart rate. In dire cases, allergic reactions can bring about a loss of consciousness and sometimes death. Food allergies are different from food intolerances. For a discussion of the differences, see page 178.

Fortunately, most people outgrow their food allergies, although allergies to fish, shellfish, and certain kinds of nuts appear to last a lifetime. Allergies can be mysterious. Most doctors who treat gastro-intestinal disease have met at least one patient who is allergic to all foods. However, according to studies conducted by Dr. Scott Sicherer of the Mt. Sinai School of Medicine, 25 percent of people who believe they have a food allergy don't really have one. Only 6 percent of children and 1 to 2 percent of adults have a genuine food allergy. And most adults who have food allergies are allergic to only four foods: peanuts, tree nuts, shellfish, and fish.

❖❖

ALLERGIES VERSUS FOOD INTOLERANCES

An allergy is a specific biological response that is mediated by the immune system. The symptoms of allergies include itching, hives, rashes, swelling, and gastrointestinal upset. The symptoms usually appear a short time after the food is consumed. Allergies can be readily identified by allergy skin testing.

Not all negative reactions to food are caused by allergies. In fact, most negative reactions are not caused by allergies but by food intolerances. Food intolerances and reactions are usually not mediated through the immune system. For that reason, they do not show up on tests that use an immunologic reaction as the basis of detection. Food intolerances are probably mediated by a number of different processes. The most likely culprits, however, are improper digestion, specific enzyme deficiencies, and bacterial fermentation in the gut.

Before you climb aboard the very expensive food allergy testing treadmill, we recommend eating a modified elimination diet to sort out your food sensitivities.

Sometimes doctors fail to consider other causes of allergies apart from food. Dust, animal dander, and molds also cause allergic reactions. High levels of histamine in foods can cause what appears to be an allergic reaction. Wine, cheese, and fish (especially mackerel and tuna) that has not been refrigerated properly are high in histamine. Food poisoning brought on by contaminated meat produces many of the same symptoms as a food allergy.

Pinpointing the foods to which they are allergic can be difficult for people who suffer from allergies. A handful of tests are available for identifying these foods:

- *Cytotoxic testing.* White blood cells are separated from the subject's blood sample and exposed to slides that are coated with various food extracts. The blood cells are examined to see whether they change shape or disintegrate upon contact with the food. The test results vary widely and are considered unreliable.

Cytotoxic testing has been discredited and is banned in some states. The test is also called the ALCAT test, Bryan's test, Metabolic Intolerance Test, and sensitivity testing.

- *Double-blind, placebo-controlled food challenges.* Subjects eat either a placebo food or the food to which they may be allergic. They are monitored for skin rashes and other changes that indicate an allergic reaction. This test is very reliable, but it is very expensive. Doctors must be present throughout the test and emergency medications must be on hand in case of violent reactions.

- *Prick-puncture skin test.* An extract of the food to which the patient may be allergic is placed on the patient's skin. Then the skin is pricked with a needle. If swelling or redness appears, the patient may indeed be allergic. This test is considered reliable only when its result is negative. A positive result is not considered proof of an allergy because positive test results are only accurate 50 percent of the time. The prick-puncture test, at a hundred years old, is the old standby test for allergies.

- *Radioallergosorbent test (RAST).* A blood sample is examined in a test tube to see whether it contains IgE antibodies for different foods. The presence of IgE antibodies means the patient has an allergy. This test is considered more reliable than the prick-puncture test, but again, a positive result is not considered proof of an allergy because test results are not accurate all the time.

According to one theory, some people deal with food allergies by becoming addicted to the foods to which they are allergic. Similar to King Mithradates, who made himself immune to poison by taking small amounts of poison every day, these people unknowingly eat the foods to which they are allergic as a way of making themselves immune to allergic reactions. Dr. James Braly originated this theory in his *Dr. Braly's Food Allergy & Nutrition Revolution* (McGraw-Hill, 1992). According to the doctor, if you crave a food, you may well be allergic to it.

If you believe you are allergic to a certain food, try this simple experiment before you go out of your way to take an expensive allergy test: Avoid the food for five days and then eat it in moderate portions when your stomach is empty. Before and after eating the food, take your pulse. If you are allergic, your pulse rate will quicken by a few beats.

Ultimately, the best way to overcome an allergy is to improve your digestive health and reinoculate your gut with beneficial intestinal flora. By doing so, you will alter the allergens—the parts of food that cause allergic reactions—in your gut in such a way that they no longer will cause allergies. Besides reinoculating the gut, the Guts and Glory program provides nutrients that help strengthen the gut mucosa. Strengthening the gut mucosa can reverse gut hyperpermeability (leaky gut syndrome) and in so doing dramatically reduce allergies and sensitivities.

Hair Mineral Analysis

In hair mineral analysis, a strand of hair is plucked from the nape of the subject's neck and sent to a laboratory to have its mineral content measured. Proponents of the test claim that trace minerals in hair reveal a lot about a person's health. For example, the analysis shows mineral deficiencies and excesses. It also shows whether the subject has been poisoned by heavy metal toxins. Some practitioners claim that hair mineral analysis reveals whether the subject of the test is predisposed to getting certain diseases.

However, critics of hair mineral analysis argue that the analysis is unreliable because too many considerations come into play. For example, the subject's age and gender have to be considered along with the growth rate of the subject's hair. Other considerations include the subject's use of shampoos and hair dyes. Critics point out that hair grows slowly. Hair in a sample may be several weeks old and not indicative of the subject's present state of health.

As early as 1974, the American Medical Association's Committee on Cutaneous Health and Cosmetics reached this conclusion about hair mineral analysis: "The state of health of the body may be entirely unrelated to the physical and chemical condition of the hair

. . . Although severe deficiency states of an essential element are often associated with low concentrations of the element in hair, there are no data that indicate that low concentrations of an element signify low tissue levels nor that high concentrations reflect high tissue stores. Therefore . . . hair metal levels would rarely help a physician select effective treatment."

Nevertheless, with the proper lab analysis and proper practitioner interpretation, useful information can be gleaned from this type of testing. Hair mineral analysis is a good way to screen for toxic exposure as well as dietary trends. The analysis appears especially useful in assessing the body's mineral status. Still, it is unusual for this type of test to be of primary diagnostic value.

Iridology and Sclerology

Iridology, also known as iris diagnosis, is the study of the iris for the purpose of diagnosing the health of the individual. Iridology is based on the idea that nerve endings in the iris are connected to specific parts of the brain and nervous system. By examining the lesions, patterns, and color variations on the iris, you can gauge the body's health. Like iridology, sclerology is the art of gazing into the patient's eye to determine his or her health. Sclerologists, however, gaze at the blood vessels on the sclera (the white portion of the eye), not at the iris. Says iridologist Bernard Jensen D.C. about his craft, "Nature has provided us with a miniature television screen showing the most remote portions of the body by way of nerve reflex responses."

Iridology was the brainchild of Ignatz Von Peczely, a nineteenth-century Hungarian physician. As a youth, Von Peczely nursed an owl with a broken leg back to health. In the course of the treatment, he noticed the black streak in a part of the owl's iris change into a white, crooked line. Thus began his life-long interest in mapping the parts of the iris to the different parts of the body.

The diagnoses made by iridologists and sclerologists are often inconclusive and off-base. Nevertheless, we include iridology and sclerology in this book because they put a strong emphasis on bowel health, which is good. Still, although the eyes are the windows of the soul, you shouldn't take much stock in the opinions of an iridologist or sclerologist.

Live Blood Cell Analysis

In live blood cell analysis, a drop of blood is drawn from the patient's fingertip and examined under a dark-field microscope. In this kind of microscope, the object is illuminated not from the rear but from the sides, so the object stands out in relief against a dark background. The patient and health practitioner examine the blood cells together often by way of a video monitor that has been hooked up to the microscope. The practitioner can supposedly tell by looking at the blood cells how well the patient is absorbing food, whether the patient has vitamin and mineral deficiencies, how stress affects the patient, and a number of other things (the promotional literature on this score is very broad indeed). After reviewing the live blood cell analysis, the practitioner may prescribe a nutritional supplement or some other treatment. Live blood cell analysis is also called nutritional microscopy, nutritional blood analysis, dry blood microscopy, live cell analysis, and dark-field video analysis.

Critics of live blood cell analysis point to a number of faults with the technique:

- A practitioner has to be very skilled to draw conclusions from observing blood cells under a microscope. Practitioners must also be highly qualified to make diagnoses and to recommend treatments based on their conclusions.
- Blood specimens are easy to mishandle. In live blood cell analysis, for example, the specimen is viewed under a glass cover slip. Unless the practitioner is careful, the blood dries quickly, especially near the perimeter of the cover slip.
- Exercise, dehydration, recently consumed fat, and others factors temporarily change the appearance of blood cells. The cells being viewed under the microscope might not be representative of the patient's blood.

➤ Practitioners sometimes point to clumping in the blood cells as evidence of ill health. But blood cells naturally clump together in the confined space of a glass cover slip. In their natural environment, blood cells are pumped at high pressure through the blood vessels and do not clump together nearly as easily.

Live blood cell analysis appears to be another technique that requires a skilled practitioner to be useful. A well-trained and scrupulous microscopist can provide a wealth of information, but the very nature of the test leaves open the opportunity for abuse. What's more, live blood cell analysis seems to be used as a means to sell products. Often the results of the analysis show an illness that can be relieved by a product that the practitioner happens to be selling! As the saying goes, "Let the buyer beware."

Nambudripad Allergy Elimination Technique

The Nambudripad allergy elimination technique (NAET) is an offshoot of applied kinesiology. Like applied kinesiologists, NAET practitioners test special identifier muscles, in this case to find out if the patient is allergic to a certain food. Like applied kinesiology, NAET borrows ideas from traditional Chinese medicine. NAET practitioners believe that allergies are caused by a blockage of Qi, the life energy that flows through the body in meridians. When the brain thinks it is being threatened by an allergen, it blocks the flow of Qi. This blocked Qi energy, unable to find an outlet, is expended as an allergic reaction.

NAET was developed by Devi S. Nambudripad, D.C., an acupuncturist and chiropractor. Afflicted throughout her life by severe allergies, Nambudripad noticed as a student that her allergies were relieved by acupressure. Later, she administered acupuncture to herself while in the presence of carrots, a food to which she was allergic. To her surprise, she ate carrots soon afterward and was not allergic to them. Without realizing it, Nambudripad had hit on a method for treating allergies. While being exposed to a food to which the patient is allergic, the patient is given acupuncture and acupressure to unblock the Qi energy and forestall the allergic reaction.

NAET practitioners test for allergies using methods borrowed from applied kinesiology. The patient holds a food to which he or she may be allergic while the practitioner tests an identifier muscle. If the test shows that the patient is allergic, he or she is given acupuncture and acupressure treatments along the spine to unlock the Qi energy. The patient must refrain from eating the food to which he or she is allergic for the next twenty-four hours. After that time, the patient is tested again to see if he or she still has the allergy. Most don't, according to NAET practitioners and testimony from many patients. Acupuncture coupled with acupressure massage cures patients of their allergies. The test is repeated to find another food to which the patient is allergic and the process begins anew.

Applied kinesiology is a tenuous procedure to begin with. Add it to Nambudripad allergy elimination, also a tenuous procedure, and you get tenuous squared. Testimonies to the benefits of NAET are easy to come by, but we are not certain whether the placebo effect or the procedure is responsible for reversing people's allergies.

The surest way to overcome an allergy is to improve your diet. By reinoculating your gut with beneficial intestinal flora, you alter the allergens—the food that causes an allergic reaction—such that your allergies either go away or are not as much of a problem. We respectfully suggest forgoing the Nambudripad allergy elimination technique and trying the Guts and Glory Program instead.

Organic Acid Urine Testing

Autism, attention deficit disorder (ADD), and other pervasive developmental disorders (PPDs) remain a mystery. No one can say for certain what causes these disorders. However, a school of thought has arisen around the idea that these disorders originate in the gut. The theory is that fungi, yeasts such as *Candida albicans,* and bacteria such as clostridium cause autism, ADD, and other PPDs. Most urine samples from children who suffer from these disorders have at least one abnormal organic acid compound. These compounds are associated with abnormal levels of certain kinds of bacteria and yeasts, including candida and clostridium.

Many laboratories, including the Great Plains Laboratories of Overland Park, Kansas, offer urine testing for organic acid compounds. Organic acids are analyzed in the urine because they are concentrated a hundred times more in the urine than in the blood serum. People who test high for organic acids can be treated with dietary restrictions and supplements to bring their intestinal flora into balance.

We have become disenchanted with these kinds of tests. Because the environment in the gut fluctuates from moment to moment, it is hard to get an accurate picture of gut health no matter what kind of test is undertaken. When test results vary, do you order a new test? Organic acid urine testing is impractical in terms of the cost, which is not covered by insurance. Rather than spend a lot of money for organic acid urine tests, spend the money on goat's milk yogurt. Spend it on healthy food that will improve your intestinal health.

Standard Blood Work

Standard blood work is included in this chapter to alert readers to the shortcomings of blood testing when it comes to bowel diseases. Knowing a patient's sedimentation rate, a measurement of inflammatory activity, can be helpful. Blood tests also reveal the level of C-reactive proteins, another a measure of inflammatory activity. Furthermore, doctors can learn about electrolytes and get an idea whether the patient is dehydrated.

Twenty-four-Hour Urinalysis

The purpose of twenty-four-hour urinalysis is to look for enzyme deficiencies. As Chapter 3 explains, enzymes are essential for digesting and absorbing food. Digestive enzymes are manufactured by the pancreas. (The enzymes in raw, uncooked food also help with digestion.) An enzyme deficiency can have any number of causes— aging, an overworked pancreas, an overgrowth of candida, a damaged intestinal lining. People who have enzyme deficiencies are liable to have fatigue and other ailments that result from undernourishment. Enzyme deficiencies have also been implicated in autism, ADD, and other PDDs.

Instead of a single urine sample, samples are taken every two hours over a twenty-four-hour period. The idea is to account for fluctuations and get a complete picture of the patient's health. To put it plainly, urine is what the body throws away. Twenty-four-hour urinalysis, by examining what has been discarded, can determine what is and isn't being properly absorbed. If nutrients that would normally be absorbed are wasted in the urine, it may signal an enzyme deficiency. Health practitioners can study the results of the urinalysis and determine which enzymes are lacking. Patients who have an enzyme deficiency can take enzyme supplements to help them properly digest and absorb their food.

This test is based upon an old but valid theory of intestinal toxemia. While the test is certainly worthwhile, finding a practitioner who can administer it may be difficult. The Guts and Glory Program includes easy-to-digest foods and the most comprehensive digestive enzyme formulations available. We have seen longstanding enzyme deficiencies clear up rapidly under the program.

❖ 8 ❖

A Summary of Sub-Par Supplements

The shelves of health-food stores and even some supermarkets these days are crowded with supplements. Among others, you will find protein supplements and colon cleansers, antioxidants, and structured water. These supplements often have unusual names. What they do to the body and how they do it can be confusing.

This chapter will help you make good choices when you purchase supplements. The title of this chapter is something of a misnomer, since we review the entire spectrum of supplements, from the recommended to the sub-par to the "avoid at all costs." In keeping with the principles of the Guts and Glory Program, we believe that whole foods and whole-food supplements are the best sources of nutrition. Most dietary supplements on the market are isolated or fractionated foods or herbs. Many are synthetic and made in laboratories much like pharmaceutical drugs are made. These supplements are often made from inferior raw materials and manufactured in facilities whose quality control is suspect. Unfortunately, many supplements attempt to provide pharmaceutical-type results, but fail miserably. Most supplements are suspect for that very reason.

A Word About Supplements

One of the premises of this book is that eating a primitive diet along with taking selected whole-food supplements provides nutrients in their most accessible form. The foods in the primitive diet are pure, whole foods. They have not been refined. They present nutrients to the body in such a way that the body recognizes them and can take full advantage of their nutritional power. Obviously, our primitive ancestors did not take the powders, capsules, and pills that we call "supplements." They obtained their nutrients from lean meat, fruit, and vegetables in their natural state.

Practitioners of alternative and complementary medicine often claim that supplements are completely natural preparations. By contrast to pharmaceutical drugs they may seem natural, but most supplements are not truly natural. The isolated materials from plants, herbs, fungi, and other organic materials that go into supplements are inert. They are devoid of the cofactors—the enzymes, minerals, and other components—that synergistically give whole food its dynamic nutritional properties. The body does not recognize most supplements as food. As food goes through the digestive process, the body selects and extracts the nutrients it needs. An isolated supplement, on the other hand, presents the body with an exorbitant number of nutrients, and the body treats the supplement like a drug. Most supplements are not the biologically active, physiologically precise nutritional complexes that are found in nature.

This does not mean that isolated supplements have no value. On the contrary, we use them on occasion. Isolated supplements, however, are a bit of a wild card. There is nothing natural or nutritional, for example, about taking 5,000 milligrams of vitamin C. No one knows what the long-term consequences of taking megadoses of a vitamin or supplement are. The body is not accustomed to taking concentrated nutrients in such large amounts. No one knows precisely how the body utilizes supplements and how much of the supplement is absorbed. Supplements, like pharmaceutical drugs, may have untoward consequences of which we are not aware.

Properly prepared, whole-food nutritional supplements are quite different from isolated supplements. Whole-food supplements are dried at low temperatures, made from high-quality foods, and delivered in easy-to-assimilate forms in therapeutic quantities. The consumption of high-quality whole-food supplements is a necessity in the Guts and Glory Program. These supplements provide high-quality vitamins, minerals, enzymes, and antioxidants that may be lacking even in the best of diets. For the supplements that we recommend taking as part of the Guts and Glory Program, see Chapter 9. For guidelines for choosing supplements, see the following chart:

GUIDELINES FOR CHOOSING SUPPLEMENTS

When you shop for a nutritional supplement, follow these guidelines:

◆ Make sure the ingredients are offered in therapeutic dose ranges. In other words, enough of an ingredient has to be in the supplement to make the ingredient effective. Sometimes ingredients are added to supplements as "window dressing." The ingredient's name is put on the label to attract buyers, but not enough of the ingredient is found in the supplement to have any effect.

◆ Make sure the ingredients are organically produced, if possible, and come from clean, uncontaminated sources.

◆ Make sure the label can be read and you know precisely what is in the supplement.

◆ Make sure the ingredients have a track record of being effective. The ingredients should have been used in the past to promote health.

◆ Make sure that scientific claims as to the effectiveness of the supplement are made for the supplement itself, not for similar supplements. Primary research is important.

◆ Make sure you buy your supplements from companies that have been audited and certified by governing bodies. The company's products should have what they say and say what they have.

Aloe Vera

As a folk remedy, aloe vera is taken the world over. Topically, it is used to soothe cuts. Orally, it is taken as a laxative. It produces its laxative effect by encouraging peristalsis and by reducing the absorption of liquids in the colon.

If possible, aloe vera should be consumed raw. Most commercial products don't contain what they say and what they contain has little significant potency. Be sure to avoid whole-leaf aloe vera products. They contain the compound aloin. This compound is a cathartic herb and can harm the digestive tract.

Amino Acids

Protein, the stuff from which the muscles, blood, hair, and internal organs are made, is composed of amino acids. There are two types of amino acids. The essential amino acids, of which there are about eight, must be obtained from food or supplements. The nonessential amino acids, of which there are about fourteen, are manufactured inside the body. The body needs protein and the amino acids from which protein is made to build muscles. Although many would argue with us, we believe that animal sources of protein are exponentially better than other sources when it comes to human nutritional needs. Beef, chicken, fish, eggs and milk are called complete proteins because they supply all of the essential amino acids. Vegetables and other protein sources (soy and rice, for example) are called incomplete proteins because they do not supply all of the essential amino acids. Unless you get enough protein, your body cannot build new cells and tissue. Many amino acid supplements are sold to athletes and bodybuilders to help them build muscle strength.

The problem with these supplements, however, is that they are a far cry from the amino acids in food. In the protein from food sources, different kinds of amino acids are bound together in long molecule chains, but in supplements the amino acids are free form, or unbound. Each type of amino acid is sold as an isolate. Research suggests that these isolate, free-form amino acids are not absorbed adequately. Cofactors present in food sources probably help the body metabolize amino acids, but those cofactors aren't present in free-form amino acids.

As long as you are getting enough protein in your food, you do not need to take amino acid supplements. Consume lacto-fermented foods and take high-quality digestive enzymes to improve your protein digestion if you feel that you are deficient in amino acids. In general, however, we do not recommend these supplements for most patients.

Antioxidants

In biochemistry, molecules called antioxidants are capable of reversing the damage that free radicals do to body tissue. A free radical is an unstable, highly reactive molecule with an unpaired electron. By nature, electrons want to occur in pairs, so unpaired free radicals steal electrons from other molecules in a process called oxidation. Oxidation provides energy, plays a role in metabolism, and kills malignant cells. In excess, however, oxidation can damage cell membranes and DNA. It can damage tissue and speed up the aging process. To put it plainly, oxidation can cause decay. Antioxidants reverse decay by neutralizing free radicals.

Vitamin A, vitamin C, vitamin E, and selenium (or ACES as they are sometimes collectively called) are the backbone of most antioxidant formulas. Before you go shopping for vitamins or antioxidant supplements, however, you should know that antioxidants can be found in abundance in most fruits and vegetables. We can't be certain whether antioxidants in pill form are useful for preventing disease. By contrast, we know for certain that people who eat adequate amounts of fruits and vegetables have lower incidences of, for example, cardiovascular disease and cancer. Instead of considering isolated antioxidant supplements, increase the amount of fruits and vegetables in your diet.

In 1999, the U.S. Department of Agriculture's Human Nutrition Research Center on Aging at Tufts University did a study to determine which fruits and vegetables have the highest antioxidant properties. In the study, fruits and vegetables were ranked according to their oxygen radical absorbency capacity (ORAC). Prunes ranked the highest among the fruits and kale the highest among the vegetables. Table 8.1 shows the results of the Tufts University study (in the table, ORAC units are per 100 grams—about 3.5 ounces).

Coauthor and Italian-American Dr. Joseph Brasco believes that garlic is the best antioxidant. He is convinced that the Tufts University study, conducted in New England, where spicy foods are underappreciated, was biased against garlic!

Bee Products

Bee products fall in the "superfood" category. They are low in calories and high in nutrition. They offer sulfur-bearing protein. Bee products are among of the best natural sources of riboflavin. Ribo-

TABLE 8.1.

Oxygen radical absorbency capacity (ORAC) of fruits and vegetables with the highest antioxidant properties

	Fruits	ORAC*	Vegetables	ORAC*
1	Prunes	5770	Kale	1770
2	Raisins	2830	Spinach	1260
3	Blueberries	2400	Brussels sprouts	980
4	Blackberries	2036	Alfalfa sprouts	930
5	Strawberries	1540	Broccoli	890
6	Raspberries	1220	Beets	840
7	Plums	949	Red bell pepper	710
8	Oranges	750	Onion	450
9	Red grapes	739	Corn	400
10	Cherries	670	Eggplant	390
11	Kiwi fruit	602		
12	Pink grapefruit	483		

*Per 100 grams or 3.5 ounces of the fruit or vegetable.

flavin, also known as vitamin B_2, is essential for energy production. The bee products include the following:

- *Propolis.* To construct and seal the hive, worker bees make a resinous "bee glue" called propolis. It is a mixture of tree sap, leaves, bark, pollen, nectar, and wax.
- *Royal jelly.* Worker bees use this jelly is used to feed the larvae of the bees that may become queens. The worker bees secrete royal jelly from their salivary glands. The substance is astringent-tasting because it contains so many nutrients and tannins.
- *Bee pollen.* As bees forage for nectar, pollen granules stick to their hairy bodies and are transferred from flower to flower. In this way, flowers and other plants are pollinated. The pollen is collected from the bees when they return to the hive and is eaten as food.

We endorse bee products for the general public, but believe that people who suffer from digestive problems should avoid them for the first few months. Propolis, royal jelly, and bee pollen should melt in your mouth when you taste it. The dry varieties do not have the same nutritional benefits. If you have allergic reactions to pollen, proceed with caution when taking bee products. Incidences of allergic reactions to bee products have been reported.

Butyrate

Butyrate is a sulfur-bearing short-chained fatty acid. This acid is very important to the colon, which uses it as an energy source. Butyrate has also shown promise as an antimicrobial. No studies that we are aware of show that butyrate taken in isolated form has any beneficial effects in the gut. It appears that butyrate taken by mouth in a pill form may never reach the colon. However, butyrate taken in an enema shows promise as a treatment for inflammatory conditions such as pouchitis, proctitis, and left-sided colitis. Unfortunately, butyrate's clinical application is limited due to its horrendous sulfur odor.

There is no reason to take a butyrate supplement when butyrate is so easy to obtain in food. Milk fat, butter, and goat's milk products are all natural sources of butyric acid. Goat's milk, in fact, has twice the butyrate as cow's milk. Coconut oil is also a source of butyrate as well as other short- and medium-chain triglycerides. Yet another way to get butyrate is to manufacture it in your gut. A healthy gut colonized with the right bacteria can break down fiber and create butyrate.

Clay

As preposterous as it may seem, clay is good for the intestines. It soothes flare-ups. It absorbs toxins in the intestines and helps remove them from the body. The theory is that clay's minerals are negatively charged while toxins are positively charged, and the clay works like a magnet to draw the toxins out. Clay is also a source of minerals.

Primitive people ate clay, sometimes on purpose and sometimes not. They weren't as fastidious as we are about cleaning their food. They ate the dirt that clung to the roots of plants. They buried their food, meat included, to preserve it and ate particles of dirt on the food after they dug it up. Many cultures still eat dirt for its medicinal properties. In his classic *Nutrition and Physical Degeneration*, Dr. Weston Price observed primitive people on three continents eating clay as late as 1930:

> Among this group in the Andes, among those in central Africa, and among the Aborigines of Australia, each knapsack contained a ball of clay, a little of which was dissolved in water. Into this they dipped their morsels of food while eating. Their explanation was to prevent "sick stomach." This is the medicine that is used by the natives in these countries for combating dysentery and food infections.

We highly recommend using clay products that are designed for human consumption. In fact, clay is a critical component of the Guts and Glory Program. It can help people move through a crisis situation. We have found it especially helpful in controlling the diarrhea that accompanies so many gut disorders. For sources of clay, see "Resources" on page 344.

Colon Cleansers

Colon cleansers include *Cascara sagrada* (the bark of the Cascara tree), aloin (a derivative of the sap of aloe), senna, triphala (a combination of three Indian fruits—amalaki, haritaki, and vibhitaki), turkey rhubarb, butternut bark, and buckthorn bark.

We believe that you should avoid colon cleansers. These substances are too harsh and abrasive on the gut. What's more, they can cause Melanosis coli, a dark pigmentation in the colonic mucosa. In and of itself, Melanosis coli is an innocuous condition. But it is a hallmark of beginning bowel dependency, also known as lazy colon syndrome. People who take colon cleansers often become addicted to them and discover that their bowels won't move unless they take the cleanser. Every morning they need the cleanser to jumpstart their bowels. Colon cleansers inhibit the natural peristalsis action of the colon.

As an occasional quick-fix, colon cleansers are a reasonable alternative to harsh pharmaceutical laxatives. However, they are obviously not an effective long-term solution to the problem of constipation.

Colostrum

Colostrum is the cloudy "pre-milk" that mammals, humans included, secrete from their breasts shortly after giving birth. Most commercially made colostrum supplements are made from cow's colostrum. Cows produce roughly nine gallons of colostrum in the thirty-six hours after they give birth.

Colostrum is very nutritious. It is rich in vitamins and minerals, as well as antibodies, the immune system proteins that fight illness and infection. Claims that the antibodies in colostrum can fight intestinal disease and parasites are overblown. Although a handful of studies have shown that colostrum is useful in the colon against some strains of bacteria, most of these studies were done with large, unrealistic doses (the equivalent to 20 grams of dried colostrum). Colostrum, however, can be an excellent multinutrient if it is obtained from goat's milk.

Colostrum is another one of those highly touted GI panaceas, but coauthor Dr. Brasco has failed to see the clinical results from this product that its manufacturers claim in their literature. He believes that the jury is still out on this one.

Deglycyrrhizinated Licorice

The licorice (*Glycyrrhiza glabra*) root and licorice root extracts have been used as folk remedies in different cultures for many, many centuries. Licorice root is used to treat indigestion and stomach ulcers. Deglycyrrhizinated licorice (DGL) is licorice with the glycyrrhizin removed. Taken in high amounts, glycyrrhizin causes hypertension and retention of potassium. With DGL, you get the benefits of licorice without the drawbacks. (By the way, the licorice sold in most candy stores no longer contains real licorice. Anis, a cousin of licorice, is usually substituted for flavoring in these products.)

DGL heals the mucosa lining of the stomach. It increases the production of prostaglandins. We think DGL is a good short-term remedy for upset stomachs, esophageal reflux, overeating, and the overconsumption of alcohol. In the long term, however, probiotics and digestive enzymes are a better remedy for indigestion.

Digestive Enzymes

You need enzymes to digest food. Digestive enzymes break down food so it can be absorbed in the small intestine. The body obtains digestive enzymes from two different sources. Endogenous enzymes are made inside the body by the pancreas. Exogenous enzymes are obtained from uncooked food or digestive enzyme supplements. These enzymes enter the body with food and help the digestive process.

We subscribe to the theories about nutrition that Dr. Edward Howell put forth in his classic *Enzyme Nutrition.* (This book occupies a prominent place in our nutritional libraries. If you have not read it, please do so. You will find the experience quite rewarding.) Dr. Howell believed that each of us is born with the ability to produce only a finite number of enzymes. If the body has to devote too many enzymes to digestion, it must curtail the production of enzymes for other purposes—for operating the brain, muscles, organs, and tissues. Because the heat used in cooking destroys the enzymes in food, Howell advocated eating more raw food and taking advantage of the digestive enzymes that raw food has to offer. Howell summarized his ideas about enzymes and enzyme depletion in his famous "enzyme nutrition axiom" (the italics are his):

> The *length of life* is inversely proportional to the *rate* of exhaustion of the *enzyme potential* of an organism. The increased use of food enzymes promotes a *decreased* rate of exhaustion of the enzyme potential.

We give a hearty "thumbs up" to digestive enzymes. We have seen tremendous results in everything from inflammatory bowel disease to chronic diarrhea with digestive enzyme supplements. Not only are the supplements an aid to digestion, they also reduce inflammation and are being used in Europe to treat sports injuries and help patients recover from surgery.

The digestive enzymes in supplements come from the pancreases of livestock animals (for example, trypsin and chymotrypsin), fungi (for example, *Aspergillus orazeae*), and plants (for example, papain from papayas and bromelain from pineapples). We prefer digestive enzymes that have been cultured from plants. Enzymes of animal origin work in a narrow pH range. If your stomach is too acidic or alkalinic, the animal-origin enzymes don't work. What's more, the source of these enzymes is usually difficult to trace. Most likely, animal-origin enzymes come from animals that died in a slaughterhouse. For that reason, it is impossible to know whether these animals were raised without steroids or antibiotics. People who object to eating pork products can never be sure if the animal-origin digestive enzymes they are getting originated with pigs.

Essential Fatty Acids

Essential fatty acids (EFAs) are fatty acids that the body cannot make on its own. We must get these important fats from the food we eat. There are two essential fatty acids:

- *Omega-3.* You can get the omega-3 fatty acids, including linolenic acid, in flaxseeds, chia seeds, and walnuts. The elongated
  forms of this fatty acid, EPA and DHA, are found in fish oils and
  can be obtained through the consumption of ocean fish such
  as salmon, tuna and sardines. Grass-fed livestock and free-range
  chicken and eggs are also excellent sources of omega-3 fatty acid.
  While the body can convert linolenic acid into EPA and DHA,
  scientists disagree about the efficiency of this process. Most agree,
  however, that caffeine, elevated insulin levels, and conditions
  such as diabetes can slow the linolenic-acid conversion process
  even further. Studies show that omega-3 fatty acids are helpful
  against blood clotting, heart disease, high blood pressure, diabetes, colitis, and inflammatory diseases.
- *Omega-6.* You can get the omega-6 fatty acids, including linoleic
  acid, in vegetable oil, sunflower oil, peanut oil, and other grain,
  nut, and seed oils. There is also an elongated form of linoleic acid
  known as gamma linoleic acid (GLA). Again, scientists disagree
  about the efficiency and the conversion, but most agree that the
  process is slowed by caffeine, high insulin levels, and conditions
  such as diabetes.

Ideally, the ratio of omega-3 to omega-6 fatty acids should be
somewhere between one to one and one to five. However, modern
agricultural techniques along with a reliance on vegetable oils for
cooking and food preservation have tilted the ratio in favor of the
omega-6 fatty acids. By some estimates, Americans consume twenty
times more omega-6 than omega-3 fatty acids. Too much omega-6
in the diet creates an imbalance and can disrupt the production
of prostaglandins. The results can be heart disease, blood clotting,
diabetes, high blood pressure, an increased prevalence for autoimmune disorders, and an increase in the risk of cancer.

For many years, fats were vilified, but people are becoming
aware of the concept of "good fats." And that's excellent news. By
far the best way to get essential fatty acids is from whole foods or
properly prepared oils. A great way to get essential fatty acids into

your diet is to combine them with various nutritious whole foods. Consume them with dairy products to get a balance of saturated and polyunsaturated fat. Eat them in salads along with a meal that includes meat.

Although the body can convert linolenic acid into EPA and DHA, you cannot obtain optimal levels of these highly desirable fats without going out of your way to include them in your diet. To include EPA and DHA, we recommend taking cod liver oil in addition to consuming fatty fish two or three times per week. By consuming grass-fed meat and free-range poultry, you can obtain another critical fat known as CLA. This nutrient is important for proper metabolism and preventing certain cancers. Another healthy supplement is GLA, which is found in borage oil, in black currant seed oil, and most popularly in primrose oil.

Balance is essential in all areas of nutrition, but especially when it comes to the essential fats. People are beginning to understand that the overconsumption of omega-6 fats can be deleterious to your health. In true American fashion, however, some people believe that "if a little is good, then a lot must be better." These people are now overcompensating by taking inordinate amounts of omega-3 fatty acids to the exclusion of their omega-6 cousins. The long-term consequences of overdoing the omega-3 oils include overthinning of the blood and mild immuno-suppression. What's more, you eventually lose friends because you end up smelling like a beached cod. Yes, there is such a thing as too much of good thing.

Fiber Products

Fiber is the undigestible carbohydrate found in plants. The body cannot digest fiber, so it is expelled along with the feces. Fiber, also known as roughage, is necessary to prevent constipation. It increases the volume of waste matter in the large intestine and puts pressure on the rectum muscles to loosen and expel waste. There are two kinds of fiber. Insoluble fiber cannot be broken down at all, whereas soluble fiber dissolves in water. Insoluble fiber is believed to reduce the risk of colon cancer.

Food sources of fiber are many. Fruits, vegetables, and grains are excellent sources of fiber. Here is a summary of three popular fiber products:

- *Psyllium.* Made from the husks of the psyllium plant. This fiber can ferment in the gut, which can cause problems for certain people with inflammatory bowel disease and irritable bowel syndrome. However, many people with digestive problems can tolerate psyllium husks with little problems.
- *Methylcellulose.* Cellulose that has been chemically altered to make it resistant to breakdown by bacteria. We don't recommend methylcellulose because it is a very refined product and its long-term effects are not well understood.
- *A combination of soluble and insoluble fiber made from predigested grains, seeds, and legumes.* For people who can tolerate fiber products (mainly people with functional bowel diseases such as chronic constipation, chronic diarrhea, and IBS), this type of products seems to be the healthiest of the bunch. However, the Guts and Glory Program provides ample amounts of fiber if it is followed correctly.

All fiber products are a mixed bag for people who have GI disorders. Some people's symptoms improve with fiber products but others experience increased gas and bloating. Each individual has to experiment with different sources and different combinations to find the right one. If you have constipation, we recommend eating whole foods that are high in fiber instead of relying solely on fiber products.

Glutamine

Glutamine is a conditionally essential amino acid. That means the body can produce glutamine on its own except during times of physical stress, when it uses it up faster than it can produce it. Glutamine figures in cell growth, muscle building, and immune system enhancement. By some estimates, 40 percent of glutamine is consumed by the cells of the small intestine, which use glutamine for repair and tissue regeneration. Glutamine is depleted during exercise, times of stress, and illness. Meat, raw eggs, dairy products, and raw goat's milk products are great natural sources of glutamine. Glutamine supplements are made as a by-product of grain fermentation.

Glutamine is a widely recommended supplement especially for people with gastrointestinal disorders. Many practitioners claim great success with this product, but neither of the authors of this book has been able to duplicate their results. In our experience, even heroic doses of glutamine to the tune of 20 to 40 grams a day are disappointing. We have not seen significant clinical benefits from the supplement, probably because it is missing the cofactors that are present in natural sources of glutamine. Glutamine has been used successfully to treat people with short bowel syndrome (a condition in which the small intestine has trouble absorbing nutrients because it is diseased or a section has been surgically removed). However, the glutamine was administered intravenously, not given in powders or gel capsules. Unfortunately, many practitioners cite these studies inappropriately to attest to glutamine's value.

Green Foods

Mothers the world over are quite correct to tell their children, "Eat your greens—they're good for you." The health benefits of green vegetables and micro-algae such as spirulina cannot be overestimated. These foods provide minerals, vitamin A, vitamin C, beta-carotene, and folate, a water-soluble B vitamin. They are high in antioxidants and phytochemicals, which help prevent cancer. Greens provide fiber. Spirulina has antiviral properties and high levels of protein.

People with digestive disorders have had excellent results from taking green-food supplements. If you have considered taking a multivitamin, consider taking cereal grass juices made from barley, oats, rye, and wheat leaves instead. These green-food supplements are preferable to multivitamins. They are easier on the digestive tract and they offer more nutrients. One serving of wheat grass, for example, has the same number of nutrients as a green salad. What's more, green-food supplements contain superoxide dismutase (SOD), a very potent antioxidant enzyme that is not found in traditional green vegetables.

Certain greens, such as spinach, are difficult to absorb. And they have to be cooked before they can be eaten. Eating green-food supplements gives you a chance to eat vegetables in their raw form when their digestive enzymes are intact (cooking destroys these enzymes). Green-food supplements are also high in folate (from the Latin for "leaf" and similar to the English word *foliage*). Folate is a form of the B vitamin folic acid that is found in food. It prevents anemia, prevents neural tube birth defects, and is an important part of the cascade of nutrients that are needed to metabolize homocysteine. (Homocysteine is a highly inflammatory compound that the body produces naturally. If homocysteine is not quickly neutralized, its can accumulate in the body. High levels of homocysteine have been implicated in cardiovascular disease.) Studies have demonstrated that the body's assimilation of folate from fresh produce is not very good. Probably our ancient ancestors had hardier GI tracts than we do and were able to get their folate from leaves. We can't eat most leaves, however, so green-food supplements are our best source of folate.

When shopping for green-food supplements, be sure to look for the predigested, fermented products, or buy them in juice form. The whole dried powders may be too hard to digest. Sometimes they contain brown rice or maltodextrin (a corn syrup yield), which make them even more difficult to digest. In our experience, the green-food formulas such as spirulina and chlorella that contain algae are a little more difficult to digest than the pure grass and vegetable juice powders.

Herbs

Stool samples reveal that one in five people harbors parasites. Nevertheless, most parasites are relatively benign. Intestinal parasites include protozoa and different kinds of worms—tapeworms, pinworms, roundworms, whipworms, and hookworms. Some health professionals have suggested that unrecognized parasites are related to every disease and malady known to humankind. However, this controversial idea is probably greatly overstated. The number of individuals whose disease is directly attributable to parasites is likely quite small.

Humans have been harboring and trying to rid themselves of parasites from the beginning. For that reason, there are many folk remedies for parasites, including ginseng root, wormwood, gentian root, cloves, garlic, quassia, and the green unripe hull of the black walnut.

Over the centuries, herbalists have also tried their hand at treating candida. This disease results when the yeast *Candida albicans* grows out of control. Candida causes vaginal infections, cramping, and thrush. Herbal remedies for candida include grapeseed extract, caprylic acid, and the olive leaf.

Promotional literature makes many claims for the herbs used to treat parasites and candida. However, our patients have had inconsistent results from using these herbs. What's more, these herbs can be harsh and may exacerbate digestive problems. People with inflammatory bowel disease and irritable bowel syndrome often cannot handle them. These herbs sometimes upset the balance of the intestinal flora—and that defeats the purpose of taking the herbs. The best medicine for parasites and candida is a balanced intestinal terrain in which parasites and candida cannot thrive. This can be achieved by consuming high-quality probiotics and lacto-fermented foods such as cultured goat's milk yogurt.

Although parasite and fungi infestations are common in intestinal disorders, we believe that parasites and fungi are more of a symptom than a cause. After the intestinal terrain is healthy, these invaders seem to diminish to manageable levels and pose little threat.

Hydrochloric Acid

Hydrochloric acid in the stomach plays a very important role in digestion. The job of hydrochloric acid is to break down protein and increase its surface area so that it can be assimilated by the digestive system. Hydrochloric acid is produced by parietal cells in the stomach lining. For reasons that are unclear, there appears to be an association between suboptimal hydrochloric acid secretion and autoimmune disorders, chronic disease, and advanced age in general. Half of people over the age of sixty cannot produce enough hydrochloric acid to properly digest protein. A deficiency of hydrochloric acid has also been implicated in food allergies. What's more, the pancreas does not start releasing digestive enzymes until hydrochloric acid passes from the stomach to the small intestine. If no hydrochloric acid is passed, you have fewer enzymes with which to digest your food.

Older people and people with the aforementioned conditions often do very well with hydrochloric acid supplements. We like to start patients off with digestive enzymes, and if they don't respond, we prescribe hydrochloric acid supplements. By the way, nature offers a certain kind of food that stimulates the production of hydrochloric acid—bitters. Bitters include dandelion leaves, artichoke leaves, borage, angelica root, and wormwood. Sometimes you can find the two popular bitter aperitifs, Angostura and Campari, in liquor stores. Try a small amount of bitters before a meal to see if this alone sufficiently improves mild gastrointestinal distress.

Immune System–Enhancing and –Modulating Products

The immune system is responsible for preventing diseases and fighting them off if they succeed in attacking the body. In a single day, your immune system may encounter literally billions of bacteria, viruses, parasites, and toxins. The immune system is also responsible for vanquishing enemies within the body such as precancerous cells. Immune system–enhancing and –modulating products are preventative medicines. They bolster the immune system. Products include the homeopathic remedy acanasia, sterols, medicinal mushroom extracts, aloe isolates, and arabinogalactan, a polysaccharide powder made from larch tree wood.

The ideal immune system is neither sluggish nor overactive, but wide awake and ready to fight off disease. A sluggish immune system makes the body susceptible to infections and cancer. An overactive immune system makes the body susceptible to allergies and autoimmune disorders such as diabetes and lupus in which the body attacks itself. Some researchers believe that inflammatory bowel disease is an autoimmune disorder. We recommend immune-modulating products that contain multiple species of mushrooms combined with key botanicals that have been predigested with probiotics.

MSM

Methylsulfonylmethane (MSM), a dietary sulfur supplement, is an isolate of sulfur. Promoters of MSM point out that sulfur is found in unprocessed protein foods and that it is required for the creation and maintenance of the connective tissue—tendons and cartilage—in the body. Because sulfur is present in the connective tissues, some MSM manufacturers claim that the supplement can be used to treat osteoarthritis, also known as degenerative joint disease. This disease is marked by the breakdown of the articular cartilage inside joints.

Anecdotal evidence to the contrary, however, there is no scientific proof that MSM helps against osteoarthritis or makes the tendons or cartilage stronger. This supplement is overrated and may very well be unstable. A better way to obtain sulfur is to dispense with high-priced supplements and eat eggs, meat, fish, and raw goat's milk products. The Guts and Glory Program provides all the sulfur you need for strong tendons and cartilage.

Peptide Products

When protein is digested, the body turns it into peptides. Peptides are small amino-acid chains. Peptide products present a way to take protein in a predigested form. The protein is predigested through a fermentation process before it is dried and placed in capsules. People who take peptide capsules get the advantages of protein the trouble of having to break down the protein digesting it. The muscles, skin, bones, heart, blood, and brains are made largely of protein. The amino acids in protein, it has been said, are the building blocks of human life. In theory, peptide products can help people with impaired digestion get the nutrients they need because the peptides are predigested and thus are easier to assimilate. Once again, however, manufacturers' claims and clinical experience do not add up. In practice, our GI patients have not seen remarkable results with peptide products, and therefore these products do not represent a first-line treatment strategy.

Prebiotics

Prebiotics are supposed to feed the friendly bacteria in the gut (don't confuse *prebiotics* with *probiotics*, the friendly bacteria itself). However, the notion that a prebiotic can feed friendly bacteria but not other bacteria is, frankly, preposterous. The problem with prebiotics is they feed friendly and unfriendly bacteria alike. The most popular prebiotic, FOS, is often made from purified sucrose. Inulin, another poplular prebiotic, is made from Jerusalem artichoke or chicory. Prebiotics can cause bloating and cramping. In our experience, they do very little to help maintain a healthy balance of microflora and can actually cause problems. We think you should avoid them. Coauthor Dr. Brasco has seen many patients become significantly worse after taking FOS and inulin.

Rather than prebiotics, eat fermented foods. These foods are both pre- and probiotics. They are prebiotics because they acidify the colon with lactic acid and make the probiotics grow at the expense of the pathogens. They are probiotics because they introduce friendly bacteria into the colon.

Probiotics

Probiotics are the friendly bacteria that live in your intestinal tract. Probiotics keep the harmful bacteria and viruses in check. They can potentially alleviate conditions such as Crohn's disease and lactose intolerance. They can be found in yogurt, kefir, properly prepared sauerkraut, and other fermented foods. Probiotic supplements— acidophilus, bifidobacteria, and HSOs, to name a few—are friendly bacteria strains that have been cultured, isolated, and placed into powders, pills, or refrigerated dairy products.

Perhaps more so than the other supplements discussed in this chapter, probiotics illustrate why whole foods are superior to supplements. Here are some drawbacks of probiotic supplements:

- The strains that are used may not have any proven clinical benefits. There are literally thousands of strains of each bacterium. New ones are cultured all the time. Some strains are better than others. Many of the known healthy strains cannot be cultured in large amounts.
- Labels tell which bacteria are in the supplement as well as the number of "live cells" in each bacterium. However, these "live cell" numbers are often meaningless because live-cell bacteria die off rapidly. Manufacturers know how high the attrition rate for bacteria is. That's why they put so many microorganisms in their products. One new probiotic supplement, for example, contains a hundred thousand times more microorganisms than can be found in a normal serving of fermented food. The numbers are so high to ensure that some of the bacterial microorganisms make it into the intestines. Be sure to check expiration dates carefully. But even if the product is within its expiration date, the number of "live cells" is probably significantly lower than the number on the label.
- When tens of billions of bacteria enter the body, which is the case with many probiotic supplements, the body may assume that it is being invaded by foreign pathogens and mount an immune system response. If that happens, the immune system kills off the bacteria and the probiotics never reach the intestines.

Research has shown that as little as 5 percent of the bacteria in some supplements actually make it into the intestines. (The exception to this rule are HSOs. HSOs are much hardier than their probiotic cousins and thus require a smaller number of microorganisms to be ingested. For this reason, HSOs are a critical component of the Gut's and Glory Program.)

In the short run, some supplements work like antibiotics and destroy harmful microbes in the gut. Overall, however, you are better off getting probiotics from live fermented foods or whole-food probiotic supplements, such as HSOs. In addition to probiotics, these foods and supplements contain the valuable cofactors that are missing from isolated probiotic supplements.

Protein Powders

Protein is the basic stuff from which the body is made. Enzymes, hormones, and antibodies are made primarily of protein. Protein fuels most biochemical activities. It increases stamina, builds muscle strength, raises energy levels, and supports the immune system. Protein powders are usually marketed to athletes and weekend warriors, the idea being that these people need more protein for muscle repair and muscle building.

However, most protein powders are highly processed. Regardless of how natural the manufacturer says its product is, protein has never been consumed in powder form in the history of humankind. Protein powder is a pharmacological agent. The long-term consequences of taking protein powders are unknown. No one knows precisely what happens when the body is bombarded by protein isolates.

We are also concerned with the way the protein powders are made and the sources from which they are made. The powders are often subject to heat processing. High temperatures kill the enzymes in the protein source and may well render the protein inert and lifeless. Most powders are made from whey, soy, rice, or a combination of those foods. Whey is a milk by-product of cheese manufacturing. Knowing where the milk was produced and whether the cows were given antibiotic feed and injected with growth hormones is nearly impossible. Therefore, all protein powders made from whey are suspect.

Protein products that contain rice and soy are to be avoided. Soy is difficult to digest. It contains compounds that interfere with the function of the thyroid gland. The phytic acid in soy keeps minerals from being properly absorbed. Soy also contains enzyme inhibitors that may depress growth. As for rice, it is a very poor protein source and certainly a problem for people with compromised digestion. The only type of protein powder that we recommend is made from goat's milk. We use this goat's milk protein product to make the Jordan Seth Smoothie (see page 331), which should be consumed during the maintenance phase of the program. (Four sources of goat's milk protein products, see "Resources" on page 333.)

Structured Water Products

Structured water is created naturally in the great outdoors as it swirls and ebbs in currents and eddies and is hurled over waterfalls. Structured water is lighter than and not as dense as conventional tap water. It has a strong electrical charge and a lower surface tension. Structured water, also known as clustered water, is water that has been processed to give it all the properties of "wild water." Some researchers attribute the good health and longevity that some societies enjoy to mineral-rich, structured-type water.

Medical doctor and researcher Dr. F. Batmanghelidj has used water alone to cure thousands of cases of peptic ulcers and indigestion. In his groundbreaking book *Your Body's Many Cries for Water* (Global Health Solution, 1995), he attributes many digestive and other diseases to simple dehydration.

Water is the supreme delivery vehicle of nutrients to the cells of the body. It also carries away toxins. For people with bowel diseases, drinking water is essential for hydration. We endorse high-quality structured water products for the extra boost they provide. (For sources of structured-water products, see "Resources" on page 333.)

Vitamins and Minerals

Again, in general we do not recommend taking vitamin and mineral supplements. These supplements are isolated in laboratories. As already discussed, vitamin and mineral supplements do not come with the full complement of cofactors that make vitamins in food effective. Vitamin and mineral isolates do not have the synergistic micronutrients that are found in natural vitamins. The body uses them in a different way and, indeed, may not use them at all when they arrive in megadoses. We have heard people call vitamins "expensive urine." Some studies show that the body absorbs as little as 15 percent of water-soluble vitamins—the rest is flushed out with the urine because it is unneeded. A healthy diet combined with whole-food supplements provides all the vitamins and minerals that the body needs. You do not need to resort to vitamin and mineral supplements if you eat properly.

To illustrate what can go wrong with taking vitamin and mineral supplements, consider the beta-carotene debacle. Beta-carotene, a vegetable-based carotenoid that under certain conditions can be converted into vitamin A, is found in broccoli, apples, carrots, sweet potatoes, and cantaloupe. For many years, beta-carotene supplements were touted as a means of preventing cancer. Recently, however, studies have shown that beta-carotene supplements can actually be dangerous in certain individuals. In one widely publicized report in the *Journal of the American Medical Association,* Finnish researchers tracked 29,000 male smokers for five to eight years. Of the smokers who took beta-carotene supplements, 18 percent more developed lung cancer. The reason for these truly unexpected results is not known, but many suspect that the synthetic source of the beta-carotene was what caused the smokers to develop cancer.

Research is still being done, but probably the interaction of the beta-carotene with other phytochemicals is what prevents disease, not the beta-carotene alone. Nowhere in nature can you take a bite from a piece of fruit and get only beta-carotene. Fruit contains hundreds of carotenoids that work in concert with each other. The

Finnish study shows that the synthetic form of beta-carotene is fundamentally different from what is found in an apple or carrot. A carrot is very rich in carotenoids, but it will never promote lung cancer in smokers. The beta-carotene debacle is an example of a vitamin isolate producing unintended consequences—bad ones in this case.

Part Two

GUTS AND GLORY
THE PRACTICE

❖ 9 ❖

The Guts and
Glory Program

This chapter is a roadmap for conquering your digestive problems. It explains the basic tenets of the Guts and Glory Program. It describes the three phases of the program, what you should eat during each phase, and what you should do during each phase to attain optimum health. Compliments of Clint Eastwood, we have divided food into four categories—The Good, The Not So Bad, The Bad, and The Ugly—to help you understand which foods to eat and which foods to avoid. Along the way, this chapter explains how to handle a flare-up, how to follow the Guts and Glory Program on a limited budget, and how to stick to the program even when the road gets bumpy.

Phase One and Phase Two of the Guts and Glory Program last seven to fourteen days each. If yours is a severe case of bowel disease and you follow the program to a tee but you do not improve after twenty-eight days, the Guts and Glory Program most likely will not work for you. By the same token, if you go through the first two phases in six days, you are not giving this program a chance. You are not giving yourself a chance, either. We formulated the Guts and Glory Program very carefully on the basis of our research and our observations in clinical practice. Give this program a chance and it will very likely work for you just as it has worked for thousands of others.

For detailed information about a certain digestive problem and instructions on how to tailor the Guts and Glory Program for that problem, see Chapter 10.

Now Is the Best Time

Complementary and alternative medicine have not consistently succeeded in treating people with chronic, degenerative diseases. Thousands of people ride the hamster wheel of alternative medicine, try hundreds of different so-called cures, and never get well. But conventional medicine has not succeeded either. The problem is that getting well from a severe, so-called incurable disease is never as easy as taking a pill or undergoing a treatment. It requires making some fundamental changes in the way you eat, the way you play, the way you exercise, and the way you live your life.

In other words, it's not easy. The diligence and discipline you need to overcome an incurable disease is similar to what a professional or Olympic athlete needs. Winter and summer, competitive swimmers from high school to the Olympic level have to wake up at five-thirty in the morning and jump into a cold pool to practice while their friends sleep in. It takes that kind of commitment to get well from a chronic or degenerative disease.

Getting well is a process. It takes a lot of time. You take three steps forward and one step back. After you have a temporary setback—and it happens to everyone—you must get right back on the wagon at the very next meal. As someone who suffers from a gastrointestinal illness, you have the opportunity to make a right or wrong decision every time you put food in your mouth. Making the right decision isn't always easy, but the point is that you are in control of your diet and thus your health. No one else decides what you eat.

If you don't make the change now, where will you be in three months? Where will you be in a year? Unless you make changes to your diet and your way of life starting today, you will remain the same. The oldest definition of "insanity" is to keep doing the same thing but expect different results.

Sometimes overcoming an illness means dropping out of your normal life for a while. It means making certain sacrifices. You may have to cut back the number of hours you work to focus on yourself. You may even have to take a leave of absence from work for a week or two. If that sounds difficult, remember that the investment you make in improving your health pays great dividends in the long run. You will have more energy and stamina. You will feel good about yourself. You will get your health back. You will be able to look back on the dark period of your life when you had an illness as something in the past that you have put behind you. Remember that famous ethos of the philsopher Friedrick Nietszche: "That which doesn't kill you makes you stronger."

Cured by Diet: A Sample Patient's Story

One of the central ideas of this book is that diet is the best way to cure a gastrointestinal disease. This brief story from coauthor Dr. Joseph Brasco's practice illustrates how intestinal disease can be cured by diet and how a poor diet can cause intestinal disease:

> I was approached by a nurse prior to the Christmas holidays in the year 2000. Her daughter, who was coming home from college in Washington State, had terrible abdominal problems that no doctor was able to diagnose or cure. She knew I practiced complementary medicine and wanted to know if I would see her daughter.
>
> The daughter came to my office for a visit. She had had a number of tests done and we reviewed them. She had had an endoscopy, a lower GI series, small bowel X-rays, CT scans, ultrasound, and all the typical lab tests. Everything came up negative, but she continued to feel bad.
>
> Her complaints alternated between constipation and diarrhea. She had severe abdominal bloating to the point where at midday or midafternoon she had to loosen her clothes or change into larger pants because her belly became so distended and uncomfortable. She had all the symptoms consistent with functional bowel disease or irritable bowel syndrome.
>
> Most of the pathological sources of her disease had already been addressed during her previous evaluations in Washington. We dove

right into some aspects of her life—her stress level, her course load at school, and of course, her diet. We spent a lot of time discussing her diet. Her boyfriend was a devout vegetarian. Along with him, she ate large amounts of grain, beans, and legumes. I felt that her diet was a large part of her problem. She did not agree to consume poultry or meat, but did agree to consume fish and eggs. We increased her intake of essential fats. We started her on an enzyme supplement and a probiotic supplement. Our visit—it was the only one we had—lasted for an hour.

I got a letter from her about three weeks later saying that she felt great and was completely symptom free. She no longer had any abdominal pain. She said that what we accomplished in an hour far outstripped any time she had spent with her other doctors. She continues to do well, although, much to my chagrin, she still consumes far too many carbohydrates, especially grains. But she is continuing to get essential fats (cod liver oil, GLA, and CLA alternately). She continues to eat more protein in the form of eggs and fish. She continues to take her probiotic supplement and digestive enzymes. Not only have her digestive problems gone away, but she reports better skin tone and overall better health. Her vegetarian boyfriend is disstressed that she continues to eat fish, and until his digestion fails and he has to start eating animal foods too, I suspect he will continue to be bothered by her healthy diet.

Phase One: Rest and Repair

Phase One is the most difficult phase of the Guts and Glory Program. We considered calling this phase "Bowel Boot Camp." Approach this phase as though you were in training for an Olympic sport or the military. Be diligent. You may not notice results right away, but you should start to feel healthier within the first week if you are disciplined and stick to the program.

Phase One lasts from seven to fourteen days. The goals of the Guts and Glory Program during this period are as follows:

◆ *To rest the bowel.* The recommended low-calorie, high-nutrient foods are easy for the body to absorb. Instead of devoting its resources to digestion, the body can devote them to repairing the damaged lining of the bowel wall.

- *To repair the lining of the bowel.* As Chapter 2 explains, damaged villi and microvilli on the intestinal wall cannot properly absorb food. Our program restores the mucus lining of the wall of the intestines to good health.

- *To reduce the total microflora.* By reducing the total population of microorganisms in the gut, you reduce the amount of harmful bacteria. As Chapter 5 explains, harmful bacteria may cause many gut diseases. Reducing the amount of bacteria leaves fewer bacteria to ferment undigested food that travels in the colon. That means less bloating and gas.

- *To reduce inflammation.* The anti-inflammatory products we recommend reduce the amount of inflammation. They also reduce the amount of pathogenic bacteria in the gut and inhibit two inflammatory-causing enzymes, cyclooxygenase-2 (COX-2) and 5-lipoxygenase (5-LOX). These products also inhibit the overproduction of inflammatory chemicals such as cortisol and tumor necrosis factor alpha (TNF alpha).

- *To rehydrate the body.* Many people, especially those coming out of the hospital with inflammatory bowel disease, are chronically or acutely dehydrated. Our program provides electrolytes to help the body rehydrate.

- *To detoxify.* The clay we recommend draws toxins out. Clay's minerals are negatively charged while toxins are positively charged. Clay works like a magnet to draw toxins out.

During Phase One, you should feel better right off the bat because your intestines will get a rest. However, you may feel somewhat weak and fatigued. Especially if you are on medications, you will feel muscle aches as your body detoxifies, but overall you will feel less pain and discomfort in your intestines. You will experience less gas and bloating. You will have fewer bowel movements and less bleeding. You may experience sweating, but that is okay. You will get more sleep and be in a better mood. At the end of Phase One, you will start to believe for the first time that you will get well.

However, if you feel a touch better but are still experiencing gas and bloating after the first week, stay on Phase One for the full fourteen days.

Phase One Foods and Supplements

The foods in Phase One are easy to absorb but also very nutritious. In this early stage, you need foods that are soothing to the bowel but also give you strength to get well. The supplements in Phase One are meant to ease the pain of inflammation and remove toxins from the bowel. Following are the foods and supplements we recommend in Phase One. Sources for these foods and supplements can be found in "Resources" on page 343. Chapter 3 explains why these foods are so nutritious. Chapter 8 describes the supplements in detail.

- *Gelatin-rich, collagen-building substances.* Supplied by Brasco Broth (see page 328 for the recipe) and anti-inflammatory supplements.
- *Protein.* Supplied by chicken in Brasco Broth.
- *Fats.* Supplied by chicken in Brasco Broth.
- *Carbohydrates and fiber.* Supplied by cooked vegetables in Brasco Broth.
- *Antimicrobial substances.* Supplied by garlic and natural anti-inflammatories and antifungals in Brasco Broth.
- *Anti-inflammatory substances.* Supplied by Brasco Broth and by anti-inflammatory supplements.
- *Anti-inflammatory formula.* For persons with Crohn's disease, ulcerative colitis, IBS, celiac disease, diverticulitis, and food allergies. Take three doses of four caplets each on an empty stomach.
- *Antifungal formula.* For persons with candidiasis, parasites, food poisoning, or chronic or acute diarrhea. Follow the instructions on the bottle for a two-week intensive protocol.
- *Detoxification clay.* Take 1 tablespoon mixed with 8 ounces of water two to four times a day on an empty stomach. Persons with constipation should not take clay. Persons with Crohn's disease,

ulcerative colitis, IBS, parasites, or candidiasis accompanied by chronic diarrhea should take 4 tablespoons of clay in 8 ounces of water until symptoms resolve and stool is formed.

◆ *Structured water additive.* Add 12 drops to 8 ounces of water. Drink at least 64 ounces of structured water per day.

Sample Three-Day Plan

Here is a sample three-day meal and supplement plan for Phase One.

◆ **Day One** ◆

- Upon rising: 1 to 2 tablespoons of detoxification clay and 12 drops of structured water additive mixed in 8 ounces of water.
- Morning supplements: four caplets of natural anti-inflammatory formula and 12 drops of structured water additive mixed in 8 ounces of water.
- Breakfast: 1 to 2 cups of Brasco Broth (see page 328 for the recipe).
- Mid-morning supplements: four caplets of natural anti-inflammatory formula and 12 drops of structured water additive mixed in 8 ounces of water.
- Lunch: 1 to 2 cups of Brasco Broth.
- Late-afternoon supplements: four caplets of natural anti-inflammatory formula and 12 drops of structured water additive mixed in 8 ounces of water.
- Dinner: 1 to 2 cups of Brasco Broth.
- Before bed: 1 to 2 tablespoons of detoxification clay and 12 drops of structured water additive mixed in 8 ounces of water.
- Beverages: Pure water with 12 drops of structured water additive mixed in each 8-ounce glass. If diarrhea is frequent, drink clay water up to four times per day on an empty stomach with 1 to 2 tablespoons of clay mixed in each 8-ounce glass.

◆ Day Two ◆

- Upon rising: 1 to 2 tablespoons of detoxification clay and 12 drops of structured water additive mixed in 8 ounces of water.
- Morning supplements: four caplets of natural anti-inflammatory formula and 12 drops of structured water additive mixed in 8 ounces of water.
- Breakfast: 1 to 2 cups of Brasco Broth.
- Mid-morning supplements: four caplets of natural anti-inflammatory formula and 12 drops of structured water additive mixed in 8 ounces of water.
- Lunch: 1 to 2 cups of Brasco Broth.
- Late afternoon supplements: four caplets of natural anti-inflammatory formula and 12 drops of structured water additive mixed in 8 ounces of water.
- Dinner: 1 to 2 cups of Brasco Broth.
- Before bed: 1 to 2 tablespoons of detoxification clay and 12 drops of structured water additive mixed in 8 ounces of water.
- Beverages: Pure water with 12 drops of structured water additive mixed in each 8-ounce glass. If diarrhea is frequent, drink clay water up to four times per day on an empty stomach with 1 to 2 tablespoons of clay mixed in each 8-ounce glass.

◆ Day Three ◆

- Upon rising: 1 to 2 tablespoons of detoxification clay and 12 drops of structured water additive mixed in 8 ounces of water.
- Morning supplements: four caplets of natural anti-inflammatory formula and 12 drops of structured water additive mixed in 8 ounces of water.
- Breakfast: 1 to 2 cups of Brasco Broth.
- Mid-morning supplements: four caplets of natural anti-inflammatory formula and 12 drops of structured water additive mixed in 8 ounces of water.
- Lunch: 1 to 2 cups of Brasco Broth.

- Late-afternoon supplements: four caplets of natural anti-inflammatory and 12 drops of structured water additive mixed in 8 ounces of water.
- Dinner: 1 to 2 cups of Brasco Broth.
- Before bed: 1 to 2 tablespoons of detoxification clay and 12 drops of structured water additive mixed in 8 ounces of water.
- Beverages: Pure water with 12 drops of structured water additive mixed in each 8-ounce glass. If diarrhea is frequent, drink clay water up to four times per day on an empty stomach with 1 to 2 tablespoons of clay mixed in each 8-ounce glass.

A word for the budgetarily challenged: The two supplements recommended in Phase One, the natural anti-inflammatory formula and the structured water concentrate, can be eliminated if your financial situation makes it necessary. You can still achieve results just by substituting higher-quality ingredients such as organic chicken and vegetables for your regular conventional nonorganic foods, but your return to good health will take longer.

Notes on Phase One

Unless you just got out of the hospital with inflammatory bowel disease (IBD) or you are having a major crisis with IBS, the first two or three days of Phase One may be all you need. You may decide to skip ahead to Phase Two and begin eating more. No matter what your state of health, don't move ahead in this program until your symptoms have improved significantly. Moving ahead prematurely to Phase Two, the reinoculation phase, can cause you discomfort if your bowel is not at least somewhat healed. The tissue lining in the bowel wall regenerates every few days. It regenerates even faster in people who have been ill. Before going ahead to the reinoculation phase, you need to accomplish Phase One's goal—to build healthy cells in your small intestine and colon and to stop the inflammatory process.

You may lose weight during Phase One. Some patients have expressed alarm at this. Their gastrointestinal disease has caused them to lose weight already and they are upset when they lose more. Don't be alarmed. Think of it this way: You are preparing the soil for recovery. In the same way that tilled soil is rugged and rough but is in fact primed to produce crops, you are preparing your bowels for health in Phase One. You are resting and repairing your bowels so they can start absorbing food again. When this phase is over, you will quickly regain the weight you lost.

Physical rest, of course, is essential for overcoming almost any disease. However, there is a difference between allowing yourself to rest and resting. If you are at home feeling guilty because you are not at work, for example, you are not truly resting. To rest, do a passive activity that you like. Read a book. Watch a great movie, a comedy perhaps, or take a warm bath. Resting puts you in a relaxed state of mind in which you start to feel that you will get well. Reaching that state of mind is a prerequisite to getting well.

We also recommend squatting to relieve yourself. As discussed in Chapter 4, squatting aligns the colon properly for elimination and allows it to empty more completely. To adapt the Western toilet for squatting, fit an elimination bench around the toilet. (For sources of elimination benches, see "Resources" on page 350.) Our patients tell us that proper elimination does wonders for them.

For a discussion of the Guts and Glory Program and your medications, see page 225.

When You're Ready for Phase Two

In Phase One, your symptoms will improve and you will have less pain, gas, and bloating. You will have fewer bowel movements per day and enjoy a better emotional state. At this point, you will be ready for Phase Two.

Phase Two: Reinoculation of the Gut

During this crucial phase of the program, the objective is to flood the body with nutrients and create an intestinal terrain that is capable of absorbing nutrients. In Phase Two, you consume cultured

WHAT ABOUT MY MEDICATIONS?

We have seen many instances in which individuals who followed the Guts and Glory Program were able to gradually reduce or even eliminate all their prescription medications. As the body begins to heal, it needs these medications less and eventually not at all. That said, always consult your doctor before lowering or discontinuing a prescription medication.

In general, the medications prescribed for IBS are to relieve the pain and other symptoms. Because the Guts and Glory Program relieves the pain and other symptoms, patients with IBS can usually quit taking the drugs after they have been on the program for a while because the drugs are no longer needed.

IBD is another matter. IBD patients should not change or quit taking their medications until they go into remission. Patients taking asacol, a relatively safe drug, can slowly stop taking the drug when they start to go into remission. The same is true of Immuran. Prednisone, however, is a powerful drug with many side effects. Our warning not to change your intake of prescription drugs without consulting your physician needs to be underscored in the case of prednisone. However, because prednisone is usually used in acute situations, many patients can slowly cease taking it as their symptoms come under control with the Guts and Glory Program.

When taking the supplements that our program recommends, be sure to take the supplements and your prescribed medications at least one hour apart. As your symptoms improve, your physician may decide to lower your medications. Make sure your physician understands that you are on the Guts and Glory Program. If not, your physician may give credit for your improvement to the medications, not the diet.

What really matters is that you return to good health. Most physicians never recommend going off prescribed medications because drugs are the only tools they know of that reduce symptoms. That said, we believe the body may never truly heal properly as long as you take medication.

dairy products in large amounts to reinoculate the gut with friendly intestinal bacteria. For the same reason, you take a high-potency probiotic product. To make sure the detoxification process continues, you keep taking the Brasco Broth and detoxification clay. Depending on your condition (see the protocols in Chapter 10 that describe how to treat the different conditions), you may continue taking a natural anti-inflammatory or natural antifungal product. To eliminate wastes, you consume more soft, thoroughly cooked vegetables. By adding a high-potency digestive enzyme to your meals, you minimize the amount of undigested food that gets into the colon. In this way, you starve the unfriendly bacteria and yeast in your gut and repopulate your gut with friendly microbes.

Phase Two lasts from seven to fourteen days. The goals of the Guts and Glory Program during this phase are as follows:

- *To lower the colonic pH.* The colonic pH should be slightly acidic to achieve optimal intestinal health. Pathogenic microbes such as *Candida albicans*, *Salmonella*, and parasites cannot live in the colon if it is properly acidified. To acidify the colon, you will eat fermented dairy products.
- *To enable the intestines to absorb nutrients.* The proper absorption of nutrients allows for the regeneration of body tissues, especially the intestinal mucosa.
- *To provide healing fats.* Healthy fats properly lubricate the intestines, reduce inflammation, and enhance immune function.

During Phase Two, you will start to see improvement. Your energy will start to come back. When you go to the bathroom, your stools will be well formed, probably for the first time in a long while. After about one week on Phase Two, your stools will not give off a putrid odor. Stool odor is the best way to tell whether the colon is slightly acidic and populated with friendly microbes. However, during the first few days, your stools may give off an extremely putrid odor, which is due to the fact that a high amount of unfriendly microorganisms are being eliminated. At the end of Phase Two, you will begin to forget that you are "ill."

Phase Two Foods and Supplements

Phase One starved or lowered the microbial population in the gut and repaired the intestinal wall. In Phase Two, you continue to consume broths with vegetables and meat as well as take anti-inflammatory preparations and clay. In this phase, however, properly fermented dairy products are added to the diet as well as digestive enzymes and probiotics. You may choose to add a whole-food mineral powder to your regime to supply your body with the crucial trace elements it needs to function properly. Following are the foods and supplements we recommend in Phase Two. Sources for these foods and supplements can be found in "Resources" on page 333. Chapter 3 explains why these foods are so nutritious. Chapter 8 describes the supplements in detail.

- *Fermented dairy products.* Supplied in the form of goat's milk yogurt or a liquid probiotic cultured in fermented whey.
- *Digestive enzymes.* Take one to three caplets every time you eat.
- *Probiotic supplement.* Take two caplets the first day, then increase the dose by one caplet per day until you are taking twelve caplets a day. Continue taking twelve caplets a day for six months, then gradually decrease to your desired maintenance dose. Take the probiotic supplement in two doses, one upon rising and one at bedtime. Take one hour before or after any medications, and at least twenty minutes before the detoxification clay.
- *Detoxification clay.* Take 2 tablespoons mixed with 8 ounces of water upon rising and at bedtime. Persons with constipation should not take clay.
- *Whole food mineral formula.* Take 2 tablespoons mixed in water or vegetable juice on an empty stomach.
- *Anti-inflammatory formula.* For persons with Crohn's disease, ulcerative colitis, IBS, celiac disease, diverticulitis, and food allergies. Take six to twelve caplets a day on an empty stomach.
- *Anti-fungal formula.* For persons with candidiasis, parasites, food poisoning, or chronic or acute diarrhea. Follow the instructions on the bottle for a two-week intensive protocol.

◆ *Structured water additive.* Add 12 drops to 8 ounces of water. Drink at least 8 ounces of structured water per day.

Sample Three-Day Plan

Here is a sample three-day meal and supplement plan for Phase Two.

◆ Day One ◆

◆ Upon rising: 16 ounces of thirty-hour cultured goat's milk yogurt or 8 ounces of fermented liquid probiotic.
◆ Morning supplements: 1 to 2 tablespoons of detoxification clay and 12 drops of structured water additive mixed in 8 ounces of water. Also, three to six caplets of natural anti-inflammatory formula and one to six caplets of a probiotic supplement.
◆ Breakfast: 1 to 2 cups of Brasco Broth (see page 328 for the recipe) with additional steamed, soft vegetables and one to three caplets of digestive enzymes.
◆ Mid-morning supplements: 8 ounces of thirty-hour cultured goat's milk yogurt or 8 ounces of fermented liquid probiotic.
◆ Lunch: 1 to 2 cups of Brasco Broth with additional steamed, soft vegetables and one to three caplets of digestive enzymes.
◆ Dinner: 1 to 2 cups of Brasco Broth with additional steamed, soft vegetables and one to three caplets of digestive enzymes.
◆ Evening supplements (1 to 2 hours after dinner): 1 to 2 tablespoons of detoxification clay and 12 drops of structured water additive mixed in 8 ounces of water. Also, three to six caplets of natural anti-inflammatory formula and one to six caplets of probiotic supplement.
◆ Before bed: 8 ounces of thirty-hour cultured goat's milk yogurt or 8 ounces of fermented liquid probiotic.
◆ Beverages: Pure water with 12 drops of structured water additive mixed in each 8-ounce glass and lacto-fermented beverages.

◆ Day Two ◆

- Upon rising: 16 ounces of thirty-hour cultured goat's milk yogurt or 8 ounces of fermented liquid probiotic.
- Morning supplements: 1 to 2 tablespoons of detoxification clay and 12 drops of structured water additive mixed in 8 ounces of water. Also, three to six caplets of natural anti-inflammatory formula and one to six caplets of probiotic supplement.
- Breakfast: 1 to 2 cups of Brasco Broth with additional steamed, soft vegetables and one to three caplets of digestive enzymes.
- Mid-morning supplements: 8 ounces of thirty-hour cultured goat's milk yogurt or 8 ounces of fermented liquid probiotic.
- Lunch: 1 to 2 cups of Brasco Broth with additional steamed, soft vegetables and one to three caplets of digestive enzymes.
- Dinner: 1 to 2 cups of Brasco Broth with additional steamed, soft vegetables and one to three caplets of digestive enzymes.
- Evening supplements (one to two hours after dinner): 1 to 2 tablespoons of detoxification clay and 12 drops of structured water additive mixed in 8 ounces of water. Also, three to six caplets of natural anti-inflammatory formula and one to six caplets of probiotic supplement.
- Before bed: 8 ounces of thirty-hour cultured goat's milk yogurt or 8 ounces of fermented liquid probiotic.
- Beverages: Pure water with 12 drops of structured water additive mixed in each 8-ounce glass and lacto-fermented beverages.

◆ Day Three ◆

- Upon rising: 16 ounces of thirty-hour cultured goat's milk yogurt or 8 ounces of fermented liquid probiotic.
- Morning supplements: 1 to 2 tablespoons of detoxification clay and 12 drops of structured water additive in with 8 ounces of water. Also, six caplets of natural anti-inflammatory formula and one to six caplets of probiotic supplement.
- Breakfast: 1 to 2 cups of Brasco Broth with additional steamed, soft vegetables and one to three caplets of digestive enzymes.

- Mid-morning supplements: 8 ounces of thirty-hour cultured goat's milk yogurt or 8 ounces of fermented liquid probiotic.
- Lunch: 1 to 2 cups of Brasco Broth with additional steamed, soft vegetables and one to three caplets of digestive enzymes.
- Dinner: 1 to 2 cups of Brasco Broth with additional steamed, soft vegetables and one to three caplets of digestive enzymes.
- Evening supplements (1 to 2 hours after dinner): 1 to 2 table-spoons of detoxification clay and 12 drops of structured water additive mixed in 8 ounces of water. Also, six caplets of natural anti-inflammatory formula and one to six caplets of probiotic supplement.
- Before bed: 8 ounces of thirty-hour cultured goat's milk yogurt, 8 ounces of fermented whey beverage, or 8 ounces of fermented liquid probiotic.
- Beverages: Pure water with 12 drops of structured water additive mixed in each 8-ounce glass and lacto-fermented beverages.

A word for the budgetarily challenged: See "Guts and Glory on a Limited Budget" on page 232.

Notes on Phase Two

During Phase Two, most people will be able to handle the properly prepared, fermented dairy products that we recommend. The thirty-hour cultured goat's milk yogurt is predigested and very easy to tolerate. However, on very rare occasions, an individual may not be able to tolerate dairy products in any form, and these people should not consume fermented dairy products or take the liquid probiotic. If you have major digestive problems—bloating, gas, mucus, and phlegm—consistently an hour after consuming dairy products, you may not be able to tolerate them. We have yet to encounter anyone, however, who cannot tolerate the thirty-hour cultured Bulgarian yogurt made from goat's milk.

Goat's milk yogurt cultured for thirty hours is an excellent addition to the diet in Phase Two. Goat's milk yogurt is one of the best whole-food sources of probiotics, the friendly bacteria in the gut that promote intestinal health. Usually, people disguise the sour taste of this yogurt by adding berries or fruit to it. However, we recommend not doing that in Phase Two, as the berries or fruit may be too difficult to digest at this time. Be sure to consume the yogurt on an empty stomach to take full advantage of its healing properties. If you can't obtain a properly fermented yogurt, try drinking a high-quality liquid acidophilus. Normally, the dose is 1 tablespoon, but patients have seen improvement by drinking the entire 16-ounce bottle each day.

Consider adding coconut oil to the Brasco Broth to obtain short-chain fatty acids, which may have potent antimicrobial properties, and to help lower your intestinal pH. You may also consume eggs that are high in omega-3 fats.

When You're Ready for Phase Three

Don't be tempted to move ahead to Phase Three until you have completed Phase Two. At the end of Phase Two, you should have a few well-formed bowel movements each day. You may feel as healthy as or healthier than before you had your disease. However, if you have noticed some improvement but are still having moderate to severe symptoms, remain in Phase Two for a longer period of time.

Phase Three: Optimal Digestive Health

The object of Phase Three is to slowly but carefully and diligently restore and maintain a state of excellent health. Phase Three builds on the success of Phases One and Two. In this phase, you make your diet work for you. You learn that the foods you eat can make you well and keep you well.

The goals of the Guts and Glory Program during this phase are as follows:

- *To quantitatively reduce your intake of carbohydrates.* Undigested carbohydrates in the gut are a source of many intestinal diseases. By reducing carbohydrates, especially grains and beans, you contribute to your intestinal health.

❖

GUTS AND GLORY ON A LIMITED BUDGET

The Guts and Glory Program can put a pinch in your pocketbook. Meat from properly raised animals costs more than conventional meat. Organic food is usually but not always more expensive.

Sticking to the Guts and Glory Program on a limited budget is more a matter of what you don't eat than what you do eat. Cut back your meat consumption and consume more eggs and canned tuna or salmon. Shop in supermarkets instead of health-food stores. Health-food stores are great, but they can't offer food at discount prices because they don't sell at high volume. In a supermarket, you can usually find food on sale.

In some food categories, organic food is not much more expensive than conventional, nonorganic food. Healthy omega-3 eggs, for example, are not much more expensive than conventional eggs. Organic fruit and vegetables when they are in season don't pinch the pocketbook too tightly. Canned tuna, canned salmon, and canned sardines in water or olive oil are relatively inexpensive. Ground beef doesn't cost as much as beef cuts. The Guts and Glory Program is very likely to turn you into a better shopper as you prowl the aisles for healthy food at bargain prices.

- *To qualitatively improve the carbohydrates you do consume.* Of course, some carbohydrates are necessary. Phase Three directs you to these carbohydrates.
- *To decrease your intake of the omega-6 fatty acids and increase your intake of the omega-3 fatty acids, SCFAs, MCTs, and CLA.*
- *To introduce beneficial gut bacteria.* This is done through probiotic supplementation and fermented foods.

Phase Three Foods and Supplements

Lists of "Good," "Not So Bad," "Bad," and "Ugly" foods follow. Obviously listing every type of food is impossible, but you can follow this rule of thumb to determine which category a food belongs in: If a food is overly processed, you can be pretty sure that it belongs in the "Bad" or "Ugly" category.

During Phase Three, do your very best to choose foods exclusively from the "Good" and the "Not So Bad" categories in a 75-percent to 25-percent ratio. Only after you are free of symptoms for at least three months can you occasionally eat foods in the "Bad" food category. Try to avoid foods in the "Ugly" category altogether. These foods do not impart any beneficial qualities and actually cause harm to the body. They should be avoided by everyone whether healthy or ill. If you deviate from the program at any time, always go back to Phase One or Two for a few days. This way, you can restore your gut to health again.

"GOOD" FOODS

Foods that fall in the "Good" category are optimal foods for optimal wellness. They supply the body with the building blocks it needs to heal itself and to maintain vibrant health. These foods are highly nutritious and life-giving. They have kept people healthy and disease-free for thousands of years. They have a low to moderate amount of calories per serving. Generally speaking, foods in the "Good" category are well tolerated even by people with gastrointestinal diseases, food allergies, and food sensitivities. These foods contain the same naturally occurring nutrients that they contained hundreds of years ago. In their organic form, they contain little or no residues from pesticides, herbicides, hormones, or antibiotics. The utmost care is taken in their growth and they are grown in accordance with self-sustaining agricultural practices. We selected each food on the "Good" list according to its level of vitamins, minerals, healthy fats, enzymes, and probiotics. These foods truly exemplify the principals of the primitive diet.

Sources of many foods in the "Good" category can be found in "Resources" on page 333. We strongly recommend re-reading Chapter 3, which explains in detail the nutritional values of these foods for people with gastrointestinal diseases.

◆ Protein. In the form of:

Organic meat and fowl. Grass-fed meat is preferable.

Game, such as venison, buffalo, and elk.

Eggs, at the very least free-range, but preferably high in the omega-3 fats.

Fish with fins and scales. Use deep-water ocean fish, not farm-raised fish. The best are salmon, halibut, tuna, cod, sea bass, and sardines. If canned, they should be packed in water or olive oil, not soy bean oil. Look for a fat content of 16 to 17 grams per serving.

Organic organ meats such as liver and heart.

◆ Fats. In the form of:

Raw, organic, chemical-free goat's-milk butter. Raw butter, particularly from goat's milk, has therapeutic properties not found in pasteurized butter. Butter made from the milk of grass-fed animals is preferable. Do not heat the butter.

Pasteurized goat's-milk butter from organically raised animals.

Organic expeller-pressed coconut oil, coconut butter, and coconut cream.

Expeller-pressed extra virgin olive oil. This is the only oil that should be used for cooking, and then just occasionally.

Unrefined expeller-pressed flax seed oil, cod liver oil, hemp seed oil, pumpkin seed oil, and hazel nut oil.

Water-packed olives, coconut, and avocado, certified organic or locally grown and/or herbicide- and pesticide-free.

◆ Dairy. In the form of:

Organic, cultured dairy products such as yogurt, crème Bulgare, and kefir made from whole goat's milk cultured for thirty hours or more.

◆ Vegetables. In the form of:

Raw, frozen, or cooked vegetables. The best are organic or un-sprayed and free of genetically modified organisms.

Unpasteurized fermented vegetables, including sauerkraut, squash (winter and summer), broccoli, artichoke (French, not Jerusalem), asparagus, beets, cauliflower, Brussels sprouts, cabbage, carrots, celery, cucumber, eggplant, pumpkin, garlic, onion, kale, collard greens, okra, lettuce and greens of all kinds, mushrooms, peas, peppers, string beans, tomatoes, turnips, watercress, and sprouts (such as broccoli, sunflower, and pea shoots). *Avoid* bean and alfalfa sprouts, corn, potatoes, yams, and sweet potatoes.

Raw vegetable juices, including wheat grass juice (field grown is preferred). If using commercially grown vegetables, wash the vegetables thoroughly to remove any pesticide residues and chemicals.

Note: Raw vegetables and vegetable juices are very healthy for most individuals, but may cause GI disturbances in people with GI problems. Once your diarrhea is under control, use raw vegetables and vegetables juices judiciously.

◆ Fruits. In the form of:

Fresh, frozen, or cooked fruits. The best are fully ripened, organic, and unsprayed. Limit intake to two to three pieces a day.

Note: Raw fruit and fruit juices are very healthy for most individuals, but may cause GI disturbances in people with GI problems. Once your diarrhea is under control, use fruits and fruit juices judiciously.

◆ Sweeteners. In the form of:

Raw, unheated, unpasteurized honey, filtered or unfiltered. Use honey in moderation.

◆ Nuts and seeds. In the form of:

Organic nuts and seeds, soaked or sprouted.

Certified organic nut and seed butters, and nut and seed flours.

Note: Because nuts and seeds, even if sprouted, can be difficult to digest, limit your consumption to 2 to 3 ounces per day. Many people cannot tolerate nuts and seeds until after they have been on the Guts and Glory Program for six months. When consuming nuts and seeds, chew them well.

- **Beverages**. In the form of:
Filtered, noncarbonated, high-mineral or catalyst-altered water.
Meat stocks and vegetable broths.
Raw vegetable juices.
Lacto-fermented beverages.

- **Condiments.** In the form of:
Celtic sea salt and Herbamare.
Lacto-fermented sauces and condiments.
Raw, homemade salsa and guacamole.
Homemade salad dressings.
Apple cider vinegar.
Organic herbs and spices.

"NOT SO BAD" FOODS

Foods in the "Not So Bad" category should be eaten sparingly, especially during your first year on the program. Be sure to reread Chapter 3. It explains which foods have nutritional value especially for people with intestinal disease.

- **Protein.** In the form of:
Nonorganic meat and poultry.
Farm-raised fresh-water fish.
Canned tuna and salmon packed in spring water.
Shellfish such as crab, lobster, shrimp, oysters, scallops, muscles, and clams, in season, from clean waters, and cooked.
Nonorganic eggs.
Fresh cold cuts such as deli turkey, chicken, and roast beef from free-range sources with no preservatives.
Smoked fish without preservatives or sugar.
Fermented soy products such as miso, natto, and wheat-free tempeh, in small amounts only.
Note: Coauthor Jordan Rubin has chosen to strictly abstain from pork, shellfish, catfish, eel, and other scavengers due to research findings, personal experience, and his spiritual beliefs.

◆ Fats. In the form of:
Expeller-pressed, unrefined, organic or chemical-free sesame oil, peanut oil, grapeseed oil, and walnut oil.
Nonorganic virgin olive oil.
Unrefined palm oil, palm kernel oil, and avocado oil.
Nonorganic coconut.
Water-packed nonorganic olives.
Nonorganic avocado.
Chicken, goose, duck, lamb, and beef fat from free-range animals.

◆ Dairy. In the form of:
Raw goat's milk.
Pasteurized, cultured dairy products such as yogurt and kefir made from whole goat's milk.
Organic hard cheeses such as cheddar, Swiss, Havarti, and Colby made from raw or pasteurized goat's milk.
Organic dry-curd cottage cheese made from goat's milk.

◆ Grains and starches. In the form of:
Certified organic, sprouted, or yeast-free sourdough whole-grain breads.
Soaked nongluten whole grains and soaked whole-grain meals and flours, including quinoa, amaranth, millet, buckwheat, and brown rice.

◆ Vegetables. In the form of:
Heated fermented vegetables such as sauerkraut and pickles with no vinegar.
Canned organic vegetables, including tomato products, sweet potatoes, yams, sea vegetables, parsnips, and jicama.

◆ Fruits. In the form of:
Raw or cooked nonorganic fruits. The best are fully ripened.
Dried organic fruits with no added sugar or sulfites.
Canned organic fruits packed in their own juices and without added sugar.

◆ Sweeteners. In the form of:
Filtered or heated honey.

◆ Legumes. In the form of:
White beans, lentils, split peas, and lima beans, soaked for 8
    hours or fermented.
Organic peanut butter.

◆ Nuts and seeds. In the form of:
Nonorganic nuts and seeds, raw, soaked, or sprouted.
Nonorganic nut and seed butters.
Blanched organic almonds.

◆ Beverages. In the form of:
Fresh raw fruit juices. *Note:* Fruit juices are very healthy for most
    individuals, but may cause GI disturbances in people with GI
    problems. Once your diarrhea is under control, use fruit juices
    judiciously.
Unpasteurized organic dry red wine.
Organic herbal teas sweetened with honey.
Green tea.
Purified water filtered by reverse osmosis.
Naturally carbonated mineral waters.

◆ Condiments. In the form of:
Organic wheat-free soy sauce (tamari).
Organic mustard.
Organic-quality mayonnaise.
Mayonnaise mixed with flax.
Fish sauce.
Ketchup.
Organic tomato sauce.
Wasabi.
Organic salsa.
Organic salad dressings.
Organic carob or cocoa powder, preferably raw.
Nonorganic spices with no added starches, sugars, or stabilizers.

"BAD" FOODS

Foods in the "Bad" category should be strictly avoided during the first six to twelve months of the program. And when the first twelve months have passed, make these foods just a small part of your diet. If you knowingly consume foods in the "Bad" category, take additional digestive enzymes with the food. By the way, we strongly recommend re-reading Chapter 3. It explains why some of the foods in this category are "bad."

- Protein. In the form of:
  Pork. *Note:* According to research, pork products contain carcinogenic substances and heat-resistant pathogenic organisms.
  Supermarket cold cuts such as nonorganic turkey breast, chicken roll, and deli roast beef.
  Health-food-store bologna, sausage, hot dogs, and turkey bacon from free-range sources. *Note:* These products contain added fat.
  Smoked ocean-caught fish.
  Natural, preservative-free, sugar-free jerky.
  Egg whites without yolks.
  Whey and milk protein powders.
  Tofu.

- Fats. In the form of:
  Cow's-milk butter and cream.
  Chicken, goose, duck, lamb, and beef fat from conventionally raised animals.
  Expeller-pressed soy, canola, sunflower, safflower, and olive oil.

- Dairy. In the form of:
  Cultured full-fat cow's milk.
  Hard and soft cheeses made from cow's milk.
  Sour cream, cream cheese, and nonorganic dry-curd cottage cheese made from cow's milk.
  Pesticide-free dairy products such as yogurt and kefir made from cow's milk, without added sweeteners.

- **Grains and starches.** In the form of:
  Unsoaked, unsprouted whole grains, whole-grain flour, and whole-grain pasta.

- **Vegetables.** In the form of:
  Canned nonorganic vegetables and tomato products.
  Organic white potatoes.
  Heated fermented vegetables with vinegar.
  Organic corn.

- **Fruits.** In the form of:
  Canned nonorganic fruits packed in their own juices with no added sugar.
  Dried nonorganic fruits with no added sugar or sulfites.

- **Sweeteners.** In the form of:
  Organic cane sugar such as Sucanat and Rapadura.
  Organic maple syrup.
  Stevia.

- **Legumes.** In the form of:
  Black-eyed peas and garbanzo, adzuki, kidney, and soy beans, soaked for 8 hours or fermented.

- **Nuts and seeds.** In the form of:
  Unsoaked nuts and seeds.
  Nonorganic nut flours.
  Roasted nuts and seeds.
  Nonorganic nut and seed butters.

- **Beverages.** In the form of:
  Distilled water.
  Freshly ground organic coffee.
  Organic black tea.
  Nonorganic herbal teas sweetened with honey.
  Pasteurized 100-percent juice not from concentrate.
  Unpasteurized beer.
  White wine.
  Carbonated beverages with added carbonation.

◆ <u>Condiments.</u> In the form of:
Condiments made with organic sugar, canola mayonnaise, unflavored gelatin, or nonorganic spices, starch, or stabilizers.

"UGLY" FOODS

Foods in the "Ugly" category should be strictly avoided by all individuals who want to attain and maintain health. Eating any of these foods will significantly increase the risk of relapse. If you do consume these foods, you would be prudent to consume extra digestive enzymes with the food and to increase your consumption of probiotics for three days afterwards. Chapter 3 explains in detail why the "ugly" foods should be avoided.

◆ <u>Protein.</u> In the form of:
Ham, nonorganic bacon, nonorganic hot dogs and sausages.
Cured meats.
Imitation shellfish.
Organ meats from conventionally raised animals.
Smoked farm-raised fish.
Smoked meats.
Nonorganic jerky.
Imitation eggs.
Soy and other vegetable proteins.
All soy imitation-protein foods, such as soy bacon, deli meats, burgers, meatloaf, and turkey.
Deep-fried and breaded chicken and fish.
Frozen prepared meals.

◆ <u>Fats.</u> In the form of:
All refined vegetable and seed oils such as corn, safflower, canola, and sunflower oil from supermarkets.
Lard.
Hydrogenated or partially hydrogenated oils, margarines, and shortenings.
Nondairy creamer.

◆ Dairy. In the form of:
All reduced-fat or nonfat dairy products.
All pasteurized or ultra-heat-treated fluid dairy products, organic or nonorganic.
All homogenized nonorganic dairy products.
Powdered milk, acidophilus milk, and buttermilk.
Imitation milk, including rice, soy, oat, and almond milk.
Sour cream.
Processed cheese products, including American cheese, processed cheese food, nonorganic cream cheese, cottage cheese, ricotta cheese, and mozzarella.
Ice cream and frozen yogurt.

◆ Grains and starches. In the form of:
Unbleached, bleached, and fortified white flour and white-flour products such as breakfast cereal, packaged grain products, grain flours, tapioca, arrowroot, and corn starch. Also, most commercially made crackers, cookies, pastries, and cakes.

◆ Vegetables. In the form of:
Deep-fried or processed vegetables.

◆ Fruits. In the form of:
Canned fruits packed in heavy or light syrup or with added sugar.
Dried fruits with added sugar or sulfites.

◆ Sweeteners. In the form of:
Malt.
Barley malt.
Corn syrup.
Sugar.
Artificial sweeteners such as aspartame, acesulfame K, sucrulose, and saccharine.
Rice syrup.
Fruit juice concentrate.
Fructose.
Glucose.
Dextrose.

FOS.
Inulin.
Dahulin.

- **Legumes.** In the form of:
Unsoaked legumes and beans.
Nonorganic peanut products.

- **Nuts and seeds.** In the form of:
Nuts and seeds roasted in vegetable oil.
Honey-roasted nuts and seeds.
Soy nut butter.

- **Beverages.** In the form of:
Concentrated fruit juices and frozen concentrates.
Carbonated soft drinks.
Tap water.
Diet drinks.
Nonorganic coffee.
Wine with sulfites.
Pasteurized beer.
Hard liquor.

- **Condiments.** In the form of:
Condiments made with sugar, preservatives, MSG, texturized
    vegetable protein (TVP), soy protein isolate, or artificial sweet-
    ener.
Pickled ginger with sugar.
Bouillon cubes.
Instant soups.
Agar.
Carrageen.
Nonorganic mayonnaise made with soybean oil.
Bean and other dips.

- **Miscellaneous items.** In the form of:
Liquid medications and elixirs that contain sugar or artificial
    sweeteners. Ask your pharmacist for help.

Sample Three-Day Plan

Here is a sample three-day meal and supplement plan for Phase Three.

◆ Day One ◆

◆ Upon rising: 1 to 2 tablespoons of detoxification clay and 12 drops of structured water additive mixed in 8 ounces of water; 1 to 2 tablespoons of detoxification clay, one serving of natural fiber product, and 12 drops of structured water additive mixed in 12 ounces of water; 8 to 16 ounces of thirty-hour cultured goat's milk yogurt; or 1 to 2 tablespoons of whole-food mineral powder mixed in 8 to 16 ounces of vegetable juice.

◆ Morning supplements: One serving of probiotic supplement and three to six caplets of natural anti-inflammatory formula.

◆ Breakfast: Synergy Smoothie (see page 331 for the recipe) and one to three caplets of digestive enzymes.

◆ Lunch: Grilled salmon with organic vegetables (broccoli, onion, yellow squash, and garlic) stir-fried in coconut oil and one to three caplets of digestive enzymes.

◆ Dinner: Green salad with High Omega-3 Salad Dressing (see page 330 for the recipe); grass-fed meatloaf with roasted or steamed vegetables; and one to three caplets of digestive enzymes.

◆ Snack: Balanced Veggie Juice (see page 327 for the recipe).

◆ Evening supplements: One serving of probiotic supplement and three to six caplets of natural anti-inflammatory formula.

◆ Before bed: 1 to 2 tablespoons of detoxification clay and 12 drops of structured water additive mixed in 8 ounces of water; 1 to 2 tablespoons of detoxification clay, one serving of natural fiber product, and 12 drops of structured water additive mixed in 12 ounces of water; 8 to 16 ounces of thirty-hour cultured goat's milk yogurt; or 1 to 2 tablespoons of whole-food mineral powder mixed in 8 to 16 ounces of vegetable juice.

◆ Beverages: Pure water with 12 drops of structured water additive mixed in each 8-ounce glass, a lacto-fermented beverage, or Balanced Veggie Juice. Drink beverages between meals.

◆ Day Two ◆

◆ Upon rising: 1 to 2 tablespoons of detoxification clay and 12 drops of structured water additive mixed in 8 ounces of water; 1 to 2 tablespoons of detoxification clay, serving of natural fiber product, and 12 drops of structured water additive mixed in 12 ounces of water; 8 to 16 ounces of thirty-hour cultured goat's milk yogurt; or 1 to 2 tablespoons of whole-food mineral powder mixed in 8 to 16 ounces of vegetable juice.

◆ Morning supplements: One serving of probiotic supplement and three to six caplets of natural anti-inflammatory formula.

◆ Breakfast: Three poached high omega-3 eggs; 2 ounces of raw sauerkraut; steamed organic vegetables topped with olive oil, coconut oil, or goat's milk butter and Celtic sea salt or Herbamare, or 2 pieces of sprouted or natural sourdough bread with Brasco Butter (see page 329 for the recipe); and one to three caplets of digestive enzymes.

◆ Lunch: Green salad with chicken, tuna, or salmon, or free-range chicken with steamed or stir-fried vegetables; and one to three caplets of digestive enzymes.

◆ Dinner: Green salad with High Omega-3 Dressing; Brasco Broth with chicken and vegetables; and one to three caplets of digestive enzymes.

◆ Snack: Creamy High Enzyme Dessert (see page 330 for the recipes).

◆ Evening supplements: One serving of probiotic supplement and three to six caplets of natural anti-inflammatory formula.

◆ Before bed: 1 to 2 tablespoons of detoxification clay and 12 drops of structured water additive mixed in 8 ounces of water; 1 to 2 tablespoons of detoxification clay, one serving of natural fiber product, and 12 drops of structured water additive mixed in 12 ounces of water; 8 to 16 ounces of thirty-hour cultured goat's milk yogurt; or 1 to 2 tablespoons of whole-food mineral powder mixed in 8 to 16 ounces of vegetable juice.

◆ Beverages: Pure water with 12 drops of structured water additive mixed in each 8-ounce glass, lacto-fermented beverage, or Balanced Veggie Juice. Drink beverages between meals.

◆ Day Three ◆

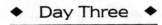

◆ Upon rising: 1 to 2 tablespoons of detoxification clay and 12 drops of structured water additive mixed in 8 ounces of water; 1 to 2 tablespoons of detoxification clay, one serving of natural fiber product, and 12 drops of structured water additive mixed in 12 ounces of water; 8 to 16 ounces of thirty-hour cultured goat's milk yogurt; or 1 to 2 tablespoons of whole-food mineral powder mixed in 8 to 16 ounces of vegetable juice.

◆ Morning supplements: One serving of probiotic supplement and three to six caplets of natural anti-inflammatory formula.

◆ Breakfast: Three eggs soft-boiled or fried in coconut oil; sliced oranges, apples, or grapefruit; 1 tablespoon each of raw nut or seed butter and honey; and one to three caplets of digestive enzymes.

◆ Lunch: Roasted chicken; carrots and onions; and one to three caplets of digestive enzymes.

◆ Dinner: Green salad with High Omega-3 Dressing or fruit and soft goat's milk *chèvre;* grilled fish (salmon, tuna, snapper, or cod); steamed or stir-fried vegetables; and one to three caplets of digestive enzymes.

◆ Snack: Raw organic carrots dipped in raw organic almond butter or organic apple slices spread with organic almond or sesame butter.

◆ Evening supplements: One serving of probiotic supplement and three to six caplets of natural anti-inflammatory formula.

◆ Before bed: 1 to 2 tablespoons of detoxification clay and 12 drops of structured water additive mixed in 8 ounces of water; 1 to 2 tablespoons of detoxification clay, one serving of natural fiber product, and 12 drops of structured water additive mixed in 12 ounces of water; 8 to 16 ounces of thirty-hour cultured goat's milk yogurt; or 1 to 2 tablespoons of whole-food mineral powder mixed in 8 to 16 ounces of vegetable juice.

- Beverages: Pure water with 12 drops of structured water additive mixed in each 8-ounce glass, lacto-fermented beverage, or Balanced Veggie Juice. Drink beverages between meals.

A word for the budgetarily challenged: If you are on a restricted budget, we recommend consuming canned tuna, sardines, and salmon instead of fresh fish. You can also eat conventionally grown fruits and vegetables that have been treated with a special produce wash. (For sources of produce washes, see "Resources" on page 333.)

Notes on Phase Three

Mercury is an issue in the case of deep-water fish. However, we feel that the benefits of eating fish outweigh the risks from mercury poisoning. Fish is rich in vitamins A and D. It contains healthy omega-3 fatty acids. Fish provide zinc and iodine, two minerals that are found in abundance in the ocean but have been depleted from the soil. Deep-water fish are not as subject to mercury poisoning because they live so far from land.

All cooking oils should be certified organic or chemical free. Processed oils are produced under high heat. They are subject to rancidity. Most include deodorizing chemicals that disguise their rancidity.

Organic fruit and vegetables are excellent, but they are also expensive. What's more, the definition of "organic" differs from person to person and from state to state. Do your best to obtain organic vegetables and fruit while staying within your budget. If you have to make compromises, we recommend compromising on organic fruits and vegetables before grass-fed meat and free-range poultry. In other words, it is better to spend the money on high-quality meat than on organic fruit and vegetables.

It is important to carry digestive enzyme supplements with you at all times. This way, when you eat at someone else's house or in a restaurant that offers only "Bad" or "Ugly" foods, you can take the enzymes and hope to digest the food properly. For additional guidelines when eating out, see page 249.

Handling a Flare-Up

During a flare-up, the old familiar symptoms of bowel disease return and you may think that you are sick again. In fact, many people who start to feel better after having been ill for a long time believe that their flare-up is going to last and they will never be well again. You must not buy into this lie. Flare-ups happen to many people. During the flare-up, you need to consume food that is easy to digest, high in nutrient density, and low in calories and volume. In other words, you need food that packs a lot of nutrients but is easy to digest. Digestion takes work. Not only does the body have to work harder to digest high-calorie food, high-calorie food also taxes the immune system, since the immune system has to run a check for pathogens on all food as it arrives.

Chicken broth is the ideal food during a flare-up. If you can't get chicken broth, then try beef broth. As the South American proverb states, "Good broth resurrects the dead." Here is a protocol for people experiencing flare ups:

- Day One: Eat chicken broth only. Make sure the chicken broth is well cooked and does not contain hard fibrous vegetables, which are difficult to digest. Move on to Day Two if you start to feel better. Otherwise, continue with the broth.
- Day Two: Eat chicken broth with well-cooked vegetables. If you start to feel better, move on to Day Three. Otherwise, continue consuming the broth with vegetables.
- Day Three: Consume thirty-hour cultured goat's milk yogurt. However, if you have a known milk allergy, substitute soft fruits and vegetables or a probiotic supplement. The object of consuming yogurt, kefir, or a probiotic supplement is to increase the beneficial bacteria in your intestines.

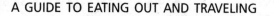

A GUIDE TO EATING OUT AND TRAVELING

Besides the usual challenge of keeping your self-discipline, sticking to the Guts and Glory Program presents a new set of difficulties when you are traveling. You don't know where the stores that sell healthy food are. You find yourself in restaurants where "Bad" and "Ugly" food is served.

When you go to restaurants on the road, stick with the proteins—fish, chicken, and beef. Ask the waiter if the food is cooked in butter or margarine and choose food items prepared in butter. Always order vegetables instead of potatoes. If your budget allows, eat at higher-end restaurants, which generally offer more "Good" and "Not So Bad" choices than, for example, fast-food restaurants. Typically, they offer the healthiest food. Most importantly, avoid bread and desert. These foods are loaded with carbohydrates and calories. Usually, the simpler the meal, the better it is for your digestive health.

Here are some meal suggestions for eating out:

◆ Breakfast: Eggs, fruit, and lean meats such as breakfast steak are the best choices. Ask the waiter if the eggs are prepared in margarine or shortening, and if they are, avoid them. Skip the ubiquitous toast and hash browns that are served at so many roadside diners.

◆ Lunch: Salads, lean meats, fish, and fresh fruit are available on most luncheon menus. Stay with olive oil dressings. That means no ranch or Thousand Island dressing.

◆ Dinner: Ask for seafood or lean meat as the main course, and remember to keep it simple. Avoid rich sauces. As a side dish, have steamed vegetables or salad.

Be sure to pack digestive enzyme supplements when you are going on the road. No matter where your travels take you and what food you eat, digestive enzymes can help you digest the food. They make it less likely that you will suffer heartburn, diarrhea, or worse.

We strongly recommend eating homemade chicken broth with whole free-range chickens, organic vegetables, and Celtic sea salt. Canned chicken soup contains large amounts of processed salt and other additives that are difficult for the bowel to handle. Moreover, a broth you make yourself contains far more nutrients, including collagen, gelatin, and vitamins A and D, as well as healthy omega-3 fats.

If you have IBS or a functional bowel disorder, your flare-up should resolve within twenty-four to thirty-six hours. People with IBD, on the other hand, may need to stay on the flare-up program longer, for three days to two weeks.

After the flare-up starts to calm down, the next step is to acidify and rebalance the flora in the gut. The best way to do that is with thirty-hour cultured goat's milk yogurt. You should also consider taking a natural anti-inflammatory formula.

Sometimes modified fasting is the best course. It depends on how sick you are. A day of fasting or semifasting for people with a gut problem is helpful because it allows the gut to rest. It also suppresses bacterial replication and reduces the total population of microflora in the gut, including the harmful bacteria. Modified fasting should be undertaken only occasionally and should be augmented with easy-to-assimilate foods such as Brasco Broth. The medication Flagyl can be beneficial for IBD especially early on and may even work because it lowers the microbial population. You can, however, suppress bacterial replication in the gut with a simple chicken broth diet and short fasts. Fasting is especially useful for those with Crohn's disease.

Foods Essential to Healing

The last part of this chapter concerns the foods that are essential to healing and good health. You are encouraged to fall in love with these foods. They can be your best friends. These foods are nutritious and soothing to the bowel. They have been eaten since primitive times for their nutritional qualities, not to mention their good flavor. Sources for these foods can be found in "Resources" on page 333.

Cereal Grass Juice

Cereal grass juice from the young leaves of wheat, oat, and barley are nutrient powerhouses. Wheatgrass juice has been consumed around the world and taken as a primary therapy for digestive disorders such as IBS, ulcers, and inflammatory bowel disease (Crohn's and ulcerative colitis). The minerals in wheatgrass are easy to assimilate. Wheatgrass contains minerals, lightweight vegetable proteins, and chlorophyll. It is nature's richest source of trace minerals. Many people with digestive sensitivities cannot handle fresh wheatgrass juice, but many do well with powder juice extracts.

Coconut Oil

Coconut oil is an extremely healthy fat. It contains large amounts of lauric acid, one of the chief fatty acids in breast milk. According to scientific and clinical research, consuming coconut oil can reduce the risk of deadly degenerative diseases such as cancer, heart disease, and diabetes. Coconut oil supports the immune system and helps prevent bacterial, viral, and fungal infections. Reportedly, it reduced the symptoms of Crohn's disease, ulcerative colitis, diverticulosis, IBS, and constipation. Coconut oil is one of the best oils to cook with because it can withstand heat without oxidation. People who suffer from digestive disorders often notice an improvement in symptoms after they substitute coconut oil for their regular cooking oil.

Cod Liver Oil

For those who can't stomach organ meats, cod liver oil is the next best thing. Cod liver oil contains large amounts of fat-soluble vitamins A and D, as well as the essential fatty acids EPA and DHA. You will be glad to know that you can obtain flavored cod liver oil that actually tastes pretty good.

Cultured Beverages

Cultured beverages such as kvass are great sources of probiotics, enzymes, and electrolytes. Consuming cultured beverages between meals strengthens the digestive tract and aids in the restoration of the proper acidic balance of the colon. Cultured beverages provide electrolytes, which help to rapidly hydrate the body.

Cultured Vegetables

Raw, cultured vegetables are a great source of naturally occurring probiotics and enzymes. Cultured vegetables can aid in the digestion of meals that contain cooked animal protein. The daily consumption of raw, cultured vegetables, including sauerkraut, can help keep the digestive tract healthy and even eliminate harmful microorganisms such as *Candida albicans*.

Fatty Fish

High-fat ocean fish such as salmon, sardines, mackarel, herring, and tuna is nature's richest source of the omega-3 fatty acids EPA and DHA. Dr. Weston Price found that cultures that relied on fish as their main source of protein were the healthiest among all the indigenous groups he studied. Fish provides easily absorbable protein and minerals. It is great for the heart. Fresh fish is best, but canned sardines and herring (with skin and bones) may be the exception to the rule. Canned sardines contain healthy levels of omega-3 fat, are high in calcium, and are one of nature's richest sources of nucleic acids.

Goat's Milk Butter

Goat's milk butter is an excellent source of the short-chain fatty acids CLA and medium-chain triglycerides. Short-chain fatty acids such as butyric acid and medium-chain triglycerides such as caprylic acid have beneficial effects on intestinal health. They lower the colonic pH and destroy harmful pathogens such as *Candida albicans.* The molecules in goat's milk butter are small than those in cow's milk. For that reason, the molecules can pass through the intestinal wall more easily and be absorbed by the body.

Rather than cook with goat's milk butter, use it as a spread on food served at room temperature or cooler. Or eat it off a spoon with some honey. Dr. Weston Price found that the butter made from animals that grazed on grass and vegetation taken along with cod liver oil provides excellent health benefits to those suffering from various illnesses, including malnutrition. We recommend consuming goat's milk butter or coconut oil instead of butter made from cow's milk.

Grass-Fed or Organic Organ Meat

Almost all of the ancient cultures that Dr. Weston Price studied prized organ meats for their ability to build strength and vitality. Organ meats are rich sources of fat-soluble vitamins A and D. They contain a great balance of the B vitamins and are among the best sources of minerals, including zinc. It is important to note that organ meats must come from organic or free-range animals. Toxins tend to concentrate in the organs of animals that are given growth hormones and pesticides. For that reason, eating organ meats from animals that were not properly raised is very harmful.

Grass-Fed Red Meat

Grass-fed red meat, including beef, buffalo, and lamb, is an excellent source of high-quality protein, vitamin $B_{12,}$ and iron. Grass-fed red meat provides protective nutrients such as CLA, carnitine, and creatine. Grass-fed meat also has a much higher omega-3 fatty acid content than grain-fed meat.

High Omega-3 Eggs

Eggs from chickens, turkeys, and ducks that are truly free to roam and eat a diet high in insects and worms, as well as eggs from chickens fed certain strains of algae, contain large amounts of the important omega-3 fatty acids. Eggs from these birds usually contain a ratio of omega-3 to omega-6 acids between one to one and one to four, whereas eggs from battery-raised hens have a ratio of omega-3 to omega-6 fatty acids of one to twenty. Studies show that omega-3 fatty acids are helpful against high blood pressure, heart disease, blood clotting, diabetes, colitis, and inflammatory diseases. So-called battery-raised hens are kept in coops where a light is always burning. This confuses the hens into thinking it is daytime, which makes them lay more eggs.

In addition to DHA, omega-3 eggs contain significant amounts of vitamins E and B_{12}, as well as the antioxidants lutein and beta-carotene. By eating two eggs high in the omega-3 fatty acids, you get as much as 150 milligrams of DHA. Eggs are healthiest when they are poached or soft boiled. Frying and scrambling eggs can damage some of the nutrients contained in the yolk. Omega-3 eggs make a wonderful addition to any diet.

Organic Berries

Berries are some of nature's richest sources of antioxidants. Organic blueberries, strawberries, raspberries, and blackberries contain powerful disease-fighting phytochemicals such as ellagic acid, quercetin, vitamin C, and anthocyanins. Berries are also high in fiber. A great way to enjoy the antioxidant power of berries is to incorporate them into smoothies, top them with yogurt, or top them with quark, a yogurt-like cheese from central Europe available in specialty food stores.

Stocks

Soup stocks properly prepared from meat, fish, or poultry contain many life-giving nutrients, including minerals, gelatin, and electrolytes from vegetables. Many people are unaware of the research that has been done on the naturally occurring gelatin found in stocks. Gelatin acts as a digestive aid. It has been used successfully in the treatment of many intestinal disorders, including nonulcerative dyspepsia (sour stomach), IBS, ulcers, and Crohn's disease. Stocks also contain cartilage and collagen, both of which have been used to aid in the health of those suffering from arthritis and other inflammatory conditions. The consumption of stocks such as chicken soup can help heal the digestive lining and reduce the inflammation that occurs in many severe digestive disorders.

❖

The Dangers of *Streptococcus Thermophilus*

We recommend choosing cultured dairy products that do not contain the bacterial strain *Streptococcus thermophilus*. Studies have shown that people who suffer from autoimmune diseases such as rheumatoid arthritis run the risk of aggravating the symptoms of their disease if they consume more than two cups of yogurt that contains *Streptococcus thermophilus*. What's more, *Streptococcus thermophilus* can cause a shift in immune function known as a Th2-dominated immune system. People with Th2-mediated immune systems have higher incidences of allergies and other illnesses. People suffering from digestive problems usually have imbalanced or weak immune systems. For this reason, avoiding products that may contribute to immune system dysfunction is wise if you have an intestinal disease.

Most commercial yogurts and probiotic supplements, even those found in health-food stores, contain *Streptococcus thermophilus*. We have found that goat's milk yogurt cultured for thirty hours that does not contain *Streptococcus thermophilus* but is cultured using *Lactobacillus bulgaricus*, *Lactobacillus acidophilus*, and other friendly strains.

Thirty-Hour Cultured Goat's Milk Products

Goat's milk yogurt that has been fermented for thirty hours is a rich source of probiotics, enzymes, and short-chain fatty acids. It is virtually free of lactose, which means that people who are lactose intolerant can consume it. It is a rich source of selenium. It does not contain *Streptococcus thermophilus,* the bacterial strain that has been known to exacerbate certain autoimmune disorders, or *Mycobacterium avium* paratuberculosis (MAP), the microorganism that some believe may be involved in the development of Crohn's disease. (For a discussion of *Streptococcus thermophilus,* see page 255.)

Not only does goat's milk yogurt have no negative effects, it is very beneficial for a healthy immune system. Anybody who can obtain this excellent healing food should take full advantage of it. Co-author Jordan Rubin has consumed cultured goat's milk products for the last seven years and believes they are one of the secrets that helped him overcome his digestive illness.

Unheated Honey

Raw, unheated honey is nature's only predigested food. Unheated honey supplies a rich array of nutrients, including amino acids and enzymes. The body uses pure honey for quick energy. Consumed in small amounts, honey does not contribute to blood sugar imbalances. Raw, unheated honey is the only sweetener we recommend. Nevertheless, you should consume it in moderation.

Vegetable Juice

Vegetable juices, especially green juices, are potent sources of enzymes, vitamins, and trace minerals. Vegetable juices are easy to assimilate. They supply many of the nutrients that are needed to rebuild health.

❖ 10 ❖

Protocols

This chapter presents protocols, or plans of treatment, for some two-dozen gastrointestinal diseases and disorders. It also describes the various gut-related diseases and disorders. Using the protocols, the vast majority of our patients have improved their digestive health. They have dramatically improved their absorption and assimilation of foods and nutrients. They have dramatically improved their elimination of waste. Many of our patients have been able to overcome longstanding symptoms and remain free of disease. They have been able to stop taking medications.

All the protocols refer to the foods and supplements in the Guts and Glory Program. For that reason, we refer often to Phase One, Phase Two, and Phase Three of the program. The three phases are explained in Chapter 9. You will also find references to "Good," "Bad," "Not So Bad," and "Ugly" foods. These foods are listed in Chapter 9.

As part of each protocol, you will find recommendations in these categories:

- *Diet.* The phases of the Guts and Glory Program to follow and how long to remain on them.
- *Therapeutic foods.* The foods that can positively enhance your body's healing response.

◆ *Supplements.* The health supplements you can take to alleviate your symptoms and improve your gut health.

The focus of this book is overcoming digestive illness, but we believe that the health of the gastrointestinal tract is fundamental for overall well-being. If you follow these protocols diligently, you should see improvement in the first month of the program. What's more, you may experience many side benefits. You will have more energy, a healthy weight loss, and improved skin tone. Your memory and ability to concentrate will improve. However, if you are suffering from a severe digestive disorder, you may not notice a significant improvement for as long as ninety days. If after that period you see little or no results and you can honestly say that you followed the program diligently, the program is unlikely to work for you. We advise you to seek help elsewhere.

Lifestyle Therapies

Throughout this chapter, we explain therapeutic foods you can eat to improve your health. We also list supplements to take. However, changing your lifestyle is another important part of conquering digestive illness. Following are some lifestyle therapies that we recommend. When a therapy requires obtaining a product of some kind, you will find sources for the product in "Resources" on page 350. Chapter 4 explains the benefits of these lifestyle therapies in detail.

◆ *Squatting for elimination.* Squatting aligns the colon properly for elimination and allows the colon to empty more completely. Using an elimination bench to raise the legs during elimination can help to fully detoxify the colon.
◆ *Exercise.* As well as toning and strengthening the muscles, exercise encourages peristalsis, the wavelike expanding and contracting of the digestive system that eliminates waste. If your condition allows it, we recommend taking some form of moderate exercise daily. Something as simple as walking can be very healthy.
◆ *Avoiding oral contraceptives (females).* Evidence shows that oral

contraceptives can lead to imbalanced intestinal flora and may contribute to yeast overgrowth (candidiasis).

- *Sunlight.* Spend approximately twenty minutes each day in the sun. Most of the vitamin D you obtain comes from sunlight. Many people with chronic diseases as well as digestive disorders have less than the optimal levels of vitamin D.
- *Breathing properly.* Doing five to fifteen minutes of deep breathing exercises can be very beneficial. Inhale through your nose for three to seven seconds and exhale quickly through your mouth. Deep breathing can enhance your oxygen utilization and improve the functioning of your immune system.
- *Sauna or steam detoxification.* Spend twenty to thirty minutes daily in a sauna or steam bath. Raising the temperature of your body helps it detoxify and expel foreign substances.
- *Detoxification baths.* Take baths with essential oils, clays, and other healing compounds. Doing so aids the body's ability to detoxify harmful chemicals. To make a clay bath, fill the tub with hot water and add a half to 1 cup of powdered clay (available in the cosmetic section of most health-food stores). Stay in the bath for five to thirty minutes. These baths may cause a temporary feeling of weakness and other detoxification symptoms, so you may have to stay in the bath for short periods of time at first. After the bath, consume 16 ounces of structured water, vegetable juice, or water mixed with 1 to 2 tablespoons of a whole-food mineral powder.
- *Skin brushing.* Skin brushing removes dead skin, improves the circulation, and aids in the detoxification of harmful chemicals.
- *Sleep.* Getting enough sleep is essential, especially if you have a digestive disorder. Nighttime is when the body detoxifies and regenerates. The time you go to sleep matters. Try to get at least one to two hours of sleep before midnight.
- *Chewing properly.* Chew each bite of food thirty to fifty times to ensure proper digestion and absorption. Slowing down to eat and chewing properly greatly decrease indigestion.
- *Eating smaller meals.* Eat small meals instead of stuffing yourself. Many foods recommended in our program greatly enhance me-

tabolism. When large portions are consumed, however, metabolism slows down, digestion is stressed, and feelings of weakness and lethargy ensue.

◆ *Avoiding ice-cold foods and beverages.* Ice-cold foods and beverages may shock your digestive tract and shut down your digestive function. The body must work very hard to raise the temperature of foods and beverages to body temperature. People in Eastern cultures never consume cold foods because they "weaken the digestive fire." Even foods from the refrigerator should be left at room temperature for ten minutes to help dispel the cold.

Allergies

See Food Allergies and Food Intolerances.

Bloating

See Intestinal Gas and Bloating.

Candidiasis

Candidiasis, also known as candida, is caused by a yeast fungus called *Candida albicans*. As a yeast, *Candida albicans* is found in many places in the body: the throat, mouth, digestive tract, and vaginal tract. It is also found on the skin. *Candida albicans* has many uses in the digestive tract. For example, the yeast recognizes and destroys harmful bacteria. However, if the yeast grows out of control, it can become aggressive and produce candidiasis, intestinal disease, vaginal infections, and thrush, an infection of the mouth. Sufferers also complain of fatigue, allergic-type reactions, and episodic occurrences of altered sensorium (better known as brain fog).

Candida is believed to contribute to a host of gastrointestinal complaints when it is out of balance with the other microbes in the gastrointestinal tract. These complaints include constipation, diarrhea, gas, bloating, and abdominal pain. Although conventional medicine does not recognize it, enough anecdotal evidence can be found to suggest the existence of a yeast overgrowth syndrome. This syndrome occurs when the by-products of yeast metabolism enter the system.

Many cases of candida occur after taking antibiotics. Antibiotics kill all bacteria, friendly and unfriendly, in the gut. Because candida is a yeast, however, it is unaffected by antibiotics. After the bacteria in the gut die, candida can take over and multiply. In susceptible individuals, a sugar-rich diet may also contribute to the development of candida because the yeast tends to favor sugar. (Interestingly, a study concerning yeast and sugar published several years ago in the *American Journal of Clinical Nutrition* found that a high-sugar diet made certain individuals worse, but did not uniformly increase the growth of candida in all individuals on the sugar diet. The authors of the study concluded that a high-sugar diet alone may not be enough to cause candida, but if you have candida or are susceptible to developing it, a high-sugar and -carbohydrate diet will likely make your candida worse.) Hormonal changes brought on by the menstrual cycle, oral contraceptives, and diabetes can also cause or exacerbate a candida infection.

The authors of this book humbly acknowledge the presence of gut candida as a true entity, but we do not think it is the scourge of humanity. In the alternative medical community, every human ill from gut aches to bad hair to global warming has been attributed to a candida infection. This pseudo-diagnosis is thrown around haphazardly, and frankly, it drives us crazy. We believe that candida overgrowth is a symptom, not a disease entity unto itself. When the gut flora are fortified and the factors that contribute to candida are properly addressed, the body should be able to heal itself of candida. Following the principles of the Guts and Glory Program, we have often successfully treated candida without having to resort to antifungal pharmaceuticals.

Diet

Phase One: one day.

Phase Two: fourteen days.

Phase Three: six to twelve months.

Restrict your consumption of grains, fruits, and sweeteners of any kind until your symptoms are gone. Candida favors the sugar in these foods.

Therapeutic Foods

These therapeutic foods will help you get well:

- *Cultured goat's milk dairy products.* Consume 8 to 32 ounces of the highest-quality cultured dairy products from goat's or sheep's milk. Try to find yogurt that does not contain the organism *Streptococcus thermophilus*, a bacterial microbe that has been implicated in the exacerbation of certain immune-system disorders.
- *Grass-fed red meat.* Red meat from grass-fed cattle, buffalo, and lamb is very healthy and can be eaten several times per week. This meat is a great source of protein, minerals, vitamin B_{12}, vitamin D, beta-carotene, omega-3 fats, and CLA.
- *Omega-3 eggs.* Consume as many as two to four eggs high in the omega-3 fatty acids each day. These eggs contain DHA, vitamins E and B_{12}, and antioxidants.
- *Coconut oil.* This oil is perhaps the healthiest of the widely available oils. We recommend cooking almost exclusively with coconut oil. Consume as much as 2 to 4 tablespoons of the oil in cooking, in smoothies, or right off the spoon. It contains large amounts of lauric acid, a potent antimicrobial and one of the chief fatty acids in breast milk.
- *Ocean-caught fish.* This type of fish is perhaps the healthiest of all the protein sources. Salmon, sardines, mackerel, herring, and tuna are high in the omega-3 fatty acids EPA and DHA. Ocean-caught fish can be consumed every day to enhance digestive and immune system health.
- *Cod liver oil.* Take 1 teaspoon of plain or flavored cod liver oil each day. Cod liver oil is a fantastic source of the omega-3 fats DHA and EPA, as well as of vitamins A and D.
- *Vegetable juice.* As long as your diarrhea is not active, consume

vegetable juices that are low in carbohydrates, such as celery and green juices, mixed with a small amount of higher-carbohydrate veggies, such as carrot or beet. Mix in some form of healthy fat with each glass of the juice. A teaspoon of cultured goat's milk, coconut milk and cream, or flaxseed oil enhances the absorption of minerals and prevents spikes in blood sugar.

◆ *Fermented vegetables.* Consume a few tablespoons of fermented vegetables such as sauerkraut with each meal to aid in digestion. Fermented vegetables are excellent sources of naturally occurring probiotics and enzymes.

◆ *Stocks.* After completing Phases One and Two of the program, consume stocks on a regular basis, especially when you have a cold or the flu. Stocks made from the bones of chicken, fish, lamb, or beef contain minerals, gelatin, cartilage, collagen, and electrolytes. Stocks help to heal the gut lining and reduce inflammation.

Supplements

Take these health supplements to alleviate your symptoms and get well:

◆ *Antifungal formula.* Follow the two-week, intensive antifungal program as directed on the label. Return to the two-week program if symptoms return.

◆ *Probiotic with HSOs.* Begin after the two-week intensive antifungal program. Take six caplets a day, adding one caplet per day until you have reached twelve. Remain at twelve caplets per day for six months or until your symptoms disappear. Then gradually reduce the dosage to three to six caplets per day for maintenance purposes.

◆ *Digestive enzymes.* Take one to three caplets with each meal and snack.

◆ *Fiber.* Along with clay (see below), consume one serving twice per day, morning and evening. Consuming a fiber supplement is essential during the first two weeks of the program. Thereafter, consume fiber as needed.

- *Clay.* Take 1 to 2 tablespoons of clay along with fiber (see above) during the initial two weeks of the program. The clay will absorb the toxins excreted by the fungi as they are destroyed. Taking clay is essential when you have a fungal infection.
- *Essential fats.* Take 1 teaspoon of flavored cod liver oil.
- *Protein digestant.* If you are over sixty years of age and you experience post-meal belching and bloating after one full month on the program, take one to five tablets at the beginning of each meal containing protein.
- *Structured mineral water.* Consume at least 64 ounces per day of a high-quality structured or high-mineral water.
- *Pet natural antimicrobial product.* We recommend giving your pets a natural antimicrobial product to minimize the chance of cross-infection by microbes.

Additional Therapies

Essential oils and aromatherapy may be helpful in eradicating fungal infections. To eradicate nail and skin fungi, look for natural antifungals made from grapefruit seed extract or other essential oils. Be sure to follow the instructions for use carefully. We believe that fungal infections of the skin and fingernails can be outward symptoms of a systemic fungal infestation. (Toenail infections, however, are often isolated and not associated with a systemic condition.) Skin and fingernail infections often improve after the internal environment is rid of yeast overgrowth. (In the case of stubborn fingernail infections, coauthor Dr. Brasco sometimes reluctantly turns to antifungal pharmaceuticals. Under close supervision, these agents are relatively safe and usually effective.)

Fungi, particularly candida, can be passed easily between partners during intercourse. Using the same bathroom regularly can also spread fungi. To successfully eliminate a chronic fungal infection, it is crucial for all members of the family to consume a probiotic with HSOs at the bare minimum.

Celiac Disease

Celiac disease, also known as gluten intolerance or sprue, is a genetic disorder in which the sufferer cannot digest gluten. Gluten is found in wheat, rye, barley, oats, and spelt. The disease affects 1 in 150 to 250 American adults, according to the University of Maryland Center for Celiac Research. The disease usually strikes people of Northern European descent and is twice as common in women than men. The symptoms include weight loss, diarrhea, constipation, bloating, abdominal cramping, and steatorrhea (gray or tan stools that are foamy and float due to their high fat content). Because celiacs have trouble absorbing food, the disease may also cause iron deficiency, anemia, malnutrition, osteopenia, and bone pain. Some researchers blame celiac disease for depression and schizophrenia as well. The disease is sometimes difficult to diagnose because certain people have mild or nonspecific symptoms that last for many years.

Most researchers trace celiac disease to a protein fraction called gliadin that is found in gluten. In certain sensitive individuals, gliadin damages the villi on the lining of the small intestine such that the villi no longer absorb food properly. This lack of absorption subsequently leads to a malabsorption syndrome and all the problems associated with it.

Diet

Phase One: seven to fourteen days (severe cases only).

Phase Two: seven to fourteen days.

Phase Three: three to six months.

If you have been diagnosed with true gluten intolerance, it is essential that you avoid all grain and legume products for up to one year on the program or until your symptoms have disappeared. After your symptoms have been gone for six months, you can try sourdough or sprouted breads, or nongluten grains such as amaranth and quinoa. Celiacs should always take high-potency digestive enzyme supplements with each meal. To remain healthy, some celiacs should never again consume grains or legumes.

Therapeutic Foods

These therapeutic foods will help you get well:

- *Cultured goat's milk dairy products.* Consume 8 to 32 ounces of the highest-quality cultured dairy products from goat's or sheep's milk. Try to find yogurt that does not contain the organism *Streptococcus thermophilus*, a bacterial microbe that has been known to make certain immune-system disorders worse. (Nearly all available yogurt brands contain *S. thermophilus*.) Look for the description "Bulgarian yogurt."
- *Grass-fed red meat.* Red meat from grass-fed cattle, buffalo, and lamb is very healthy and can be eaten several times per week. This meat is a great source of protein, minerals, vitamin B_{12}, vitamin D, beta-carotene, omega-3 fats, and CLA.
- *Omega-3 eggs.* Consume as many as two to four eggs high in the omega-3 fatty acids each day. These eggs contain DHA, vitamins E and B_{12}, and antioxidants.
- *Coconut oil.* This oil is perhaps the healthiest of the widely available oils. We recommend cooking almost exclusively with coconut oil. Consume as much as 2 to 4 tablespoons of the oil in cooking, in smoothies, or right off the spoon. It contains large amounts of lauric acid, a potent antimicrobial and one of the chief fatty acids in breast milk.
- *Ocean-caught fish.* This type of fish is perhaps the healthiest of all the protein sources. Salmon, sardines, mackerel, herring, and tuna are high in the omega-3 fatty acids EPA and DHA. Ocean-caught fish can be consumed every day to enhance digestive and immune system health.
- *Cod liver oil.* Take 1 teaspoon of plain or flavored cod liver oil each day. Cod liver oil is a fantastic source of the omega-3 fats DHA and EPA, as well as of vitamins A and D.

- *Vegetable juice.* As long as your diarrhea is not active, consume vegetable juices that are low in carbohydrates, such as celery and green juices, mixed with a small amount of higher-carbohydrate veggies, such as carrot or beet. Mix in some form of healthy fat with each glass of the juice. A teaspoon of cultured goat's milk, coconut milk and cream, or flaxseed oil enhances the absorption of minerals and prevents spikes in blood sugar.
- *Fermented vegetables.* Consume a few tablespoons of fermented vegetables such as sauerkraut with each meal to aid in digestion. Fermented vegetables are excellent sources of naturally occurring probiotics and enzymes.
- *Stocks.* After completing Phases One and Two of the program, consume stocks on a regular basis, especially when you have a cold or flu. Stocks made from the bones of chicken, fish, lamb, or beef contain minerals, gelatin, cartilage, collagen, and electrolytes. Stocks help to heal the gut lining and reduce inflammation.

Supplements

Take these health supplements to alleviate your symptoms and get well:

- *Probiotic with HSOs.* Begin taking during Phase Two and work up to six to twelve caplets per day for six months. Then gradually reduce the dosage to three to six caplets per day for maintenance purposes.
- *Digestive enzymes.* Take one to three caplets per meal. Take more when consuming grains or legumes.
- *Whole-food mineral powder.* Take 1 to 2 tablespoons twice daily on an empty stomach to enhance your mineral absorption. The absorption of minerals is often hindered by gluten intolerance.
- *Essential fats.* Take 1 teaspoon per day of cod liver oil.
- *Protein digestant.* If you are over sixty years of age and you experience post-meal belching and bloating after one full month on the program, take one to five tablets at the beginning of each meal containing protein.

◆ *Structured mineral water.* Consume at least 64 ounces per day of a high-quality structured water.

Chronic Constipation

It seems that everyone gets constipation now and then. Constipation is defined as difficulty in voiding the bowels. Straining to relieve yourself, producing hard pellet-like stools, and going more than three days without elimination are all signs of constipation. Chronic constipation is defined as being constipated for at least one year and requiring laxatives or enemas to relieve yourself of waste matter. Women are more likely than men to suffer from chronic constipation. Seniors are afflicted more often than others. Constipation is a very common disorder. Americans spend about $725 million per year on laxatives. Some researchers believe that nearly 80 percent of the population suffers from some form of constipation. Many health experts believe that the bowels should move two to three times per day, which is the number of times the bowels move in healthy individuals who live in primitive cultures.

A number of factors can cause constipation. A lack of fiber in the diet is the chief cause. Essentially, fiber is plant material that the human body cannot digest. It comes from plant stems, leaves, and seeds. Fiber increases the volume of waste matter in the large intestine and puts pressure on the muscles of the rectum to loosen and expel waste. A lack of beneficial microorganisms in the digestive tract is another major cause of constipation. Lack of exercise and dehydration can also contribute. Some medications, including antihistamines, can be the culprit, too. Ironically, relying on laxatives causes constipation in the long run, because laxatives cause the bowel to grow lazy and fail to expel waste.

Including fibrous and enzyme-rich foods—vegetables, fruits, raw fermented foods, a high-quality probiotic, and digestive enzyme supplements—in your diet is the best way to relieve constipation. Drink plenty of water as well. Another way to prevent constipation is to exercise regularly. Exercise massages the intestines and encourages peristalsis, the rhythmic expanding and contracting of the digestive tract that pushes waste matter out of the body.

Diet

<u>Phase Three:</u> three or more months or until easy elimination occurs two to three times per day for six or more weeks.

Therapeutic Foods

These therapeutic foods will help you get well:

- *Cultured goat's milk dairy products.* Consume 8 to 32 ounces of the highest-quality cultured dairy products from goat's or sheep's milk. Try to find yogurt that does not contain the organism *Streptococcus thermophilus*, a bacterial microbe that has been known to make certain immune-system disorders worse.
- *Grass-fed red meat.* Red meat from grass-fed cattle, buffalo, and lamb is very healthy and can be eaten several times per week. This meat is a great source of protein, minerals, vitamin B_{12}, vitamin D, beta-carotene, omega-3 fats, and CLA.
- *Omega-3 eggs.* Consume as many as two to four eggs high in the omega-3 fatty acids each day. These eggs contain DHA, vitamins E and B_{12}, and antioxidants.
- *Coconut oil.* This oil is perhaps the healthiest of the widely available oils. We recommend cooking almost exclusively with coconut oil. Consume as much as 2 to 4 tablespoons of the oil in cooking, in smoothies, or right off the spoon. It contains large amounts of lauric acid, a potent antimicrobial and one of the chief fatty acids in breast milk.
- *Ocean-caught fish.* This type of fish is perhaps the healthiest of all the protein sources. Salmon, sardines, mackerel, herring, and tuna are high in the omega-3 fatty acids EPA and DHA. Ocean-caught fish can be consumed every day to enhance digestive and immune system health.
- *Cod liver oil.* Take 1 teaspoon of plain or flavored cod liver oil

each day. Cod liver oil is a fantastic source of the omega-3 fats DHA and EPA, as well as of vitamins A and D.

- *Vegetable juice.* As long as your diarrhea is not active, consume vegetable juices that are low in carbohydrates, such as celery and green juices, mixed with a small amount of higher-carbohydrate veggies, such as carrot or beet. Mix in some form of healthy fat with each glass of the juice. A teaspoon of cultured goat's milk, coconut milk and cream, or flaxseed oil enhances the absorption of minerals and prevents spikes in blood sugar.
- *Fermented vegetables.* Consume a few tablespoons of fermented vegetables such as sauerkraut with each meal to aid in digestion. Fermented vegetables are excellent sources of naturally occurring probiotics and enzymes.
- *Stocks.* After completing Phase One and Two of the program, consume stocks on a regular basis, especially when you have a cold or flu. Stocks made from the bones of chicken, fish, lamb, or beef contain minerals, gelatin, cartilage, collagen, and electrolytes. Stocks help to heal the gut lining and reduce inflammation.

Supplements

Take these health supplements to alleviate your symptoms and get well:

- *Probiotic with HSOs.* Consume six to twelve caplets per day for three to six months. After regularity is achieved, consume three to six caplets daily.
- *Digestive enzymes.* Take one to three caplets with each meal or snack.
- *Fiber.* Consume one serving twice per day, morning and evening.
- *Essential fats.* Take 1 teaspoon per day of cod liver oil.
- *Protein digestant.* If you are over sixty years of age and you experience post-meal belching and bloating after one full month on the program, take one to five tablets at the beginning of each meal containing protein.
- *Structured mineral water.* Consume at least 64 ounces per day of a high-quality structured or high-mineral water.

Additional Therapies

Colon hydrotherapy can be beneficial in cases of chronic constipation. Find a colon hydrotherapist who is properly trained and certified by a recognized certifying body. Colon hydrotherapy treatments can wash away friendly bacteria as well as putrefied waste material in the colon. For that reason, take six to twelve caplets of a high-quality probiotic with HSOs immediately following the colonic.

Colitis

See Irritable Bowel Syndrome *and* Ulcerative Colitis.

Crohn's Disease

Crohn's disease is a severe inflammation of the intestinal wall in which the inflammation extends deep into the tissue. Crohn's disease usually occurs in the small intestine, but it can occur throughout the digestive tract, in the esophagus, stomach, large intestine, and anus.

The symptoms include cramping, diarrhea, fever, rectal bleeding, and acute abdominal pain, often in the ileum, the lower part of the small intestine near the appendix. For this reason, the disease is sometimes misdiagnosed as appendicitis. The disease may form abscesses called fistulas that tunnel into surrounding tissue. Crohn's disease causes swelling and scar tissue on the walls of the intestine. This swelling and scarring can block the passage of waste in the intestines.

Because the small intestine's ability to absorb food is gravely impaired, Crohn's disease is often accompanied by weight loss, generalized weakness, and nutritional deficiencies. The disease can go into remission and flare up without notice.

The causes of Crohn's disease remain mysterious. Some researchers believe that the disease is an autoimmune reaction in which the immune system reacts mistakenly to what it thinks is a virus or bacterium in the bowel. Others think the disease is caused by a food sensitivity or an allergic reaction. Many researchers are now examining alterations in the gut microbe ecology to see if it helps cause the disease.

Diet

Phase One: seven to fourteen days, depending on the severity of the symptoms and until elimination improves.

Phase Two: seven to fourteen days, depending on severity (by the end of Phase Two, the symptoms should have significantly improved).

Phase Three: six to twelve months with extreme diligence.

After the symptoms are completely gone for at least three months, you can gradually add foods from the "Bad" category if you desire. Because people with Crohn's disease appear to have a predisposed weakness in their intestinal tracts, we strongly recommend that they adhere to a diet of foods in the "Good" and "Not So Bad" categories for the rest of their lives. If a relapse, or flare-up, occurs, go back to Phases One and Two until the symptoms improve and are eliminated.

Therapeutic Foods

These therapeutic foods will help you get well:

- *Cultured goat's milk dairy products.* Consume 8 to 32 ounces of the highest-quality cultured dairy products from goat's or sheep's milk. Try to find yogurt that does not contain the organism *Streptococcus thermophilus*, a bacterial microbe that has been known to make immune-system disorders worse.
- *Grass-fed red meat.* Red meat from grass-fed cattle, buffalo, and lamb is very healthy and can be eaten several times per week. This meat is a great source of protein, minerals, vitamin B_{12}, vitamin D, beta-carotene, omega-3 fats, and CLA.
- *Omega-3 eggs.* Consume as many as two to four eggs high in the omega-3 fatty acids each day. These eggs contain DHA, vitamins E and B_{12}, and antioxidants.

- *Coconut oil.* This oil is perhaps the healthiest of the widely available oils. We recommend cooking almost exclusively with coconut oil. Consume as much as 2 to 4 tablespoons of the oil in cooking, in smoothies, or right off the spoon. It contains large amounts of lauric acid, a potent antimicrobial and one of the chief fatty acids in breast milk.
- *Ocean-caught fish.* This type of fish is perhaps the healthiest of all the protein sources. Salmon, sardines, mackerel, herring, and tuna are high in the omega-3 fatty acids EPA and DHA. Ocean-caught fish can be consumed every day to enhance digestive and immune system health.
- *Cod liver oil.* Take 1 teaspoon of plain or flavored cod liver oil each day. Cod liver oil is a fantastic source of the omega-3 fats DHA and EPA, as well as vitamins A and D.
- *Vegetable juice.* As long as your diarrhea is not active, consume vegetable juices that are low in carbohydrates, such as celery and green juices, mixed with a small amount of higher-carbohydrate veggies, such as carrot or beet. Mix in some form of healthy fat with each glass of the juice. A teaspoon of cultured goat's milk, coconut milk and cream, or flaxseed oil the enhances the absorption of minerals and prevents spikes in blood sugar.
- *Fermented vegetables.* Consume a few tablespoons of fermented vegetables such as sauerkraut with each meal to aid in digestion. Fermented vegetables are excellent sources of naturally occurring probiotics and enzymes.
- *Stocks.* After completing Phases One and Two of the program, consume stocks on a regular basis, especially when you have a cold or flu. Stocks made from the bones of chicken, fish, lamb, or beef contain minerals, gelatin, cartilage, collagen, and electrolytes. Stocks help to heal the gut lining and reduce inflammation.

Supplements

Take these health supplements to alleviate symptoms and get well:

- *Probiotic with HSOs.* Start with one caplet per day and work up to 12 caplets per day for six to twelve months. Then gradually reduce intake to three to six caplets per day for life.

- *Digestive enzymes.* Starting in Phase Two, take one to three caplets with each meal or snack.
- *Clay.* Take 1 tablespoon of clay mixed in 8 ounces of water four times per day until your diarrhea is relieved. Thereafter, take 1 tablespoon of clay in 8 ounces of water morning and evening to promote ongoing detoxification.
- *Anti-inflammatory.* In Phase One, take four caplets three times per day for one to four weeks, followed by six caplets per day for three to six months, and then reduce to a maintenance level of three caplets per day. If a relapse, or flare-up, occurs, take twelve caplets per day for at least one week or until the symptoms are under control.
- *Whole-food mineral powder.* Starting in Phase Two, take 1 to 2 tablespoons once or twice daily with 8 ounces of water.
- *Essential fats.* Take 1 teaspoon per day of cod liver oil.
- *Structured mineral water.* Consume at least 64 ounces per day of a high-quality structured or high-mineral water.
- *Pet natural antimicrobial product.* We recommend giving your pets a natural antimicrobial product to minimize the chance of cross-infection. People with Crohn's have weakened immune systems and are more liable to be infected by microbes from pets.

Additional Therapies

For people who have or may have imbalanced intestinal flora, avoiding contact with chlorinated water is of the utmost importance. That includes bathing water and drinking water. Chlorine kills bacteria, friendly and unfriendly, in the colon. It can be absorbed through the skin. We recommend installing a shower filter to remove chlorine. Avoid swimming in chlorinated water as well.

Diarrhea (Chronic and Acute)

Everyone gets diarrhea now and then. Short-term diarrhea has many causes—diet, medications, food poisoning, stress, and drinking water contaminated with bacteria. In some cases, diarrhea is the body's way of getting rid of a microbe, toxin, or disagreeable foreign substance. In a healthy bowel, the large intestine absorbs much of the water so that waste material can solidify and form stools. In people with diarrhea, the colon for a variety of reasons does not or is unable to reclaim this water. Transit time (the amount of time that food is in the digestive tract) is then speeded up, and the stool is runny.

Acute diarrhea usually occurs suddenly and is self-limited. The symptoms subside generally within forty-eight to seventy-two hours. Diarrhea is considered chronic if it lasts for more than two weeks. Sometimes food isn't properly absorbed. At the very least, people who have diarrhea become dehydrated. For this reason, weakness and nutritional deficiencies can accompany chronic diarrhea. People who have diarrhea need to drink ten glasses of water a day to restore the water they lose.

Diarrhea is a symptom of many different bowel diseases. If you have prolonged diarrhea, it may be a sign that you are suffering from an intestinal disorder. Diarrhea accompanies lactose intolerance, irritable bowel syndrome, Crohn's disease, ulcerative colitis, celiac disease, parasites, and other bowel diseases. Consult your doctor for a proper diagnosis if you have prolonged diarrhea.

Diet

Phase One: one day (for acute diarrhea, stay in Phase One until your symptoms subside, then move directly into Phase Three when you feel better.)

Phase Two: seven to fourteen days.

Phase Three: three to six months or until your symptoms have been gone for more than three months.

Stick to the foods in the "Good" and "Not So Bad" category. After you have not had diarrhea for three months, you may gradually add foods from the "Bad" and "Ugly" categories if you desire.

Therapeutic Foods

These therapeutic foods will help you get well:

- *Cultured goat's milk dairy products.* Consume 8 to 32 ounces of the highest-quality cultured dairy products from goat's or sheep's milk. Try to find yogurt that does not contain the organism *Streptococcus thermophilus,* a bacterial microbe that has been known to make certain immune-system disorders worse.
- *Grass-fed red meat.* Red meat from grass-fed cattle, buffalo, and lamb is very healthy and can be eaten several times per week. This meat is a great source of protein, minerals, vitamin B_{12}, vitamin D, beta-carotene, omega-3 fats, and CLA.
- *Omega-3 eggs.* Consume as many as two to four eggs high in the omega-3 fatty acids each day. These eggs contain DHA, vitamins E and B_{12}, and antioxidants.
- *Coconut oil.* This oil is perhaps the healthiest of the widely available oils. We recommend cooking almost exclusively with coconut oil. Consume as much as 2 to 4 tablespoons of the oil in cooking, in smoothies, or right off the spoon. It contains large amounts of lauric acid, a potent antimicrobial and one of the chief fatty acids in breast milk.
- *Ocean-caught fish.* This type of fish is perhaps the healthiest of all the protein sources. Salmon, sardines, mackerel, herring, and tuna are high in the omega-3 fatty acids EPA and DHA. Ocean-caught fish can be consumed every day to enhance digestive and immune system health.
- *Cod liver oil.* Take 1 teaspoon of plain or flavored cod liver oil each day. Cod liver oil is a fantastic source of the omega-3 fats DHA and EPA, as well as of vitamin A and D.
- *Vegetable juice.* As long as your diarrhea is not active, consume vegetable juices that are low in carbohydrates, such as celery and green juices, mixed with a small amount of higher-carbohydrate veggies, such as carrot or beet. Mix in some form of healthy fat with each glass of the juice. A teaspoon of cultured goat's milk, coconut milk and cream, or flaxseed oil enhances the absorption of minerals and prevents spikes in blood sugar.

- *Fermented vegetables.* Consume a few tablespoons of fermented vegetables such as sauerkraut with each meal to aid in digestion. Fermented vegetables are excellent sources of naturally occurring probiotics and enzymes.
- *Stocks.* After completing Phases One and Two of the program, consume stocks on a regular basis, especially when you have a cold or flu. Stocks made from the bones of chicken, fish, lamb, or beef contain minerals, gelatin, cartilage, collagen, and electrolytes. Stocks help to heal the gut lining and reduce inflammation.

Supplements

Take these health supplements to alleviate symptoms and get well:

- *Probiotic with HSOs.* Consume six to twelve caplets per day for three months, then gradually reduce the dosage to three to six caplets per day for maintenance purposes.
- *Clay.* Take 1 tablespoon of clay mixed in 8 ounces of water two to four times per day on an empty stomach until your symptoms subside. Taking clay is especially helpful when you have acute diarrhea.
- *Digestive enzymes.* Take one to three caplets with each meal or snack.
- *Fiber.* Consume 1 serving twice per day, morning and evening.
- *Antifungal supplement.* Follow the two-week, intensive antifungal program as directed on the label.
- *Essential fats.* Take 1 teaspoon per day of cod liver oil.
- *Protein digestant.* If you are over sixty years of age and you experience post-meal belching and bloating after one full month on the program, take one to five tablets at the beginning of each meal containing protein.
- *Structured mineral water.* Consume at least 64 ounces per day of a high-quality structured or high-mineral water.

Diverticular Disease

The cause of diverticular disease is not well understood, but many believe the disease is related to the lack of fiber in the Western diet.

Over many years, as the muscles of the colon strain harder to push out feces, the extra pressure blows out parts of the intestinal wall. As a result, pouches called diverticula form in the lining of the intestine. About 10 percent of Americans over the age of forty have diverticulosis. About half of people over 60 have it, and 80 percent of Americans who reach age 80 have diverticular disease. Many have the disease without knowing it.

If the pouches become inflamed or infected, the condition is called diverticulitis. Rectal bleeding and cramping associated with fever and left-sided abdominal pain are symptoms of diverticulitis. Diverticulitis, an acute medical condition, can develop into bowel perforation and peritonitis. If you believe you have diverticulitis, do not attempt to treat the disease on your own. Seek medical attention immediately.

Diverticulitis is usually an acute condition. Although nothing is impossible, cases of chronic diverticulitis are highly unusual. Most people who suffer from chronic, nagging, lower-left-sided abdominal pain are suffering from diverticulosis, a more indolent, nonacute condition. The Guts and Glory Program is geared toward diverticulosis suffers.

Diet

Many doctors and dieticians prescribe the "diverticular diet." In this diet, patients are encouraged to avoid nuts and seeds. Unfortunately, patients on the diverticular diet often stop eating many of the foods that would improve their condition. We see *no* merit in the conventional diverticular diet. Instead of that diet, we strongly encourage you to undertake the protocol we describe in this book.

Diverticulitis (only mild cases that can be managed as an outpatient)

<u>Phase One:</u> seven to fourteen days.

<u>Phase Two:</u> seven to fourteen days.

Phase Three: six to twelve months.

Diverticulosis

Phase One: one to five days.

Phase Two: seven to fourteen days.

Phase Three: three to six months.

After you are free of symptoms for at least six weeks, you can gradually begin eating foods from the "Bad" list if you desire. However, for optimal health, we recommend that most of your diet be composed of foods on the "Good" and "Not So Bad" lists.

Therapeutic Foods

These therapeutic foods will help you get well:

- *Cultured goat's milk dairy products.* Consume 8 to 32 ounces of the highest-quality cultured dairy products from goat's or sheep's milk. Try to find yogurt that does not contain the organism *Streptococcus thermophilus*, a bacterial microbe that has been known to make certain immune-system disorders worse.
- *Grass-fed red meat.* Red meat from grass-fed cattle, buffalo, and lamb is very healthy and can be eaten several times per week. This meat is a great source of protein, minerals, vitamin B_{12}, vitamin D, beta-carotene, omega-3 fats, and CLA.
- *Omega-3 eggs.* Consume as many as two to four eggs high in the omega-3 fatty acids each day. These eggs contain DHA, vitamins E and B_{12}, and antioxidants.
- *Coconut oil.* This oil is perhaps the healthiest of the widely available oils. We recommend cooking almost exclusively with coconut oil. Consume as much as 2 to 4 tablespoons of the oil in cooking, in smoothies, or right off the spoon. It contains large amounts of lauric acid, a potent antimicrobial and one of the chief fatty acids in breast milk.
- *Ocean-caught fish.* This type of fish is perhaps the healthiest of

all the protein sources. Salmon, sardines, mackerel, herring, and tuna are high in the omega-3 fatty acids EPA and DHA. Ocean-caught fish can be consumed every day to enhance digestive and immune system health.

- *Cod liver oil.* Take 1 teaspoon of plain or flavored cod liver oil each day. Cod liver oil is a fantastic source of the omega-3 fats DHA and EPA, as well as of vitamin A and D.
- *Vegetable juice.* As long as your diarrhea is not active, consume vegetable juices that are low in carbohydrates, such as celery and green juices, mixed with a small amount of higher-carbohydrate veggies, such as carrot or beet. Mix in some form of healthy fat with each glass of the juice. A teaspoon of cultured goat's milk, coconut milk and cream, or flaxseed oil enhances the absorption of minerals and prevents spikes in blood sugar.
- *Fermented vegetables.* Consume a few tablespoons of fermented vegetables such as sauerkraut with each meal to aid in digestion. Fermented vegetables are excellent sources of naturally occurring probiotics and enzymes.
- *Stocks.* After completing Phases One and Two of the program, consume stocks on a regular basis, especially when you have a cold or flu. Stocks made from the bones of chicken, fish, lamb, or beef contain minerals, gelatin, cartilage, collagen, and electrolytes. Stocks help to heal the gut lining and reduce inflammation.

Supplements

Take these health supplements to alleviate symptoms and get well:

- *Probiotic with HSOs.* After completing Phase Two, take six to twelve caplets per day for six months. Then gradually reduce the dosage to three to six caplets per day for maintenance purposes.
- *Digestive enzymes.* Take one to three caplets per meal. Take more when consuming grains or legumes.
- *Fiber.* Choose from the recommended fiber sources and take one serving morning and evening as directed on the product label.
- *Anti-inflammatory (diverticulitis only).* Consume twelve caplets

per day in three divided doses for one month. Consume six caplets per day in two divided doses for the following two months. After three months, reduce your intake to three caplets per day.

- ◆ *Whole-food mineral powder.* Take 1 to 2 tablespoons twice daily on an empty stomach to enhance mineral absorption.
- ◆ *Essential fats.* Take 1 teaspoon per day of cod liver oil.
- ◆ *Protein digestant.* If you are over sixty years of age and you experience post-meal belching and bloating after one full month on the program, take one to five tablets at the beginning of each meal that contains protein.
- ◆ *Structured mineral water.* Consume at least 64 ounces per day of a high-quality structured or high-mineral water.

Dyspepsia

See Gastritis *and* Nonulcerative Dyspepsia.

Food Allergies and Food Intolerances

Many patients confuse food allergies and food intolerances. What's more, the conventional medical community has been slow to acknowledge the existence of food intolerances.

Classic food allergies, the kind that are caused by an immune-system response, are rarely seen in adults and are in fact quite unusual. Food allergies are caused by an immunologic reaction in which the immune system is overstimulated and mistakenly attacks the body. If the body believes that a certain kind of food is an allergen, it manufactures immunoglobulin E (IgE) antibodies. In turn, these antibodies react to the food and make the immune system release histamines and mediator chemicals. The result is an allergic reaction. Food allergies can cause bloating, diarrhea, constipation, difficulty breathing, rashes, vomiting, a swelling of the throat, as well as loss of consciousness and death. Food allergies are relatively easy to diagnose by skin testing. If you have a history of severe allergic reactions to a particular food, avoid the food at all costs.

When you test for the allergy, do so in the presence of trained medical personnel in case you have a severe reaction.

Far more common than food allergies are food intolerances. With the exception of respiratory problems and anaphylaxis, the symptoms of a food intolerance are similar to those of a food allergy. Food intolerances, however, are not mediated through the IgE pathway. In other words, they are not caused by an immune-system response. For that reason, they can be elusive and often do not react to tests that use an immunologic standard. The best way to determine if you have a food intolerance is through a detailed examination of your dietary history or the elimination diet. The first two phases of the Guts and Glory Program are essentially a modified elimination diet.

Diet

Phase One: one to seven days or depending on the severity of your symptoms.

Phase Two: seven to fourteen days.

Phase Three: three to six months, avoiding your known offending foods until your symptoms are greatly improved.

After your symptoms are gone for at least three months, you can reintroduce the foods to which you were formerly allergic. If no symptoms appear after six months, gradually introduce foods from the "Bad" and "Ugly" groups if you desire. However, we strongly recommend consuming a diet of foods predominantly from the "Good" and "Not So Bad" groups. This way, you maintain optimal health and avoid future allergies and intolerances. If your allergies and intolerances start to recur, repeat Phases One and Two until the symptoms subside.

Therapeutic Foods

These therapeutic foods will help you get well:

◆ *Cultured goat's milk dairy products.* Consume 8 to 32 ounces of the highest-quality cultured dairy products from goat's or sheep's milk. Try to find yogurt that does not contain the organism *Strep-tococcus thermophilus*, a bacterial microbe that has been known to make certain immune-system disorders worse. (Many people with true food allergies are allergic to milk. Moreover, this allergy is often specific to cow's milk, not goat's milk. Goat's milk is certainly worth trying if you are allergic to dairy products, but you must try it under the supervision of a health professional.)

- *Grass-fed red meat.* Red meat from grass-fed cattle, buffalo, and lamb is very healthy and can be eaten several times per week. This meat is a great source of protein, minerals, vitamin B_{12}, vitamin D, beta-carotene, omega-3 fats, and CLA.

- *Omega-3 eggs.* Consume as many as two to four eggs high in the omega-3 fatty acids each day. These eggs contain DHA, vitamins E and B_{12}, and antioxidants. (Many people with true food allergies are allergic to eggs. Interestingly, these people show no symptoms when they eat noncommercial eggs. Omega-3 eggs are therefore worth trying. Again, however, you should try them only under the strict supervision of medical personnel.)

- *Coconut oil.* This oil is perhaps the healthiest of the widely available oils. We recommend cooking almost exclusively with coconut oil. Consume as much as 2 to 4 tablespoons of the oil in cooking, in smoothies, or right off the spoon. It contains large amounts of lauric acid, a potent anti-microbial and one of the chief fatty acids in breast milk.

- *Ocean-caught fish.* This type of fish is perhaps the healthiest of all the protein sources. Salmon, sardines, mackerel, herring, and tuna are high in the omega-3 fatty acids EPA and DHA. Ocean-caught fish can be consumed every day to enhance digestive and immune system health. (Many people with true food allergies are allergic to fish. Obviously, if you are allergic to fish, you should omit it from your diet. If you want to reintroduce fish, you should do so in a controlled setting.)

- *Cod liver oil.* Take 1 teaspoon of plain or flavored cod liver oil each day. Cod liver oil is a fantastic source of the omega-3 fats DHA and EPA, as well as of vitamins A and D.

- *Vegetable juice.* As long as your diarrhea is not active, consume vegetable juices that are low in carbohydrates, such as celery and green juices, mixed with a small amount of higher-carbohydrate veggies, such as carrot or beet. Mix in some form of healthy fat with each glass of the juice. A teaspoon of cultured goat's milk, coconut milk and cream, or flaxseed oil enhances the absorption of minerals and prevents spikes in blood sugar.
- *Fermented vegetables.* Consume a few tablespoons of fermented vegetables such as sauerkraut with each meal to aid in digestion. Fermented vegetables are excellent sources of naturally occurring probiotics and enzymes.
- *Stocks.* After completing Phases One and Two of the program, consume stocks on a regular basis, especially when you have a cold or flu. Stocks made from the bones of chicken, lamb, or beef contain minerals, gelatin, cartilage, collagen, and electrolytes. Stocks help to heal the gut lining and reduce inflammation.

Supplements

Take these health supplements to alleviate your symptoms and get well:

- *Probiotic with HSOs.* Take six to twelve caplets per day for three to six months, then take three to six caplets per day for life.
- *Digestive enzymes.* Take one to three caplets with meals and snacks. Take more if you are consuming known allergens.
- *Fiber (if needed).* Consume one serving twice per day, morning and evening.
- *Anti-inflammatory.* Consume twelve caplets per day while in Phases One and Two. Consume six caplets per day thereafter or until your symptoms subside. After that, consume three caplets per day for three months.
- *Whole-food mineral powder.* Take 1 to 2 tablespoons twice daily on an empty stomach.
- *Essential fats.* Take 1 teaspoon per day of cod liver oil.
- *Protein digestant.* If you are over sixty years of age and you expe-

rience post-meal belching and bloating after one full month on the program, take one to five tablets at the beginning of each meal containing protein.

- *Structured mineral water.* Consume at least 64 ounces per day of a high-quality structured or high-mineral water.
- *Pet natural antimicrobial product.* We recommend giving your pets a natural antimicrobial product to minimize the chance of cross-infection by microbes.

Food Poisoning

The symptoms of food poisoning include headaches, nausea, diarrhea, vomiting, and fever. Many people who think they have a twenty-four-hour flu bug actually have a mild case of food poisoning. Food poisoning is caused by bacteria and bacterial toxins in food. Food that is left at room temperature for two to three hours or stored improperly may cause food poisoning, as bacteria are allowed to grow on the food.

Diet

Phase One: three to seven days.

Phase Two: seven to fourteen days.

Supplements

Take these health supplements to alleviate your symptoms and get well:

- *Probiotic with HSOs.* Take three caplets per day.
- *Clay.* Take 1 tablespoon of clay mixed in 8 ounces of water four times per day until your symptoms subside.
- *Fiber.* Consume one serving twice per day, morning and evening.
- *Antifungal supplement.* Take for two weeks. Follow the directions on the bottle.

◆ *Structured mineral water.* Consume at least 64 ounces per day of a high-quality structured or high-mineral water.

Functional Bowel Disease

See Irritable Bowel Syndrome.

Fungal Infections

See Candidiasis.

Gastritis

The term *gastritis* is often used quite loosely by physicians and their patients to describe nonspecific pain, discomfort, nausea, and bloating in the epigastrium (the upper abdominal region right below the rib cage). These symptoms, however, are more accurately caused by dyspepsia. Moreover, dyspepsia may or may not be associated with gastritis. Gastritis actually has a strict pathologic definition. It refers to an inflammation of the stomach that is accompanied by an infiltration of white blood cells in the gastric lining. Some of the entities normally associated with gastritis—tobacco, alcohol, and nonsteroidal anti-inflammatory drugs (NSAIDs) such as aspirin and ibuprofen—actually do not cause gastritis but cause what is known as a gastropathy. This condition is an irritation of the stomach in the absence of white blood cells. The one true gastritis that is relatively common is an infection of the stomach by the bacterium *Helicobacter pylori* (*H. pylori*).

As little as a decade ago, the theory that a bacterium such as *H. pylori* could infect the stomach was considered ridiculous by the medical community at large. Today, the theory is an unequivocal fact. The vast majority of people infected with *H. pylori*, for reasons not yet understood, show no symptoms whatsoever of gastritis. However, a significant minority are at risk for the development of chronic duodenal ulcers. More troubling, some people with a chronic *H. pylori* infection can develop a type of gastric lymphoma.

More troubling still, an association between *H. pylori* infection and gastric cancer has recently been reported. Notice, however, that we used the word "association"—*H. pylori* may not specifically be the cause of gastric cancer. If you have symptoms of chronic dyspepsia, being checked for *H. pylori* is probably worthwhile. Your doctor can do this with a simple blood test.

Diet

Phase One: three to seven days.

Phase Two: three to seven days.

Phase Three: three months or more, until your symptoms subside.

Therapeutic Foods

These therapeutic foods will help you get well:

- *Cultured goat's milk dairy products.* Consume 8 to 32 ounces of the highest-quality cultured dairy products from goat's or sheep's milk. Try to find yogurt that does not contain the organism *Streptococcus thermophilus*, a bacterial microbe that has been known to make immune-system disorders worse. (Not eating yogurt with *Streptococcus thermophilus* may be particularly effective in treating *H. pylori*.)
- *Grass-fed red meat.* Red meat from grass-fed cattle, buffalo, and lamb is very healthy and can be eaten several times per week. This meat is a great source of protein, minerals, vitamin B_{12}, vitamin D, beta-carotene, omega-3 fats, and CLA.
- *Omega-3 eggs.* Consume as many as two to four eggs high in the omega-3 fatty acids each day. These eggs contain DHA, vitamins E and B_{12}, and antioxidants.
- *Coconut oil.* This oil is perhaps the healthiest of the widely available oils. We recommend cooking almost exclusively with coconut oil. Consume as much as 2 to 4 tablespoons of the oil in cooking, in smoothies, or right off the spoon. It contains large

amounts of lauric acid, a potent antimicrobial and one of the chief fatty acids in breast milk.

- *Ocean-caught fish.* This type of fish is perhaps the healthiest of all the protein sources. Salmon, sardines, mackerel, herring, and tuna are high in the omega-3 fatty acids EPA and DHA. Ocean-caught fish can be consumed every day to enhance digestive and immune system health.
- *Cod liver oil.* Take 1 teaspoon of plain or flavored cod liver oil each day. Cod liver oil is a fantastic source of the omega-3 fats DHA and EPA, as well as of vitamins A and D.
- *Vegetable juice.* As long as your diarrhea is not active, consume vegetable juices that are low in carbohydrates, such as celery and green juices, mixed with a small amount of higher-carbohydrate veggies, such as carrot or beet. Mix in some form of healthy fat with each glass of the juice. A teaspoon of cultured goat's milk, coconut milk and cream, or flaxseed oil enhances the absorption of minerals and prevents spikes in blood sugar.
- *Fermented vegetables.* Consume a few tablespoons of fermented vegetables such as sauerkraut with each meal to aid in digestion. Fermented vegetables are excellent sources of naturally occurring probiotics and enzymes. These fermented foods may be particularly useful in fighting *H. pylori*.
- *Stocks.* After completing Phases One and Two of the program, consume stocks on a regular basis, especially when you have a cold or flu. Stocks made from the bones of chicken, fish, lamb, or beef contain minerals, gelatin, cartilage, collagen, and electrolytes. Stocks help to heal the gut lining and reduce inflammation.

Supplements

Take these health supplements to alleviate your symptoms and get well:

- *Probiotic with HSOs.* Take three to six caplets per day.
- *Digestive enzymes.* Take one to three caplets with each meal and snack. Take more when consuming grains or legumes. Digestive

enzymes may be particularly helpful for people suffering from nonspecific dyspepsia. We believe that poor digestion is the major underlying cause of the condition.

- *Hydrochloric acid.* Because hydrochloric acid is another agent that enhances digestion, it can be quite effective in the treatment of dyspepsia. One problem with taking hydrocloric acid supplements, however, is that dyspepsia is sometimes a symptom of an occult ulcer, and using hydrocloric acid supplements if you have an ulcer is not healthy. First try digestive enzymes, and if the enzymes don't solve the problem completely, try a tablespoon of apple cider vinegar (a natural source of hydrocloric acid) with each meal. If the apple cider vinegar seems to improve your symptoms, you may move on to a low-dose hydrocloric acid supplement. If any of these recommendations worsen your symptoms, stop taking the supplement and seek medical attention.
- *Essential fats.* Take 1 teaspoon per day of cod liver oil.
- *Alkalizing upper GI blend.* Take 1 to 2 tablespoons mixed in water upon rising and before bed. This supplement can be taken to relieve the pain during an episode.
- *Mastic gum.* Mastic gum is a tree resin that is known to have excellent antimicrobial properties. It is known to be particularly effective in eradicating *H. pylori* infections. Coauthor Dr. Brasco has used mastic gum extensively in his practice and has found it to be as effective as triple therapy (two antibiotics and a potent acid-blocking agent, the conventional approach to *H. pylori* therapy). What's more, taking mastic gum has no side effects.
- *Structured mineral water.* Consume at least 64 ounces per day of a high-quality structured or high-mineral water. To relieve gastritis pain, drink 8 ounces of a structured water followed by a second 8-ounce glass ten minutes later.

Obviously, you should avoid the agents that can precipitate dyspepsia: nicotine, caffeine, and alcohol.

Gastroesophageal Reflux Disease

When the acidic juices of the stomach splash upward into the esophagus, the result is heartburn. Normally, a ring of muscles called the esophageal sphincter prevents stomach acid from entering the esophagus. But if the muscles relax or open under pressure from the acidic juices in the stomach, heartburn may result. Everyone gets heartburn from time to time, but severe, persistent heartburn that occurs two or more times per week is called gastroesophageal reflux disease, or GERD. Chronic GERD has the potential to scar and damage the lining of the esophagus. It can also lead to a condition called Barrett's esophagus, which carries the risk of developing esophageal cancer.

Heartburn has many different causes. Heartburn may be caused by overeating, stress, wearing clothes that fit too tightly, and lying down soon after eating. Alcohol, nicotine, and caffeine relax the esophageal sphincter and allow stomach acid to enter the esophagus. Certain kinds of spicy food can also cause heartburn in some people. Poor digestion is another major contributor to GERD.

Diet

Phase Two: three to seven days.

Phase Three: three to six months or more until your symptoms are
    gone for at least six weeks.

Therapeutic Foods

These therapeutic foods will help you get well:

- *Cultured goat's milk dairy products.* Consume 8 to 32 ounces of the highest-quality cultured dairy products from goat's or sheep's milk. Try to find yogurt that does not contain the organism *Streptococcus thermophilus*, a bacterial microbe that has been known to make certain immune-system disorders worse.
- *Grass-fed red meat.* Red meat from grass-fed cattle, buffalo, and lamb is very healthy and can be eaten several times per week. This meat is a great source of protein, minerals, vitamin B_{12}, vitamin D, beta-carotene, omega-3 fats, and CLA.
- *Omega-3 eggs.* Consume as many as two to four eggs high in the

omega-3 fatty acids each day. These eggs contain DHA, vitamins E and B_{12}, and antioxidants.

- *Coconut oil.* This oil is perhaps the healthiest of the widely available oils. We recommend cooking almost exclusively with coconut oil. Consume as much as 2 to 4 tablespoons of the oil in cooking, in smoothies, or right off the spoon. It contains large amounts of lauric acid, a potent antimicrobial and one of the chief fatty acids in breast milk.
- *Ocean-caught fish.* This type of fish is perhaps the healthiest of all the protein sources. Salmon, sardines, mackerel, herring, and tuna are high in the omega-3 fatty acids EPA and DHA. Ocean-caught fish can be consumed every day to enhance digestive and immune system health.
- *Cod liver oil.* Take 1 teaspoon of plain or flavored cod liver oil each day. Cod liver oil is a fantastic source of the omega-3 fats DHA and EPA, as well as of vitamins A and D.
- *Vegetable juice.* As long as your diarrhea is not active, consume vegetable juices that are low in carbohydrates, such as celery and green juices, mixed with a small amount of higher-carbohydrate veggies, such as carrot or beet. Mix in some form of healthy fat with each glass of the juice. A teaspoon of cultured goat's milk, coconut milk and cream, or flaxseed oil enhances absorption of minerals and prevents spikes in blood sugar.
- *Fermented vegetables.* Consume a few tablespoons of fermented vegetables such as sauerkraut with each meal to aid in digestion. Fermented vegetables are an excellent source of naturally occurring probiotics and enzymes.
- *Stocks.* After completing Phases One and Two of the program, consume stocks on a regular basis, especially when you have a cold or flu. Stocks made from the bones of chicken, fish, lamb, or beef contain minerals, gelatin, cartilage, collagen, and electrolytes. Stocks help to heal the gut lining and reduce inflammation.

Supplements

Take these health supplements to alleviate your symptoms and get well:

- *Probiotic with HSOs.* Take three to six caplets per day.
- *Digestive enzymes.* Take one to three caplets with each meal and snack. You can also take enzymes to treat an acute attack of heartburn, but prevention is always the best approach. Sometimes taking digestive enzymes alone cures GERD.
- *Hydrocloric acid.* Hydrocloric acid is another way to improve overall digestion. Although taking hydrocloric acid to treat an acid-related problem may seem paradoxical, it can actually be quite effective. In spite of popular misconceptions, increased acid output is *not* generally associated with acid reflux disease. Taking hydrocloric acid will improve many people's digestion and subsequently improve their reflux symptoms.
- *Deglycyrrhizinated licorice.* DGL isn't curative, but you can use it to effectively control the symptoms caused by occasional bouts of heartburn. It is much healthier than many over-the-counter and prescription preparations.
- *Essential fats.* Take 1 teaspoon per day of cod liver oil.
- *Alkalizing upper GI blend.* Take 1 to 2 tablespoons mixed in water upon rising and before bed. This supplement can be taken to relieve the pain during an episode.
- *Structured mineral water.* Consume at least 64 ounces per day of a high-quality structured or high-mineral water. To relieve gastritis pain, drink 8 ounces of structured water followed by a second 8-ounce glass ten minutes later.

GERD

See Gastroesophageal Reflux Disease.

Gluten Intolerance

See Celiac Disease.

Heartburn

See Gastroesophageal Reflux Disease.

Helicobacter Pylori

See Gastritis.

Hemorrhoids

Hemorrhoids, also known as piles, are actually swollen blood vessels similar to varicose veins that form inside the anus and under the skin around the outside of the anus. These soft, purplish lumps can be very painful. Half of Americans over 50 years of age have hemorrhoids.

Hemorrhoids are caused by activities that put undue pressure on the blood vessels near the anus—straining during bowel movements, heavy lifting, sitting for long periods of time, and not getting enough exercise. A lack of fiber in the diet causes hemorrhoids. Pregnant women are especially subject to hemorrhoids because hormonal changes during pregnancy cause the blood vessels to expand and the fetus causes intra-abdominal pressure to increase. The symptoms of hemorrhoids include bloody stools, soreness, and itching.

Diet

<u>Phase Three:</u> three or more months or until your symptoms are gone for six or more weeks.

Therapeutic Foods

These therapeutic foods will help you get well:

- *Cultured goat's milk dairy products.* Consume 8 to 32 ounces of the highest-quality cultured dairy products from goat's or sheep's milk. Try to find yogurt that does not contain the organism *Streptococcus thermophilus*, a bacterial microbe that has been known to worsen certain immune-system disorders.
- *Grass-fed red meat.* Red meat from grass-fed cattle, buffalo, and lamb is very healthy and can be eaten several times per week.

This meat is a great source of protein, minerals, vitamin B_{12}, vitamin D, beta-carotene, omega-3 fats, and CLA.

◆ *Omega-3 eggs.* Consume as many as two to four eggs high in the omega-3 fatty acids each day. These eggs contain DHA, vitamins E and B_{12}, and antioxidants.

◆ *Coconut oil.* This oil is perhaps the healthiest of the widely available oils. We recommend cooking almost exclusively with coconut oil. Consume as much as 2 to 4 tablespoons of the oil in cooking, in smoothies, or right off the spoon. It contains large amounts of lauric acid, a potent antimicrobial and one of the chief fatty acids in breast milk.

◆ *Ocean-caught fish.* This type of fish is perhaps the healthiest of all the protein sources. Salmon, sardines, mackerel, herring, and tuna are high in the omega-3 fatty acids EPA and DHA. Ocean-caught fish can be consumed every day to enhance digestive and immune system health.

◆ *Cod liver oil.* Take 1 teaspoon of plain or flavored cod liver oil each day. Cod liver oil is a fantastic source of the omega-3 fats DHA and EPA, as well as of vitamins A and D.

◆ *Vegetable juice.* As long as your diarrhea is not active, consume vegetable juices that are low in carbohydrates, such as celery and green juices, mixed with a small amount of higher-carbohydrate veggies, such as carrot or beet. Mix in some form of healthy fat with each glass of the juice. A teaspoon of cultured goat's milk, coconut milk and cream, or flaxseed oil enhances the absorption of minerals and prevents spikes in blood sugar.

◆ *Fermented vegetables.* Consume a few tablespoons of fermented vegetables such as sauerkraut with each meal to aid in digestion. Fermented vegetables are excellent sources of naturally occurring probiotics and enzymes.

◆ *Stocks.* After completing Phases One and Two of the program, consume stocks on a regular basis, especially when you have a cold or flu. Stocks made from the bones of chicken, fish, lamb, or beef contain minerals, gelatin, cartilage, collagen, and electrolytes. Stocks help to heal the gut lining and reduce inflammation.

Supplements

Take these health supplements to alleviate your symptoms and get well:

- *Probiotic with HSOs.* Take six to twelve caplets per day for three to six months. After your elimination has improved and the swelling is down, consume three to six caplets per day for maintenance purposes.
- *Digestive enzymes.* Take one to three caplets with each meal and snack.
- *Fiber.* Consume 1 serving twice per day, morning and evening.
- *Essential fats.* Take 1 teaspoon per day of cod liver oil.
- *Protein digestant.* If you are over sixty years of age and you experience post-meal belching and bloating after one full month on the program, take one to five tablets at the beginning of each meal that contains protein.
- *Structured mineral water.* Consume at least 64 ounces per day of a high-quality structured or high-mineral water.

Indigestion

Indigestion is a burning sensation in the pit of the stomach. Indigestion covers a range of symptoms: heartburn, bloating, gassiness, nausea, and occasionally vomiting. Usually, indigestion is caused by a poor diet accompanied by poor digestion, although stress may also be a factor. If indigestion persists, it may be the symptom of a gastrointestinal disease, in which case you should have it diagnosed properly by a doctor.

Diet

Phase Two: three to seven days.

Phase Three: three months or more, until your symptoms subside.

Therapeutic Foods

These therapeutic foods will help you get well:

- *Cultured goat's milk dairy products.* Consume 8 to 32 ounces of the highest-quality cultured dairy products from goat's or sheep's milk. Try to find yogurt that does not contain the organism *Streptococcus thermophilus*, a bacterial microbe that has been known to make certain immune-system disorders worse.
- *Grass-fed red meat.* Red meat from grass-fed cattle, buffalo, and lamb is very healthy and can be eaten several times per week. This meat is a great source of protein, minerals, vitamin B_{12}, vitamin D, beta-carotene, omega-3 fats, and CLA.
- *Omega-3 eggs.* Consume as many as two to four eggs high in the omega-3 fatty acids each day. These eggs contain DHA, vitamins E and B_{12}, and antioxidants.
- *Coconut oil.* This oil is perhaps the healthiest of the widely available oils. We recommend cooking almost exclusively with coconut oil. Consume as much as 2 to 4 tablespoons of the oil in cooking, in smoothies, or right off the spoon. It contains large amounts of lauric acid, a potent antimicrobial and one of the chief fatty acids in breast milk.
- *Ocean-caught fish.* This type of fish is perhaps the healthiest of all the protein sources. Salmon, sardines, mackerel, herring, and tuna are high in the omega-3 fatty acids EPA and DHA. Ocean-caught fish can be consumed every day to enhance digestive and immune system health.
- *Cod liver oil.* Take 1 teaspoon of plain or flavored cod liver oil each day. Cod liver oil is a fantastic source of the omega-3 fats DHA and EPA, as well as of vitamins A and D.
- *Vegetable juice.* As long as your diarrhea is not active, consume vegetable juices that are low in carbohydrates, such as celery and green juices, mixed with a small amount of higher-carbohydrate veggies, such as carrot or beet. Mix in some form of healthy fat with each glass of the juice. A teaspoon of cultured goat's milk, coconut milk and cream, or flaxseed oil enhances the absorption of minerals and prevents spikes in blood sugar.

- *Fermented vegetables.* Consume a few tablespoons of fermented vegetables such as sauerkraut with each meal to aid in digestion. Fermented vegetables are excellent sources of naturally occurring probiotics and enzymes.
- *Stocks.* After completing Phases One and Two of the program, consume stocks on a regular basis, especially when you have a cold or flu. Stocks made from the bones of chicken, fish, lamb, or beef contain minerals, gelatin, cartilage, collagen, and electrolytes. Stocks help to heal the gut lining and reduce inflammation.

Supplements

Take these health supplements to alleviate your symptoms and get well:

- *Probiotic with HSOs.* Take three to six caplets per day.
- *Digestive enzymes.* Take one to three caplets with each meal and snack.
- *Hydrocloric acid.* Because hydrocloric acid is another agent that enhances digestion, it can be quite effective in the treatment of indigestion. One problem with taking hydrocloric acid supplements, however, is that indigestion is sometimes a symptom of an occult ulcer, and using hydrocloric acid supplements if you have an ulcer is not healthy. First try digestive enzymes, and if the enzymes don't solve the problem completely, try a tablespoon of apple cider vinegar (a natural source of hydrocloric acid) with each meal. If the apple cider vinegar seems to improve your digestion, you may move on to a low-dose hydrocloric acid supplement. If any of these recommendations worsen your symptoms, stop taking the supplement and seek medical attention.
- *Essential fats.* Take 1 teaspoon per day of cod liver oil.
- *Alkalizing upper GI blend.* Take 1 to 2 tablespoons mixed in water upon rising and before bed. This supplement can be taken to relieve the pain during an episode.
- *Structured mineral water.* Consume at least 64 ounces per day of a high-quality structured or high-mineral water.

- *Fiber.* If elimination is not optimal, consume one serving twice per day, morning and evening, as directed by the product label.
- *Protein digestant.* If you are over sixty years of age and you experience post-meal belching and bloating after one full month on the program, take one to five tablets at the beginning of each meal that contains protein.

Intestinal Gas and Bloating

Everyone has gas now and then. Most people pass gas ten to twelve times a day. A number of different factors contribute to excess gas. Swallowing air contributes to increased intestinal gas. In the diet, milk products, beans, and cruciferous vegetables—broccoli, cabbage, watercress, bok choy—can cause gas. Uncomfortable intestinal gas, the kind that causes bloating and shooting pains in the abdomen, is usually caused by undigested food that ferments in the colon. All poorly digested food can ferment in the gut, but excessive dietary carbohydrates are more susceptible to ferment and are more often the cause of intestinal cause. Gas is also a side effect of unhealthy gut ecology and bad bugs. Persistent, malodorous gas is almost always a sign that something is wrong with your digestion.

Diet

Phase One: one to four days, depending on the severity of your symptoms and until your elimination improves.

Phase Two: seven to fourteen days, depending on the severity of your symptoms (by the end of Phase Two, your symptoms should have significantly improved).

Phase Three: three to six months with extreme diligence.

Once your symptoms are completely gone for at least one month, you can gradually add foods from the "Bad" category.

Therapeutic Foods

These therapeutic foods will help you get well:

- *Cultured goat's milk dairy products.* Consume 8 to 32 ounces of the highest-quality cultured dairy products from goat's or sheep's milk. Try to find yogurt that does not contain the organism *Streptococcus thermophilus*, a bacterial microbe that has been implicated in the worsening of certain immune-system disorders.
- *Grass-fed red meat.* Red meat from grass-fed cattle, buffalo, and lamb is very healthy and can be eaten several times per week. This meat is a great source of protein, minerals, vitamin B_{12}, vitamin D, beta-carotene, omega-3 fats, and CLA.
- *Omega-3 eggs.* Consume as many as two to four eggs high in the omega-3 fatty acids each day. These eggs contain DHA, vitamins E and B_{12}, and antioxidants.
- *Coconut oil.* This oil is perhaps the healthiest of the widely available oils. We recommend cooking almost exclusively with coconut oil. Consume as much as 2 to 4 tablespoons of the oil in cooking, in smoothies, or right off the spoon. It contains large amounts of lauric acid, a potent antimicrobial and one of the chief fatty acids in breast milk.
- *Ocean-caught fish.* This type of fish is perhaps the healthiest of all the protein sources. Salmon, sardines, mackerel, herring, and tuna are high in the omega-3 fatty acids EPA and DHA. Ocean-caught fish can be consumed every day to enhance digestive and immune system health.
- *Cod liver oil.* Take 1 teaspoon of plain or flavored cod liver oil each day. Cod liver oil is a fantastic source of the omega-3 fats DHA and EPA, as well as of vitamins A and D.
- *Vegetable juice.* As long as your diarrhea is not active, consume vegetable juices that are low in carbohydrates, such as celery and green juices, mixed with a small amount of higher-carbohydrate veggies, such as carrot or beet. Mix in some form of healthy fat with each glass of the juice. A teaspoon of cultured goat's milk, coconut milk and cream, or flaxseed oil enhances the absorption of minerals and prevents spikes in blood sugar.

- *Fermented vegetables.* Consume a few tablespoons of fermented vegetables such as sauerkraut with each meal to aid in digestion. Fermented vegetables are excellent sources of naturally occurring probiotics and enzymes.
- *Stocks.* After completing Phases One and Two of the program, consume stocks on a regular basis, especially when you have a cold or flu. Stocks made from the bones of chicken, fish, lamb, or beef contain minerals, gelatin, cartilage, collagen, and electrolytes. Stocks help to heal the gut lining and reduce inflammation.

Supplements

Take these health supplements to alleviate your symptoms and get well:

- *Probiotic with HSOs.* Follow the instructions on the product label and work up to six to twelve caplets per day for three months. Then reduce the dosage to 3 caplets per day for life.
- *Digestive enzymes.* Take one to three caplets with each meal or snack.
- *Hydrocloric acid.* Hydrocloric acid is way to improve overall digestion as well as the symptoms caused by intestinal gas. One problem with taking hydrocloric acid supplements, however, is that taking HCl supplements if you have an ulcer is not healthy. First try digestive enzymes, and if the enzymes don't solve the problem completely, try a tablespoon of apple cider vinegar (a natural source of hydrocloric acid) with each meal. If the apple cider vinegar seems to improve your digestion, you may move on to a low-dose hydrocloric acid supplement. If any of these recommendations worsen your symptoms, stop taking the supplement and seek medical attention.
- *Fiber.* Some individuals with gas and bloating can benefit by adding a natural fiber supplement to their program. Start slowly and work up to one serving morning and evening as directed on the product label.
- *Whole food-mineral powder.* Take 1 to 2 tablespoons once or

twice per day with 8 ounces of water. People who suffer from intestinal distress can benefit from high-quality alkalizing minerals.

- *Essential fats.* Take 1 teaspoon per day of cod liver oil.
- *Structured mineral water.* Consume at least 64 ounces per day of a high-quality structured or high-mineral water.

Intestinal Parasites

Humans have been harboring parasites and trying to get rid of them from the beginning. An old joke claims that the oldest and shortest poem is about parasites and it goes like this:

Adam
Had 'em

Worms—tapeworms, pinworms, roundworms, whipworms, and hookworms—are the most common intestinal parasites. Protozoa also live in the intestines in a parasitical relationship. Many parasites are benign, although intestinal parasites can cause abdominal cramps, symptoms similar to those of irritable bowel syndrome, diarrhea, and anal itching. One theory says that parasites are responsible for allergies. According to this theory, parasites can cause disruption in the intercellular glue (the stuff that holds cells together), which in turn can permit large molecules to enter the bloodstream. This, in turn, can trigger an allergic response. However, the theory that parasites cause allergies is controversial and more research needs to be done.

Parasitical infection is another one of those diagnoses that is given far too much airplay in the world of alternative medicine. We acknowledge the existence of parasites, but we believe that parasites are not the source of all evil in the universe. Parasites are a symptom more so than a distinct disease entity. Clean up your diet, improve your gut ecology, and your body will do the rest.

Diet

<u>Phase One</u>: one day.

<u>Phase Two</u>: fourteen days.

Phase Three: six to twelve months.

Restrict your consumption of grains, fruits, and sweeteners of any kind until your symptoms are gone.

Therapeutic Foods

These therapeutic foods will help you get well:

- *Cultured goat's milk dairy products.* Consume 8 to 32 ounces of the highest-quality cultured dairy products from goat's or sheep's milk. Try to find yogurt that does not contain the organism *Streptococcus thermophilus*, a bacterial microbe that is known to make certain immune-system disorders worse.
- *Grass-fed red meat.* Red meat from grass-fed cattle, buffalo, and lamb is very healthy and can be eaten several times per week. This meat is a great source of protein, minerals, vitamin B_{12}, vitamin D, beta-carotene, omega-3 fats, and CLA.
- *Omega-3 eggs.* Consume as many as two to four eggs high in the omega-3 fatty acids each day. These eggs contain DHA, vitamins E and B_{12}, and antioxidants.
- *Coconut oil.* This oil is perhaps the healthiest of the widely available oils. We recommend cooking almost exclusively with coconut oil. Consume as much as 2 to 4 tablespoons of the oil in cooking, in smoothies, or right off the spoon. It contains large amounts of lauric acid, a potent antimicrobial and one of the chief fatty acids in breast milk.
- *Ocean-caught fish.* This type of fish is perhaps the healthiest of all the protein sources. Salmon, sardines, mackerel, herring, and tuna are high in the omega-3 fatty acids EPA and DHA. Ocean-caught fish can be consumed every day to enhance digestive and immune system health.
- *Cod liver oil.* Take 1 teaspoon of plain or flavored cod liver oil each day. Cod liver oil is a fantastic source of the omega-3 fats DHA and EPA, as well as of vitamins A and D.
- *Vegetable juice.* As long as your diarrhea is not active, consume vegetable juices that are low in carbohydrates, such as celery and

green juices, mixed with a small amount of higher-carbohydrate veggies, such as carrot or beet. Mix in some form of healthy fat with each glass of the juice. A teaspoon of cultured goat's milk, coconut milk and cream, or flaxseed oil enhances the absorption of minerals and prevents spikes in blood sugar.

➤ *Fermented vegetables.* Consume a few tablespoons of fermented vegetables such as sauerkraut with each meal to aid in digestion. Fermented vegetables are excellent sources of naturally occurring probiotics and enzymes.

➤ *Stocks.* After completing Phases One and Two of the program, consume stocks on a regular basis, especially when you have a cold or flu. Stocks made from the bones of chicken, fish, lamb, or beef contain minerals, gelatin, cartilage, collagen, and electrolytes. Stocks help to heal the gut lining and reduce inflammation.

Supplements

Take these health supplements to alleviate your symptoms and get well:

➤ *Antifungal/antimicrobial.* Follow the two-week program as directed by the instructions on the product label. Repeat the two-week program if your symptoms return.

➤ *Probiotic with HSOs.* After the two-week intensive antifungal program, consume six caplets per day, adding one caplet per day until you reach twelve. Remain at twelve for six months or until your symptoms resolve. Then gradually reduce the dosage to three to six caplets per day for maintenance purposes.

➤ *Digestive enzymes.* Take one to three caplets with each meal or snack.

➤ *Fiber.* Along with clay (see below), consume 1 serving twice per day, morning and evening. Consuming a fiber supplement is essential during the first two weeks of the program. Thereafter, consume fiber as needed, morning and evening.

➤ *Clay.* Take 1 to 2 tablespoons of clay along with fiber (see above) during the initial two weeks of the program. The clay will absorb the toxins excreted by the fungi as they are destroyed. Taking clay is essential when you have intestinal parasites.

◆ *Essential fats.* Take 1 teaspoon of cod liver oil.

◆ *Protein digestant.* If you are over sixty years of age and you experience post-meal belching and bloating after one full month on the program, take one to five tablets at the beginning of each meal that contains protein.

◆ *Structured mineral water.* Consume at least 64 ounces per day of a high-quality structured or high-mineral water.

◆ *Pet natural antimicrobial product.* We recommend giving your pets a natural antimicrobial product to minimize the chance of cross-infection by microbes.

Irritable Bowel Syndrome

Irritable bowel syndrome (IBS) is a general intestinal disorder that is said to afflict 10 to 20 percent of American adults. Twice as many women as men have IBS. (This statistic may reflect a reporting bias, since men are less likely to seek medical attention for bowel-disorder symptoms. Many experts suspect that IBS afflicts equal numbers of men and women.) IBS is characterized by an array of symptoms: constipation alternating with diarrhea (with one of the two usually predominating), cramping, bloating, excessive gas, and an urge to move the bowels without being able to do so. Over the years, IBS has been inappropriately called colitis, mucous colitis, nervous stomach, and spastic colon. IBS is sometimes referred to as functional bowel disease.

No one is certain precisely what causes IBS. In recent years, however, researchers have demonstrated that many IBS sufferers have a more reactive/sensitive enteric nervous system than normal. A number of studies from Europe have also implicated bad gut ecology as a possible cause. To be frank, IBS is likely a group of many disorders that have been clumped under one name because we don't understand the individual disorders clearly enough. Fortunately, IBS responds quite well to the Guts and Glory Program regardless of its etiology. Restricting dietary carbohydrates and simultaneously improving your gut ecology provides the greatest degree of improvement.

Diet

Phase One: seven to fourteen days depending on the severity of your symptoms and until your elimination improves.

Phase Two: seven to fourteen days depending on the severity of your symptoms (by the end of Phase Two, your symptoms should have significantly improved).

Phase Three: six to twelve months with extreme diligence. After your symptoms have completely disappeared for at least three months, you can gradually add foods from the "Bad" category. If you experience a relapse, or flare-up, return to Phases One and Two until your symptoms are eliminated.

Therapeutic Foods

These therapeutic foods will help you get well:

- *Cultured goat's milk dairy products.* Consume 8 to 32 ounces of the highest-quality cultured dairy products from goat's or sheep's milk. Try to find yogurt that does not contain the organism *Streptococcus thermophilus*, a bacterial microbe that may make certain immune-system disorders worse.
- *Grass-fed red meat.* Red meat from grass-fed cattle, buffalo, and lamb is very healthy and can be eaten several times per week. This meat is a great source of protein, minerals, vitamin B_{12}, vitamin D, beta-carotene, omega-3 fats, and CLA.
- *Omega-3 eggs.* Consume as many as two to four eggs high in the omega-3 fatty acids each day. These eggs contain DHA, vitamins E and B_{12}, and antioxidants.
- *Coconut oil.* This oil is perhaps the healthiest of the widely available oils. We recommend cooking almost exclusively with coconut oil. Consume as much as 2 to 4 tablespoons of the oil in

cooking, in smoothies, or right off the spoon. It contains large amounts of lauric acid, a potent antimicrobial and one of the chief fatty acids in breast milk.

- *Ocean-caught fish.* This type of fish is perhaps the healthiest of all the protein sources. Salmon, sardines, mackerel, herring, and tuna are high in the omega-3 fatty acids EPA and DHA. Ocean-caught fish can be consumed every day to enhance digestive and immune system health.
- *Cod liver oil.* Take 1 teaspoon of plain or flavored cod liver oil each day. Cod liver oil is a fantastic source of the omega-3 fats DHA and EPA, as well as of vitamins A and D.
- *Vegetable juice.* As long as your diarrhea is not active, consume vegetable juices that are low in carbohydrates, such as celery and green juices, mixed with a small amount of higher-carbohydrate veggies, such as carrot or beet. Mix in some form of healthy fat with each glass of the juice. A teaspoon of cultured goat's milk, coconut milk and cream, or flaxseed oil enhances the absorption of minerals and prevents spikes in blood sugar.
- *Fermented vegetables.* Consume a few tablespoons of fermented vegetables such as sauerkraut with each meal to aid in digestion. Fermented vegetables are excellent sources of naturally occurring probiotics and enzymes.
- *Stocks.* After completing Phases One and Two of the program, consume stocks on a regular basis, especially when you have a cold or flu. Stocks made from the bones of chicken, fish, lamb, or beef contain minerals, gelatin, cartilage, collagen, and electrolytes. Stocks help to heal the gut lining and reduce inflammation.

Supplements

Take these health supplements to alleviate your symptoms and get well:

- *Probiotic with HSOs.* After completing Phase Two, take twelve caplets per day for six to twelve months. Then gradually reduce the dosage to three to six caplets per day for life.

- *Digestive enzymes.* Starting in Phase Two, take one to three caplets with each meal or snack.
- *Hydrocloric acid.* Hydrocloric acid is a great way to improve your overall digestion. Taking hydrocloric acid will improve many people's digestion and subsequently alleviate some of the symptoms of IBS. One problem, however, is that taking hydrocloric acid supplements if you have an ulcer is not healthy. First try digestive enzymes, and if the enzymes don't solve the problem completely, try a tablespoon of apple cider vinegar (a natural source of hydrocloric acid) with each meal. If the apple cider vinegar seems to improve your digestion, you may move on to a low-dose hydrocloric acid supplement. If any of these recommendations worsen your symptoms, stop taking the supplement and seek medical attention.
- *Fiber.* Some individuals can benefit by adding a natural fiber supplement to their program. Start slowly and gradually increase the dosage. If you experience unpleasant gas or bloating even after two weeks on the product, discontinue it. People suffering from IBS who have constipation or diarrhea often improve if they start a fiber supplement slowly and work up to one serving morning and evening as directed on the product label.
- *Whole-food mineral powder.* Starting in Phase Two, take 1 to 2 tablespoons once or twice daily with 8 ounces of water.
- *Essential fats.* Take 1 teaspoon per day of cod liver oil.
- *Structured mineral water.* Consume at least 64 ounces per day of a high-quality structured or high-mineral water.
- *Protein digestant.* If you are over sixty years of age and you experience post-meal belching and bloating after one full month on the program, take one to five tablets at the beginning of each meal that contains protein.

Additional Therapies

For people who have or may have imbalanced intestinal flora, avoiding contact with chlorinated water is of the utmost importance. That includes bathing water and drinking water. Chlorine kills bacteria, friendly and unfriendly, in the colon. It can be absorbed through the skin. We recommend installing a shower filter to remove chlorine. Avoid swimming in chlorinated water as well.

Lactose Intolerance

Lactose intolerance is the inability to digest dairy products. To be specific, it is the inability to digest lactose, the milk sugar found in dairy products. People who are lactose intolerant do not produce enough lactase, the enzyme that is responsible for breaking down milk sugar in the small intestine so it can be absorbed in the bloodstream. An estimated 30 to 50 percent of Americans are lactose intolerant. As a matter of fact, for adults the ability to digest lactose can be considered an anomaly. Most adults do not have this ability and are lactose intolerant to one degree or another.

The symptoms of lactose intolerance include gas, diarrhea, bloating, cramps, and nausea. These symptoms are present thirty minutes to two hours after eating a food item that contains lactose. Lactose intolerance can itself be a symptom of an intestinal disease. If Crohn's disease or celiac disease, for example, sufficiently damages the villi of the small intestine, the villi may cease producing digestive enzymes such as lactase, and lactose intolerance may result. It is also not uncommon for lactose intolerance to develop after acute gastroenteritis.

Diet

Phase One: one to four days depending on the severity of your symptoms and until your elimination improves.

Phase Two: seven to fourteen days depending on the severity of your symptoms (by the end of Phase Two, your symptoms should have significantly improved).

Phase Three: three to six months with extreme diligence. After your symptoms are completely gone for at least 1 month, you may gradually add foods in the "Bad" category. Most people who are lactose intolerant do very well with fermented dairy products such as properly prepared 30-hour cultured yogurt. If you know you are lactose intolerant, consume only 30-hour cultured goat's milk yogurt.

Therapeutic Foods

These therapeutic foods will help you get well:

- *Cultured goat's milk dairy products.* Consume 8 to 32 ounces of the highest-quality cultured dairy products from goat's or sheep's milk. Try to find yogurt that does not contain the organism *Streptococcus thermophilus*, a bacterial microbe that has been implicated in the exacerbation of certain immune-system disorders.
- *Grass-fed red meat.* Red meat from grass-fed cattle, buffalo, and lamb is very healthy and can be eaten several times per week. This meat is a great source of protein, minerals, vitamin B_{12} vitamin D, beta-carotene, omega-3 fats, and CLA.
- *Omega-3 eggs.* Consume as many as two to four eggs high in the omega-3 fatty acids each day. These eggs contain DHA, vitamins E and B_{12}, and antioxidants.
- *Coconut oil.* This oil is perhaps the healthiest of the widely available oils. We recommend cooking almost exclusively with coconut oil. Consume as much as 2 to 4 tablespoons of the oil in cooking, in smoothies, or right off the spoon. It contains large amounts of lauric acid, a potent antimicrobial and one of the chief fatty acids in breast milk.
- *Ocean-caught fish.* This type of fish is perhaps the healthiest of all the protein sources. Salmon, sardines, mackerel, herring, and tuna are high in the omega-3 fatty acids EPA and DHA. Ocean-caught fish can be consumed every day to enhance digestive and immune system health.
- *Cod liver oil.* Take 1 teaspoon of plain or flavored cod liver oil each day. Cod liver oil is a fantastic source of the omega-3 fats DHA and EPA, as well as of vitamins A and D.
- *Vegetable juice.* As long as your diarrhea is not active, consume

vegetable juices that are low in carbohydrates, such as celery and green juices, mixed with a small amount of higher-carbohydrate veggies, such as carrot or beet. Mix in some form of healthy fat with each glass of the juice. A teaspoon of cultured goat's milk, coconut milk and cream, or flaxseed oil enhances the absorption of minerals and prevents spikes in blood sugar.

- *Fermented vegetables.* Consume a few tablespoons of fermented vegetables such as sauerkraut with each meal to aid in digestion. Fermented vegetables are excellent sources of naturally occurring probiotics and enzymes.
- *Stocks.* After completing Phases One and Two of the program, consume stocks on a regular basis, especially when you have a cold or flu. Stocks made from the bones of chicken, fish, lamb, or beef contain minerals, gelatin, cartilage, collagen, and electrolytes. Stocks help to heal the gut lining and reduce inflammation.

Supplements

Take these health supplements to alleviate your symptoms and get well:

- *Probiotic with HSOs.* Follow the instructions on the product label and work up to six to twelve caplets per day for three months. Then reduce your intake to three caplets per day for life.
- *Digestive enzymes.* With each meal and snack, take one to three caplets of a comprehensive plant enzyme formula that is high in lactase, the enzyme that helps digest milk sugar. If you are consuming dairy products that contain lactose, take more enzymes.
- *Fiber.* Some individuals with lactose intolerance benefit from a natural fiber supplement. Start slowly and work up to one serving morning and evening as directed on the product label.
- *Whole-food mineral powder.* Take 1 to 2 tablespoons once or twice daily with 8 ounces of water. People with intestinal distress can benefit from the high-quality alkalizing minerals.
- *Essential fats.* Take 1 teaspoon per day of cod liver oil.
- *Structured mineral water.* Consume at least 64 ounces per day of a high-quality structured or high-mineral water.

Microscopic Colitis

Microscopic colitis is a relatively new term in the medical lexicon. *Colitis* refers to inflammation of the colon. Microscopic colitis is a type of colitis that is not apparent on visual inspection and can be diagnosed only by a colon biopsy. The two predominant types of microscopic colitis are collangeous colitis and lymphocytic colitis. Collangeous colitis is far more common in women than men. It usually develops in middle age and can be caused by the use of nonsteroidal anti-inflammatory drugs (NSAIDs) such as aspirin and ibuprofen. Lymphocytic colitis affects both sexes equally and is associated with celiac disease. Both conditions are associated with chronic watery diarrhea.

The cause of microscopic colitis is not known but the disease is believed to be a type of inflammatory bowel disease. Coauthor Dr. Brasco has successfully treated many individuals with this condition by using the Guts and Glory Program. Restricting dietary carbohydrates and simultaneously improving your gut ecology provide the greatest degree of improvement.

Diet

Phase One: seven to fourteen days depending on the severity of your symptoms and until your elimination improves.

Phase Two: seven to fourteen days depending on the severity of your symptoms (by the end of Phase Two, your symptoms should have significantly improved).

Phase Three: six to twelve months with extreme diligence.

After symptoms are completely gone for at least three months, you can gradually add foods from the "Bad" category if you desire. Because people with microscopic colitis appear to have a predisposed weakness in their intestinal tracts, we strongly recommend that they adhere to a diet of foods in the "Good" and "Not So Bad" categories for the rest of their lives. If a relapse, or flare-up, occurs, go back to Phases One and Two until your symptoms improve and are eliminated.

Therapeutic Foods

These therapeutic foods will help you get well:

- *Cultured goat's milk dairy products.* Consume 8 to 32 ounces of the highest-quality cultured dairy products from goat's or sheep's milk. Try to find yogurt that does not contain the organism *Streptococcus thermophilus*, a bacterial microbe that has been known to make certain immune-system disorders worse.
- *Grass-fed red meat.* Red meat from grass-fed cattle, buffalo, and lamb is very healthy and can be eaten several times per week. This meat is a great source of protein, minerals, vitamin B_{12}, vitamin D, beta-carotene, omega-3 fats, and CLA.
- *Omega-3 eggs.* Consume as many as two to four eggs high in omega-3 fatty acids each day. These eggs contain DHA, vitamins E and B_{12}, and antioxidants.
- *Coconut oil.* This oil is perhaps the healthiest of the widely available oils. We recommend cooking almost exclusively with coconut oil. Consume as much as 2 to 4 tablespoons of the oil in cooking, in smoothies, or right off the spoon. It contains large amounts of lauric acid, a potent antimicrobial and one of the chief fatty acids in breast milk.
- *Ocean-caught fish.* This type of fish is perhaps the healthiest of all the protein sources. Salmon, sardines, mackerel, herring, and tuna are high in the omega-3 fatty acids EPA and DHA. Ocean-caught fish can be consumed every day to enhance digestive and immune system health.
- *Cod liver oil.* Take 1 teaspoon of plain or flavored cod liver oil each day. Cod liver oil is a fantastic source of the omega-3 fats DHA and EPA, as well as of vitamins A and D.
- *Vegetable juice.* As long as your diarrhea is not active, consume vegetable juices that are low in carbohydrates, such as celery and green juices, mixed with a small amount of higher-carbohydrate

veggies, such as carrot or beet. Mix in some form of healthy fat with each glass of the juice. A teaspoon of cultured goat's milk, coconut milk and cream, or flaxseed oil enhances the absorption of minerals and prevents spikes in blood sugar.

- *Fermented vegetables.* Consume a few tablespoons of fermented vegetables such as sauerkraut with each meal to aid in digestion. Fermented vegetables are excellent sources of naturally occurring probiotics and enzymes.
- *Stocks.* After completing Phases One and Two of the program, consume stocks on a regular basis, especially when you have a cold or flu. Stocks made from the bones of chicken, fish, lamb, or beef contain minerals, gelatin, cartilage, collagen, and electrolytes. Stocks help to heal the gut lining and reduce inflammation.

Supplements

Take these health supplements to alleviate your symptoms and get well:

- *Probiotic with HSOs.* After completing Phase Two, take twelve caplets per day for six to twelve months. Then reduce the dosage to three to six caplets per day for life.
- *Digestive enzymes.* Starting in Phase Two, take one to three caplets with each meal and snack.
- *Clay.* Take 1 tablespoon of clay mixed in 8 ounces of water four times per day until your diarrhea is relieved. Thereafter, take 1 tablespoon of clay in 8 ounces of water morning and evening to promote ongoing detoxification.
- *Anti-inflammatory.* Take 12 caplets per day in three divided doses for one to four weeks. Then reduce to a maintenance level of three caplets per day for three to six months. If a relapse, or flare-up, occurs, take twelve caplets per day for at least one week or until your symptoms are under control.
- *Whole-food mineral powder.* Starting in Phase Two, take 1 to 2 tablespoons once or twice daily with 8 ounces of water.
- *Essential fats.* Take 1 teaspoon per day of cod liver oil.

- *Structured mineral water.* Consume at least 64 ounces per day of a high-quality structured or high-mineral water.
- *Pet natural antimicrobial product.* We recommend giving your pets a natural antimicrobial product to minimize the chance of cross-infection by microbes.

Mucous Colitis

See Irritable Bowel Syndrome.

Nausea and Vomiting

Nausea is an unpleasant wavelike sensation in the throat or stomach. Nausea sometimes culminates in vomiting or retching. Motion sickness, emotional anxiety, and stomach ailments can cause nausea. Chemotherapy and certain kinds of drugs can produce nausea as well. Nausea is a symptom of many different diseases. If you experience nausea for more than three days, consult a physician to find out what is causing your nausea.

Diet

Phase One: one day.

Phase Two: fourteen days.

Phase Three: three to six months until your symptoms are eliminated.

Therapeutic Foods

These therapeutic foods will help you get well:

- *Cultured goat's milk dairy products.* Consume 8 to 32 ounces of the highest-quality cultured dairy products from goat's or sheep's milk. Try to find yogurt that does not contain the organism *Streptococcus thermophilus*, a bacterial microbe that has been implicated in the exacerbation of certain immune-system disorders.

- *Grass-fed red meat.* Red meat from grass-fed cattle, buffalo, and lamb is very healthy and can be eaten several times per week. This meat is a great source of protein, minerals, vitamin B_{12}, vitamin D, beta-carotene, omega-3 fats, and CLA.

- *Omega-3 eggs.* Consume as many as two to four eggs high in omega-3 fatty acids each day. These eggs contain DHA, vitamins E and B_{12}, and antioxidants.

- *Coconut oil.* This oil is perhaps the healthiest of the widely available oils. We recommend cooking almost exclusively with coconut oil. Consume as much as 2 to 4 tablespoons of the oil in cooking, in smoothies, or right off the spoon. It contains large amounts of lauric acid, a potent antimicrobial and one of the chief fatty acids in breast milk.

- *Ocean-caught fish.* This type of fish is perhaps the healthiest of all the protein sources. Salmon, sardines, mackerel, herring, and tuna are high in the omega-3 fatty acids EPA and DHA. Ocean-caught fish can be consumed every day to enhance digestive and immune system health.

- *Cod liver oil.* Take 1 teaspoon of plain or flavored cod liver oil each day. Cod liver oil is a fantastic source of the omega-3 fats DHA and EPA, as well as of vitamins A and D.

- *Vegetable juice.* As long as your diarrhea is not active, consume vegetable juices that are low in carbohydrates, such as celery and green juices, mixed with a small amount of higher-carbohydrate veggies, such as carrot or beet. Mix in some form of healthy fat with each glass of the juice. A teaspoon of cultured goat's milk, coconut milk and cream, or flaxseed oil enhances the absorption of minerals and prevents spikes in blood sugar.

- *Fermented vegetables.* Consume a few tablespoons of fermented vegetables such as sauerkraut with each meal to aid in digestion. Fermented vegetables are excellent sources of naturally occurring probiotics and enzymes.

- *Stocks.* After completing Phases One and Two of the program, consume stocks on a regular basis, especially when you have a cold or flu. Stocks made from the bones of chicken, fish, lamb, or beef contain minerals, gelatin, cartilage, collagen, and electrolytes. Stocks help to heal the gut lining and reduce inflammation.

Supplements

Take these health supplements to alleviate your symptoms and get well:

- *Antifungal/antimicrobial.* Follow the two-week program as directed by the instructions on the product label. Repeat to the two-week program if your symptoms return.
- *Probiotic with HSOs.* After the two-week intensive antifungal program, consume six caplets per day, adding one caplet per day until you reach twelve. Remain at twelve for three months or until your symptoms are resolved. Then gradually reduce the dosage to three caplets per day for maintenance purposes.
- *Digestive enzymes.* Take one to three caplets with each meal and snack.
- *Clay.* When nausea or vomiting are severe, take 1 tablespoon of clay with 8 ounces of water two to four times per day until the symptoms subside.
- *Protein digestant.* If you are over sixty years of age and you experience post-meal belching and bloating after one full month on the program, take one to five tablets at the beginning of each meal containing protein.
- *Structured mineral water.* Consume at least 64 ounces per day of a high-quality structured or high-mineral water.

Nonulcerative Dyspepsia

Nonulcerative dyspepsia, also known as functional dyspepsia, describes an assortment of symptoms that are not caused by ulcers, including nausea (with occasional vomiting), bloating, belching, upper abdominal pain, and abdominal distension. These symptoms usually occur shortly after eating. Current medical research with this condition is focusing on abnormalities with regard to gastric motility. However, we believe the cause can mostly be assigned to poor digestive function and a bad diet. The symptoms associated with nonulcerative dyspepsia may be caused by other more serious conditions. See your doctor for a proper diagnosis.

Diet

Phase Two: three to seven days.

Phase Three: three to six months or more until your symptoms subside.

Therapeutic Foods

These therapeutic foods will help you get well:

- *Cultured goat's milk dairy products.* Consume 8 to 32 ounces of the highest-quality cultured dairy products from goat's or sheep's milk. Try to find yogurt that does not contain the organism *Streptococcus thermophilus*, a bacterial microbe that has been implicated in the exacerbation of certain immune-system disorders.
- *Grass-fed red meat.* Red meat from grass-fed cattle, buffalo, and lamb is very healthy and can be eaten several times per week. This meat is a great source of protein, minerals, vitamin B_{12}, vitamin D, beta-carotene, omega-3 fats, and CLA.
- *Omega-3 eggs.* Consume as many as two to four eggs high in the omega-3 fatty acids each day. These eggs contain DHA, vitamins E and B_{12}, and antioxidants.
- *Coconut oil.* This oil is perhaps the healthiest of the widely available oils. We recommend cooking almost exclusively with coconut oil. Consume as much as 2 to 4 tablespoons of the oil in cooking, in smoothies, or right off the spoon. It contains large amounts of lauric acid, a potent antimicrobial and one of the chief fatty acids in breast milk.
- *Ocean-caught fish.* This type of fish is perhaps the healthiest of all the protein sources. Salmon, sardines, mackerel, herring, and tuna are high in the omega-3 fatty acids EPA and DHA. Ocean-

caught fish can be consumed every day to enhance digestive and immune system health.

- *Cod liver oil.* Take 1 teaspoon of plain or flavored cod liver oil each day. Cod liver oil is a fantastic source of the omega-3 fats DHA and EPA, as well as of vitamins A and D.
- *Vegetable juice.* As long as your diarrhea is not active, consume vegetable juices that are low in carbohydrates, such as celery and green juices, mixed with a small amount of higher-carbohydrate veggies, such as carrot or beet. Mix in some form of healthy fat with each glass of the juice. A teaspoon of cultured goat's milk, coconut milk and cream, or flaxseed oil enhances the absorption of minerals and prevents spikes in blood sugar.
- *Fermented vegetables.* Consume a few tablespoons of fermented vegetables such as sauerkraut with each meal to aid in digestion. Fermented vegetables are excellent sources of naturally occurring probiotics and enzymes.
- *Stocks.* After completing Phases One and Two of the program, consume stocks on a regular basis, especially when you have a cold or flu. Stocks made from the bones of chicken, fish, lamb, or beef contain minerals, gelatin, cartilage, collagen, and electrolytes. Stocks help to heal the gut lining and reduce inflammation.

Supplements

Take these health supplements to alleviate your symptoms and get well:

- *Probiotic with HSOs.* Take three to six caplets per day.
- *Digestive enzymes.* Take one to three caplets with each meal or snack.
- *Essential fats.* Take 1 teaspoon per day of cod liver oil.
- *Alkalizing upper GI blend.* Take 1 to 2 tablespoons mixed in water upon rising and before bed. This supplement can be taken to relieve the pain during an episode.
- *Structured mineral water.* Consume at least 64 ounces per day of a high-quality structured or high-mineral water.

- *Fiber.* If elimination is not optimal, consume a natural fiber supplement. Take one serving twice per day, morning and evening.
- *Protein digestant.* If you are over sixty years of age and you experience post-meal belching and bloating after one full month on the program, take one to five tablets at the beginning of each meal containing protein.

Parasites

See Intestinal Parasites.

Spastic Colon

See Irritable Bowel Syndrome.

Sprue

See Celiac Disease.

Ulcerative Colitis

Ulcerative colitis causes inflammation and ulceration to occur in the large intestine. The ulcerations appear where the inflammation has damaged cells on the lining of the colon. Usually, the inflammatory process occurs in the rectum or lower part of the large intestine, but the ulcerations can sometimes occur in the entire colon. The inflamed colon lining can bleed and may produce pus. The most noteworthy symptoms of ulcerative colitis are abdominal pain and bloody diarrhea. Other symptoms include weight loss, fatigue, and rectal bleeding. While most people can be treated in a doctor's office, this disease can sometimes evolve into a very serious and even life-threatening condition that requires hospitalization.

Researchers are not certain what causes ulcerative colitis. Some believe that the inflammation is caused by an autoimmune reaction. A growing body of research shows that this response may be stimulated by the presence of a particular or group of bacteria in the large bowel. The exact mechanism is not well known or understood. Ulcerative colitis clearly demonstrates a genetic predilection and tends to cluster in families. Undoubtedly, consuming junk food and excessive carbohydrates can contribute to ulcerative colitis.

Diet

Phase One: seven to fourteen days depending on the severity of your symptoms and until your elimination improves.

Phase Two: seven to fourteen days depending on the severity of your symptoms (by the end of Phase Two, your symptoms should have significantly improved).

Phase Three: six to twelve months with extreme diligence.

After your symptoms are completely gone for at least three months, you can gradually add foods from the "Bad" category if you desire. Because people with ulcerative colitis appear to have a predisposed weakness in their intestinal tracts, we strongly recommend that they adhere to a diet of foods in the "Good" and "Not So Bad" categories for the rest of their lives. If a relapse, or flare-up, occurs, go back to Phases One and Two until your symptoms improve and are eliminated.

Therapeutic Foods

These therapeutic foods will help you get well:

- *Cultured goat's milk dairy products.* Consume 8 to 32 ounces of the highest-quality cultured dairy products from goat's or sheep's milk. Try to find yogurt that does not contain the organism *Streptococcus thermophilus*, a bacterial microbe that has been implicated in the exacerbation of certain immune-system disorders.
- *Grass-fed red meat.* Red meat from grass-fed cattle, buffalo, and lamb is very healthy and can be eaten several times per week.

This meat is a great source of protein, minerals, vitamin B_{12}, vitamin D, beta-carotene, omega-3 fats, and CLA.

◆ *Omega-3 eggs.* Consume as many as two to four eggs high in the omega-3 fatty acids each day. These eggs contain DHA, vitamins E and B_{12}, and antioxidants.

◆ *Coconut oil.* This oil is perhaps the healthiest of the widely available oils. We recommend cooking almost exclusively with coconut oil. Consume as much as 2 to 4 tablespoons of the oil in cooking, in smoothies, or right off the spoon. It contains large amounts of lauric acid, a potent antimicrobial and one of the chief fatty acids in breast milk.

◆ *Ocean-caught fish.* This type of fish is perhaps the healthiest of all the protein sources. Salmon, sardines, mackerel, herring, and tuna are high in the omega-3 fatty acids EPA and DHA. Ocean-caught fish can be consumed every day to enhance digestive and immune system health.

◆ *Cod liver oil.* Take 1 teaspoon of plain or flavored cod liver oil each day. Cod liver oil is a fantastic source of the omega-3 fats DHA and EPA, as well as of vitamins A and D.

◆ *Vegetable juice.* As long as your diarrhea is not active, consume vegetable juices that are low in carbohydrates, such as celery and green juices, mixed with a small amount of higher-carbohydrate veggies, such as carrot or beet. Mix in some form of healthy fat with each glass of the juice. A teaspoon of cultured goat's milk, coconut milk and cream, or flaxseed oil enhances the absorption of minerals and prevents spikes in blood sugar.

◆ *Fermented vegetables.* Consume a few tablespoons of fermented vegetables such as sauerkraut with each meal to aid in digestion. Fermented vegetables are excellent sources of naturally occurring probiotics and enzymes.

◆ *Stocks.* After completing Phases One and Two of the program, consume stocks on a regular basis, especially when you have a cold or flu. Stocks made from the bones of chicken, fish, lamb, or beef contain minerals, gelatin, cartilage, collagen, and electrolytes. Stocks help to heal the gut lining and reduce inflammation.

Supplements

Take these health supplements to alleviate your symptoms and get well:

- *Probiotic with HSOs.* Begin taking during Phase Two and work up to twelve caplets per day for six to twelve months. Then reduce the dosage to three to six caplets per day for life.
- *Digestive enzymes.* Starting in Phase Two, take one to three caplets with each meal or snack.
- *Clay.* Take 1 tablespoon of clay mixed in 8 ounces of water four times per day until your diarrhea is relieved. Thereafter, take 1 tablespoon of clay in 8 ounces of water morning and evening to promote ongoing detoxification.
- *Anti-inflammatory.* Consume twelve caplets per day in three divided doses for one to four weeks. For the following three to six months, reduce to a maintenance level of three caplets per day. If a relapse, or flare-up, occurs, take twelve caplets per day for at least 1 week or until your symptoms are under control.
- *Whole-food mineral powder.* Starting in Phase Two, take 1 to 2 tablespoons once or twice daily with 8 ounces of water.
- *Essential fats.* Take 1 teaspoon per day of cod liver oil.
- *Structured mineral water.* Consume at least 64 ounces per day of a high-quality structured or high-mineral water.
- *Pet natural antimicrobial product.* We recommend giving your pets a natural antimicrobial product to minimize the chance of cross-infection by microbes.

Ulcers (Peptic and Duodenal)

A layer of mucus protects the stomach and the duodenum (the upper portion of the small intestine) from the corrosive effects of the gastric juices. However, if this mucosal layer fails to do its job, pepsin and the gastric juices produced by the stomach can burn the lining of the stomach or the duodenum. The result is chronic inflammation and ulcers. Failure to produce enough bicarbonate is another cause of ulcers. Normally, the stomach produces this chemical to neutralize stomach acid, but a failure to do so can contribute to ulcers. Ulcers produce a burning pain in the abdomen, loss of appetite, nausea, and vomiting.

One cause of ulcers is the habitual use of nonsteroidal anti-inflammatory drugs (NSAIDs) such as aspirin and ibuprofen. These drugs interfere with the production of mucus and bicarbonate in the stomach. Ulcers can also be caused by the bacterium *Helicobacter pylori*, which burrows into the lining of the stomach and causes inflammation.

Diet

<u>Phase One:</u> three to seven days (severe cases).

<u>Phase Two:</u> three to seven days.

<u>Phase Three:</u> three months or more until your symptoms subside.

Therapeutic Foods

These therapeutic foods will help you get well:

- *Cultured goat's milk dairy products.* Consume 8 to 32 ounces of the highest-quality cultured dairy products from goat's or sheep's milk. Try to find yogurt that does not contain the organism *Streptococcus thermophilus*, a bacterial microbe that is believed to make certain immune-system disorders worse.
- *Grass-fed red meat.* Red meat from grass-fed cattle, buffalo, and lamb is very healthy and can be eaten several times per week. This meat is a great source of protein, minerals, vitamin B_{12}, vitamin D, beta-carotene, omega-3 fats, and CLA.
- *Omega-3 eggs.* Consume as many as two to four eggs high in the omega-3 fatty acids each day. These eggs contain DHA, vitamins E and B_{12}, and antioxidants.
- *Coconut oil.* This oil is perhaps the healthiest of the widely available oils. We recommend cooking almost exclusively with coconut oil. Consume as much as 2 to 4 tablespoons of the oil in

cooking, in smoothies, or right off the spoon. It contains large amounts of lauric acid, a potent antimicrobial and one of the chief fatty acids in breast milk.

- *Ocean-caught fish.* This type of fish is perhaps the healthiest of all the protein sources. Salmon, sardines, mackerel, herring, and tuna are high in the omega-3 fatty acids EPA and DHA. Ocean-caught fish can be consumed every day to enhance digestive and immune system health.
- *Cod liver oil.* Take 1 teaspoon of plain or flavored cod liver oil each day. Cod liver oil is a fantastic source of the omega-3 fats DHA and EPA, as well as of vitamins A and D.
- *Vegetable juice.* As long as your diarrhea is not active, consume vegetable juices that are low in carbohydrates, such as celery and green juices, mixed with a small amount of higher-carbohydrate veggies, such as carrot or beet. Mix in some form of healthy fat with each glass of the juice. A teaspoon of cultured goat's milk, coconut milk and cream, or flaxseed oil enhances the absorption of minerals and prevents spikes in blood sugar.
- *Fermented vegetables.* Consume a few tablespoons of fermented vegetables such as sauerkraut with each meal to aid in digestion. Fermented vegetables are excellent sources of naturally occurring probiotics and enzymes.
- *Stocks.* After completing Phases One and Two of the program, consume stocks on a regular basis, especially when you have a cold or flu. Stocks made from the bones of chicken, fish, lamb, or beef contain minerals, gelatin, cartilage, collagen, and electrolytes. Stocks help to heal the gut lining and reduce inflammation.

Supplements

Take these health supplements to alleviate your symptoms and get well:

- *Probiotic with HSOs.* Take three to six caplets per day.
- *Digestive enzymes.* Take one to three caplets with each meal and snack.

- *Essential fats.* Take 1 teaspoon per day of cod liver oil.
- *Alkalizing upper GI blend.* Take 1 to 2 tablespoons mixed in water upon rising and before bed. Use this supplement to relieve the pain during an episode by taking 1 tablespoon in 8 ounces of water and repeating ten minutes later.
- *Structured mineral water.* Consume at least 64 ounces per day of a high-quality structured or high-mineral water.
- *Fiber.* Take one serving twice per day, morning and evening as directed on the product label.
- *Mastic gum.* Mastic gum is a tree resin that is known to have excellent antimicrobial properties. It is known to be particularly effective in eradicating *H. pylori* infections. Coauthor Dr. Brasco has used mastic gum extensively in his practice and has found it to be as effective as triple therapy (two antibiotics and a potent acid-blocking agent, the conventional approach to *H. pylori* therapy). What's more, taking mastic gum has no side effects.

Vomiting

See Nausea and Vomiting.

Yeast Infection

See Candidiasis.

❖ 11 ❖

Recipes

The following recipes will make your road to wellness an easier one. Each ingredient was carefully selected for its ability to improve gut health. Try your best to include these meals, beverages, and snacks as a regular part of your diet.

Please don't take shortcuts with these recipes. The ingredients in them contain healing compounds. Do your best to obtain the ingredients as they are listed. "Resources" on page 333 lists sources for these foods. The Brasco Broth recipe (page 328), for example, is not just chicken soup out of a can. It is specifically designed to deliver micronutrients and minerals that will assist the healing process. Especially when making the broth, following the recipe to a tee is necessary. For more great recipes, read *Nourishing Traditions* by Sally Fallon.

Balanced Veggie Juice

As long as you are not suffering from diarrhea, vegetable juices are wonderful sources of essential nutrients. Here is a great staple vegetable juice blend.

1 cup fresh carrot juice
$^1/_2$ cup fresh celery juice

1/4 cup fresh beet juice

1/4 cup fresh parsley or other green juice

1–2 tablespoons enzyme-enhanced, whole-food mineral
    blend (optional)

1 teaspoon thirty-hour goat's milk yogurt, quark, *crème
    Bulgare,* or full-fat coconut milk (milk and cream)
    (optional)

Combine all the ingredients in a tall glass and mix until well blended.

YIELD: 2 cups.

The use of a quality fat like yogurt, quark, crème Bulgare, or coconut milk helps to insure balanced blood sugar levels. However, if your blood sugar levels are negatively affected anyway, adjust the ingredients so that there is more green juice than carrot and beet juices.

Brasco Broth

3 quarts filtered water

1/2 ounce structured water additive

1 tablespoon apple cider vinegar

4–6 tablespoons coconut oil

1 medium organic, free-range or kosher whole chicken,
    cleaned and cut into pieces (if you wish, you can
    substitute beef or another type of poultry for the
    chicken)

2–4 chicken feet

8 organic carrots, sliced

6 stalks of organic celery, sliced

2–4 organic zucchinis, sliced

3 medium-size organic white or yellow onions, peeled and
    diced

4 inches ginger, grated

5 cloves garlic, peeled and diced (omit if you have upper GI
    problems or severe heartburn)

2–4 tablespoons moist high-mineral Celtic sea salt
1 large bunch parsley

Place the filtered water in a large stainless steel pot, add the structured water additive and apple cider vinegar, and let stand for 10 minutes. Add the oil, chicken, chicken feet, vegetables, ginger, garlic, and sea salt; and bring to a boil over high heat. Let boil for 60 seconds, then lower the heat and simmer for 12 to 24 hours. About 30 minutes before removing soup from the heat, add the parsley.

Remove the soup from the heat. Remove and discard the chicken feet. Remove the chicken meat from the bones; place the chicken meat back in the soup and discard the bones. Ladel into soup bowls and serve hot.

For acute situations with high inflammation, allow the soup to cool, then puree it in batches in a high-powered blender or food processor. Some people with extremely severe conditions may want to discard the chicken and vegetables and consume only the broth.

YIELD: 3 quarts.

Each ingredient in Brasco Broth is very important to the success of Phase One of the Guts and Glory Program. Most of the ingredients in the broth are available in supermarkets. However, if you are on a restricted budget, using nonorganic vegetables and kosher or conventional chicken instead of free-range chicken is acceptable. You may also substitute sea salt for the moist Celtic sea salt.

Brasco Butter

⅓ cup cold-pressed flaxseed oil
⅓ cup high-quality goat's milk butter, softened at room temperature
⅓ cup coconut oil or coconut butter, softened at room temperature

In a bowl, combine the flaxseed oil with the goat's milk butter and the coconut oil or coconut butter. Place in the refrigerator and allow to harden. Use as a spread in place of cow's milk butter or margarine.

YIELD: 1 cup.

Creamy High-Enzyme Dessert

4 ounces quark
1 tablespoon unheated honey
1 teaspoon cold-pressed flaxseed oil
1/2 cup organic fresh or frozen berries

Mix the quark, honey, and flaxseed oil, and top with the berries.

YIELD: One serving.

Fermented Veggie Drink

8 red beets, juiced
6 carrots, juiced
1 ounce ginger, juiced
2–4 tablespoons fermented whey
1 teaspoon sea salt

Place the beet, carrot, and ginger juice in a 1-quart glass container with a seal. Add the whey and salt, and stir well. Cover and let sit at room temperature for 2 to 3 days, then transfer to the refrigerator. The taste should be sour but pleasant. If the drink smells offensive, discard it and start over.

YIELD: 1 quart.

This drink is a great source of probiotics and enzymes and can be consumed several times per day.

High Omega-3 Salad Dressing

8 ounces cold-pressed flaxseed oil
8 ounces extra virgin olive oil

2 tablespoons apple cider vinegar
1 teaspoon lemon juice
Sea salt or spice blend to taste

Combine all the ingredients in a medium-size bowl and mix slowly until well blended. Keep refrigerated and use as a salad dressing or marinade.

YIELD: 2 cups.

Synergy Smoothie

10 ounces 30-hour, cultured goat's milk yogurt, *crème Bulgare*, or full-fat coconut milk (milk and cream)
1–2 omega-3 eggs
1–2 tablespoons unheated honey
1 tablespoon coconut oil
1 tablespoon cold-pressed flaxseed oil
1 tablespoon goat's milk protein powder (optional if using goat's milk yogurt or *crème Bulgare*)
1–2 scoops high-potency digestive enzyme powder (optional if using goat's milk yogurt or *crème Bulgare*)
1/2–1 cup fresh or frozen organic fruit (such as berries, bananas, or pineapple)
Vanilla extract (optional)

Place the following ingredients in a high-speed blender and mix well. Pour into a tall glass and drink immediately. Refrigerate any leftover and drink within twenty-four hours.

YIELD: 3 cups.

Properly prepared, this smoothie is an extraordinary source of easy-to-absorb nutrition. It contains large amounts of "live" enzymes, probiotics, and vitally important "live" proteins, and a full spectrum of essential fatty acids. It can be consumed one to two times per day. It should be consumed within twenty-four hours after it is blended.

For those who are underweight and wasting, it is best to use 10 ounces of *crème Bulgare* or 5 ounces of thirty-hour yogurt and 5 ounces of full-fat coconut milk as the first ingredient in the smoothie. We have seen people who were severely undernourished consume this smoothie on a daily basis and gain much-needed weight.

During coauthor Jordan Rubin's healing process, he consumed this smoothie one to two times per day with raw eggs. (Popular belief to the contrary, eggs from healthy free-range chickens are almost always free of pathogenic salmonella. However, before consuming raw eggs, it is best to thoroughly wash the shell with a mild alcohol or hydrogen peroxide solution.) For those with compromised digestion, it is best to add a high-potency enzyme powder to the smoothie. The protein-digesting enzymes contained in the product will destroy any unwanted pathogens, as will the pathogen-fighting fatty acids contained in the cultured dairy and coconut oil. For those who can't stand the thought of consuming raw eggs, the smoothie can still be beneficial without the eggs. (Did you know that egg yolks are one of the secrets of Häagen-Dazs ice cream's great taste?) However, it may take longer to see positive results.

Lactic Acid Wine

> 2 quarts freshly pressed juice from organic dark grapes
> 4–6 ounces 30-hour cultured goat's milk yogurt or liquid
>   acidophilus

Pour the grape juice and the yogurt or liquid acidophilus into a glass mason jar and mix. Cover and let stand at room temperature for 4 to 6 days, then transfer to the refrigerator. The taste should be slightly sweet and sour, the beverage should be slightly carbonated. The alcoholic content should be kept to a minimum. If the juice is fermented for too long, the alcoholic content will increase.

YIELD: 2 quarts.

This lactic acid wine is believed to be similar to the "new wine" consumed during Biblical times. It is very refreshing and extremely healthy.

For More Information

The following books, organizations, and websites may be of interest to people with gastrointestinal diseases. You are also invited to peer into the last part of this book, which lists all the reference sources we used to write this book. There, you will find the names of many more articles and books that pertain to gastrointestinal health.

Books

Batmanghelidj, F. *Your Body's Many Cries for Water*. Vienna, VA: Global Health Solutions, 1995.

Douglass, William Campbell. *The Milk Book*. Atlanta, GA: Second Opinion Publishing, 1994.

Enig, Mary. *Know Your Fats*. Bethesda, MD: Bethesda Press, 2000.

Fallon, Sally, and Mary Enig, Ph.D. *Nourishing Traditions*. Washington, DC: New Trends Publishing, 1999.

Gottschall, Elaine. *Breaking the Vicious Cycle*. Baltimore, Ontario, Canada: The Kirkton Press, 2000.

Howell, Edward. *Enzyme Nutrition*. Wayne, NJ: Avery Publishing Group, 1985.

Price, Weston A. *Nutrition and Physical Degeneration*. Los Angeles: Price-Pottenger Foundation, 1997.

Schmid, Ronald. *Native Nutrition*. Rochester, VT: Healing Arts Press, 1995.

Organizations

DESIGNS FOR HEALTH INSTITUTE
5345 Arapahoe Avenue
Boulder, CO 80303
Tel: 303-415-0229

Fax: 303-415-9154
www.dfhi.com

PRICE-POTTENGER NUTRITION FOUNDATION
P.O. Box 2614
La Mesa, CA 91943-2614
Tel: 619-462-7600
Fax: 619-433-3136

WESTON A. PRICE FOUNDATION
PMB 106-380
4200 Wisconsin Avenue, NW
Washington, DC 20016
Tel: 202-333-4325
www.westonaprice.org

Websites

WWW.DFHI.COM
The website of the Designs for Health Institute. It includes essays and information about health.

WWW.ENZYMEUNIVERSITY.COM
A website that presents everything you ever wanted to know about enzymes and digestion.

WWW.MERCOLA.COM
A health website maintained by Dr. Joseph Mercola. It includes an archive of Dr. Mercola's weekly health newsletters, as well as *Dr. Mercola's Online Cookbook* and articles such as "Reaching for Optimal Wellness."

WWW.POWERHEALTH.NET
A website maintained by Dr. Stephen Byrnes. It teaches you "how to make naturopathy, natural nutrition, and alternative medicine a vital force in your life." It includes *Stephen Byrnes' Whole Food Cookbook.*

WWW.WESTONAPRICE.ORG
The website of the Weston A. Price Foundation. It offers numerous essays about the nutritional philosophy of Dr. Weston A. Price.

References

INTRODUCTION

Everhart J E (Ed) (1994) Digestive diseases in the United States: Epidemiology and impact. (NIH Publication No. 94-1447). U.S. Department of Health and Human Services, National Institutes of Health, National Institute of Diabetes and Digestive and Kidney Diseases. Washington, DC: U.S. Government Printing Office.

Lipski E (2000) Digestive Wellness. Keats Publishing. Lincolnwood, IL.

CHAPTER 2

Aymard JP et al (1988) Haematological adverse effects of histamine H_2-receptor antagonists. *Med Toxicol Adverse Drug Exp* 3:430–48.

Hathcock JN (1985) Metabolic mechanisms of drug-nutrient interactions. *Fed Proc* 44(1): 124.

Koo J et al (2001) Antacid increases survival of *Vibrio vulnificus* and *Vibrio vulnificus phage* in a gastrointestinal model. *Applied and Environmental Microbiology*. 67:2895–902.

Moss SF et al (1998) Consensus statement for management of gastro-esophageal reflux disease: Results of a workshop meeting at Yale University School of Medicine, Department of Surgery, November 16 and 17, 1997. *J Clin Gastroenterol* 7 (27):6–12.

Salmeron J et al (2001) Dietary fat intake and risk of type 2 diabetes in women. *Am J Clin Nutr* Jun 73(6):1019–26.

Sturniolo GC et al (1991) Inhibition of gastric acid secretion reduces zinc absorption in man. *J Am Coll Nutr* 4:372–75.

CHAPTER 3

Arteca R (1996) Plant Growth Substances: Principles and Applications. Chapman & Hall. New York, NY.

Billings T (1999) Comparative anatomy and physiology brought up to date: Are humans natural frugivores/vegetarians, or omnivores/fauni-vores? *Beyond Vegetarianism* www.beyondveg.com.

Blaylock R (1996) Excitotoxins: The Taste That Kills. Health Press. Santa Fe, NM.

Bogart L et al (1966) Nutrition and Physical Fitness, 8th Edition. W. B. Saunders Co. Philadelphia, PA.

Cleave T (1974) The Saccharine Disease. Bristol John Wright & Sons Ltd. London.

Cohen MN (1989) The significance of long-term changes in diet and food economy. In Food and Evolution: Toward a Theory of Human Food Habits; Harris M et al eds. Temple University Press. Philadelphia, PA.

Cohen P et al (1991) Insulin-like growth factors (IGFs), IGF receptors, and IGF-binding proteins in primary cultures of prostate epithelial cells. *Journal of Clinical Endocrinology and Metabolism* 73(2): 401–7.

Cordain L (1999) Cereal grains: Humanity's double-edged sword. *World Rev Nutr Diet* 84:20–73.

Cordain L (2002) The Paleo Diet. John Wiley & Sons. New York, NY.

De Bakey M et al (1964) Serum cholesterol values in patients treated surgically for atherosclerosis. *JAMA* 189(9): 655–59.

DeLangre J (1992) Seasalt's Hidden Powers. Happiness Press. Magnoia, CA.

Diamond J (1993) The Third Chimpanzee: The Evolution and the Future of the Human Animal. Harper Perennial. New York, NY.

Douglass WC (1994) The Milk Book. Second Opinion Publishing. Atlanta, GA.

Dunn FL (1968) Epidemiological factors: Health and disease in hunter-gatherers. In Man the Hunter; Lee RB et al eds. Aldine Publishing, Chicago, IL.

Eaton S et al (1996) An evolutionary perspective enhances understanding of human nutritional requirements. *Journal of Nutrition.* 126:1732–40.

Eaton SB et al (1994) Women's reproductive cancers in evolutionary context. *The Quarterly Review of Biology* 69:353–67.

Enig M (2000) Know Your Fats. Bethesda Press. Bethesda, MD.

Enig M (1995) Trans Fatty Acids in the Food Supply: A Comprehensive

Report Covering Sixty Years of Research, 2nd Edition. Enig Associates Inc., Silver Springs, MD.

Fallon S (1999) Nourishing Traditions, 2nd Edition. New Trends Publishing. Washington, DC.

Fallon S et al (1997) Out of Africa: What Dr. Price and Dr. Burkett discovered in their studies of sub-Saharan tribes. *PPNF Health Journal.* 21(1):1–5.

FDA (1990) FDA pesticide program, residues in foods, 1989. *Journal of the Association of Official Analytical Chemists* 73(5):127A–46A.

Grady D (March 8, 1999). A move to limit antibiotic use in animal feed. *New York Times.* A1.

Heaton K (1990) Dietary factors in the etiology off inflammatory bowel disease. In Inflammatory Bowel Diseases; Allan R et al eds. Churchill Livingstone. New York, NY.

Hobbes T (1982) [1651] Leviathan. Viking Press. New York, NY.

Howell E (1985) Enzyme Nutrition. Avery Publishing Group. Wayne, NJ.

Jensen B (1994) Goat Milk Magic: One of Life's Greatest Healing Foods. Bernard Jensen International. Escondido, CA.

Larsen R (1999) Milk and the cancer connection. *International Health News.* http://vvv.com/healthnews/milk.html.

Lehninger A (1982) Principles of Biochemistry. Worth Publishers. New York, NY.

Lindeberg S et al (1993) Apparent absence of stroke and ischaemic heart disease in a traditional Melanesian island: A clinical study in Kitava. *J Intern Med* 233:269–75.

Lindeberg S et al (1994) Cardiovascular risk factors in a Melanesian population apparently free from stroke and ischaemic heart disease—The Kitava study. *J Intern Med* 236:331–40.

Lipski E (2000). Digestive Wellness, Second Edition. Keats Publishing. Lincoln, IL.

Nabhan G (1987) Gathering the Desert. University of Arizona Press. Prescott, AZ.

O'Dea K (1984) Marked improvement in carbohydrate and lipid metabolism in diabetic Australian Aborigines after temporary reversion to traditional lifestyle. *Lipids* 33:596–603.

O'Dea K (1991) Traditional diet and food preferences of Australian Aboriginal hunter-gatherers. *Philosophical Transactions of the Royal Society of London, Series B* 334:233–41.

Price W (1997) [1939] Nutrition and Physical Degeneration, Sixth Edition. Price-Pottenger Foundation. Los Angeles, CA.

Price W (1933) Why dental caries with modern civilization? *Dental Digest.* 89:94, 147.

Ravnskov U (1999) The Cholesterol Myths. New Trends Publishing. Washington, DC.

Robinson J (2000) Why Grassfed Is Best! Vashon Island Press. Vashon, WA.

Schaeffer O (1981) Eskimos (Inuit). In Western Diseases: Their Emergence and Prevention; Trowell H et al eds. Harvard University Press. Cambridge, MA.

Schmid R (1995) Native Nutrition. Healing Arts Press. Rochester, VT.

Schweitzer A. Preface to Berglas A (1957) Cancer: Nature, Cause and Cure. Pasteur Institute. Paris.

Stefanson V (1960) Cancer: Disease of Civilization. Hill and Wang, New York, NY.

Stefansson V (1993) The Fat of the Land. The MacMillan Co, New York, NY.

Walker M (June 2001) Goatein provides optimal amounts of absorbable protein. *Townsend Letter for Doctors & Patients* 215.

Williams WR (1908) The Natural History of Cancer, With Special Reference to its Causation and Prevention. New York: William Wood.

CHAPTER 4

Aaland M (1988) Sweat: An Illustrated History of the Sauna and Sweatbath in Finland and Other Cultures. Borgo Press. San Bernardino, CA.

Batmanghelidj F (1995) Your Body's Many Cries for Water. Global Health Solutions. Vienna, VA.

Boyle T (1994) The Road to Wellville. Penguin Books. New York, NY.

Dimmer C et al (1996) Squatting for the prevention of hemorrhoids? *Townsend Letter for Doctors & Patients* 159: 66–70.

Gaul D et al (1975) Relationship between eating rates and obesity. *Journal of Consulting and Clinical Psychology* 43(2): 123–25.

Greene B (June 17, 2000) Baseball star with an unknown name. *Abilene Reporter*. http://www.reporternews.com/2000/opinion/gree0617.html.

Leigh S (2001) Sleep protects against aging & disease. *MyPrimeTime.com*. http://www.myprimetime.com/health/fearless_aging/content/ sleep_deficit/ind ex.shtml.

Michrowski A et al (1996) Canada Mortgage and Housing Corporation, Survey of EMF Levels in Canadian Housing.

Pope A et al (2002) Lung cancer, cardiopulmonary mortality, and long-term exposure to fine particulate air pollution. *JAMA* 287:1132–41.

Valentine T (1995) Hidden hazards of microwave cooking. *Nexus New Times Magazine* 2:25.

CHAPTER 5

Bocci V (1992) The neglected organ: Bacterial flora has a crucial immuno-stimulatory role. *Persp Biol Med* 35: 251–60.

Chin J et al (2000) Immune response to orally consumed antigens and probiotic bacteria. *Immunol Cell Biol* 78(1):55–66.

Fallon S (1999) Nourishing Traditions. New Trends Publishing. Washington, DC.

Gibson G et al (1995) Dietary modulation of the human colonic microbiota: Introducing the concept of probiotics. *Journal of Nutrition* 125(6): 1401–12.

Gittleman A (1998) Beyond Probiotics. Keats Publishing. Los Angeles, CA.

Gittleman A (1993) Guess What Came to Dinner: Parasites and Your Health. Avery Publishing. Garden City Park, NY.

Halpern G (March 14, 2002) Telephone conversation regarding gut-associated lymphatic tissue.

Hamdan I et al (1974) Acidolin: An antibiotic produced by *Lactobacillus acidophilus*. *Journal of Antibiotics*. 8; 631–36.

Klebanoff S et al (1991) Viricidal effect of *Lactobacillus acidophilus* on human immunodeficiency virus type 1: Possible role in heterosexual transmission. *The Rockefeller University Press Journal* 174: 289–92.

Lipski E (2000) Digestive Wellness. Keats Publishing. Los Angeles, CA.

Loren C (1997) Evolutionary aspects of diet: Old genes, new fuels. Nutritional changes since agriculture. *World Review of Nutrition and Dietetics* 81.

Macfarlane G (1999) Probiotics and prebiotics: Can regulating the activities of intestinal bacteria benefit health? *Brit Med J* 318;129–34.

Metchnikoff E (1907) The Prolongation of Life. William Heinemann. London.

Moore W et al (1975) Discussion of current bacteriological investigations of the relationships between intestinal flora, diet, and colon cancer. *Cancer Research* 35:3418–20.

Raeburn P (December 3, 2001) Down in the dirt, wonders beckon: Soil and sea yield unknown lodes of useful microbes. *Business Week.*

Rothschild P (1993) Critters! Soil-based organisms and the immune function. *Bio/Tech News.*

Rothschild P (2000) Health repair and life extension with soil-based-microorganisms (SBMOs). *Blasts of Life That Last for Life* 1:1.

Sanders M (1998) Overview of functional foods: Emphasis on probiotic bacteria. *International Dairy Journal* 8; 341–47.

Sehnert K (1989) The garden within. *Health World Magazine* 9.

Steinman D (1999) Dirt & health. *Doctors' Prescription for Healthy Living.* 5:10.

Tamime AY (1997) Fermented milks: Historical food with modern applications. *Danone Symposium Abstract.*

Tannock GW (1999) Probiotics: A critical review. *Horizon Scientific Press.* Wymondham, Norfolk, UK.

Tilg H (1997) New insights into the mechanisms of interferon alfa: An immunoregulatory and anti-inflammatory cytokine. *Gastroenterology* 112: 1017-21.

Trenev N (1998) Probiotics: Nature's Internal Healers. Avery Publishing Group. New York, NY.

Walker M (1997) Soil-based organisms support the immune system from the ground up. *Townsend Letter for Doctors and Patients.* Aug./Sept.

Walker M (2000) Homeostatic soil organisms for one's primal defense. *Townsend Letter for Doctors and Patients.* Feb./Mar.

Weekes D (1993). Management of herpes simplex and virostatic bacterial agent. *EENT Diges* 25.

CHAPTER 6

Atkins R (1992) Dr. Atkin's New Diet Revolution. Avon Books. New York, NY.

DeCava JA (1997). The Real Truth About Vitamins & Anti-oxidants. Printery. West Yarmouth, MA.

Douglas, WC (1996) Into the Light: Tomorrow's Medicine Today. Second Opinion Publishing. Atlanta, GA.

Dunne L (2001) The Nutrition Almanac, 5th Edition. McGraw Hill. New York, NY.

Farr CH (1988) Physiological and biochemical responses to intravenous hydrogen peroxide. *Man J Adv Med* 1:113–29.

Goggins et al (1994) Celiac disease and other nutrient related injuries to the gastrointestinal tract. *American Journal of Gastroenterology.* 89(8): S2–S13.

Gottschall E (2000) Breaking the Vicious Cycle: Intestinal Health Through Diet. The Kirkton Press. Baltimore, Ontario, Canada.

Green S (1998). Oxygenation therapy: Unproven treatments for cancer and AIDS. *Sci Rev Alt Med* 2:6–12.

Itoh M et al (1985) Role of oxygen-derived free radicals in hemorrhagic shock-induced gastric lesions in the rat. *Gastroenterology* 88:1126–67.

Lynes B (1987) The Cancer Cure That Worked: Fifty Years of Suppression. Marcus Books. Queensville, Ontario, Canada.

Muir M (1996) DMSO: Many uses, much controversy. *Alternative & Complementary Therapies.* July/Aug.: 230–35.

Murry RP (1982) Natural versus synthetic. *Biomedical Nitty-Gritty* 3:1.

Sandstrom B et al (1989) Effect of protein level and protein source on zinc absorption in humans. *J Nutr* 119(1): 48–53.

Wagner RD et al (1997) Biotherapeutic effects of probiotic bacteria on *Candidiasis* in immunodeficient mice. *Infection and Immunity* 65(10):4165–72.

CHAPTER 7

Barrett S (1985) Commercial hair analysis: Science or scam? *JAMA* 254:1041–45.

Barrie S (1999) Comprehensive digestive stool analysis, in A Textbook of Natural Medicine, Pizzorno J et al eds. Churchill Livingstone. Sidcup, Kent, UK.

Howell E (1985) Enzyme Nutrition: The Food Enzyme Concept. Avery Publishing. Wayne, NJ.

Inselman P (1998) Is there any other way besides Ritalin? *The American Chiropractor* May/June.

Lazar P (1974) Hair analysis: What does it tell us? *JAMA* 229:1908-9.

Nambudripad D (1999) Say Goodbye to Illness. Delta Publishing Company. Buena Park, CA.

Seidel S et al (2001) Assessment of commercial laboratories performing hair mineral analysis *JAMA* 285:67–72.

Simon A et al (1979) An evaluation of iridology *JAMA* 242:1385–87.

Valentine T et al (1987) Applied kinesiology: Muscle response in diagnosis, therapy and preventive medicine. Thorsons Publishers. Rochester, VT.

Versendaal DA et al (1998) Contact reflex analysis & applied clinical nutrition: An effective analytical tool for the alternative health care professional. *The American Chiropractor*. March/April.

CHAPTER 8

Angerer P et al (2000) n-3 polyunsaturated fatty acids and the cardiovascular system. *Curr Opin Lipidol* 11(1):57–63.

Antonio J et al (1999) Glutamine: A potentially useful supplement for athletes. *Can J Appl Physiol* 24:1-14.

Bailey LB (2000) New standard for dietary folate intake in pregnant women. *Am J Clin Nutr* 71(5 Suppl):1304S–7S.

Batmanghelidj F (1995) Your Body's Many Cries for Water. Global Health Solutions. Vienna, VA.

Beltz S et al (1993) Efficacy of nutritional supplements used by athletes. *Clin Pharm* 12(12):900–8.

Braly J et al (1992) Dr. Braly's Food Allergy and Nutrition Revolution. McGraw-Hill. New York, NY.

Brusick D et al (1997) Assessment of the genotoxic risk from laxative senna products. *Environmental and Molecular Mutagenesis* 29:1–9.

Chin J et al (2000) Immune response to orally consumed antigens and probiotic bacteria. *Immunol Cell Biol* 78(1):55–66.

Connor WE (2000) Importance of n-3 fatty acids in health and disease. *Am J Clin Nutr* 71(1 Suppl):171S–75S.

Dudov IA (1994) Antioxidant system of rat erythrocytes under conditions of prolonged intake of honeybee flower pollen load. *WMJ* Nov-Dec;66(6):94–96.

Fallon S (1996) Tripping lightly down the prostaglandin pathways. *Price-Pottenger Nutrition Foundation Health Journal* 20(3):5–8.

Joseph J (1999) Reversals of age-related declines in neuronal signal transduction, cognitive, and motor behavioral deficits with blueberry, spinach, or strawberry dietary supplementation. *Journal of Neuroscience* 19(18): 8114–21.

Kelly et al (2000) Survival of anti-*Clostridium difficile* bovine immunoglobulin concentrate in the human gastrointestinal tract. *Antimicrobial Agents and Chemother* 41:236–41.

Lacey JM et al (1990) Is glutamine a conditionally essential amino acid? *Nutr Rev* 48:297–309.

Lemon PW (1996) Is increased dietary protein necessary or beneficial for individuals with a physically active lifestyle? *Nutr Rev* Apr 54(4 Pt 2):S169–75.

Lipski E (2000) Digestive Wellness. Keats Publishing. Los Angeles, CA.

Millward DJ (1999) Optimal intakes of protein in the human diet. *Proc Nutr Soc* 58(2):403–13.

Mitsuoka T et al (1987) Effect of fructo-oligosaccharides on intestinal microflora. *Nahrung* 31(5–6):427–36.

Pain O (2000) MSM: Does it work? *Harv Health Lett* 25(10):7.

Price W (1997) [1939] Nutrition and Physical Degeneration; Sixth Edition. Price-Pottenger Foundation. Los Angeles, CA.

Thomas P et al (2001) Dietary bioactive peptides in maintaining intestinal integrity and function. *Am J Gastroenterol* 96(9):S311.

U.S. Department of Health and Human Services, public Health Service, National Institutes of Health (1994) Digestive diseases in the United States: Epidemiology and impact. Publication 94-1447. Washington, DC.

von Schacky C (2000) n-3 fatty acids and the prevention of coronary atherosclerosis. *Am J Clin Nutr* 71(1 Suppl):224S–27S.

Warny et al (1999) Bovine immunoglobulins concentrate *Clostridium difficile* retains *C. difficile* toxin neutralizing activity after passage through the human stomach and small intestine. *Gut* 44:212–17.

Index